The International Library

THE PSYCHOANALYTIC
METHOD

Founded by C. K. Ogden

The International Library of Psychology

PSYCHOANALYSIS
In 28 Volumes

THE PSYCHOANALYTIC METHOD

OSKAR PFISTER

Introduction by Sigmund Freud

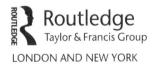

Routledge
Taylor & Francis Group

LONDON AND NEW YORK

First published in 1917
by Routledge
2 Park Square, Milton Park, Abingdon, Oxfordshire OX14 4RN
711 Third Avenue, New York, NY 10017

First issued in paperback 2014

Routledge is an imprint of the Taylor and Francis Group, an informa business

British Library Cataloguing in Publication Data
A CIP catalogue record for this book
is available from the British Library

The Psychoanalytic Method
ISBN 0415-21103-4
Psychoanalysis: 28 Volumes
ISBN 0415-21132-8
The International Library of Psychology: 204 Volumes
ISBN 0415-19132-7

ISBN 13: 978-1-138-87567-8 (pbk)
ISBN 13: 978-0-415-21103-1 (hbk)

INTRODUCTION

By Sigmund Freud (Vienna).

Psychoanalysis originated on a medical basis as a method of treatment for certain nervous maladies which are called functional and in which there is recognized with constantly increasing certainty the result of disturbances of the affectivity. It attains its object of removing the expressions of such disturbances, the symptoms, by presupposing that these symptoms may not be the only possible and final outcome of certain mental processes, and with that in view, exposes the history of the development of the symptoms in the memory, reawakens the processes lying underneath these symptoms and affords them a more favorable outlet under the guidance of the physician. Psychoanalysis has set up the same therapeutic goal as the hypnotic treatment, which, introduced by Liebault and Bernheim, after a long and hard struggle had acquired a place in the technique of neurologists. It goes far deeper, however, into the structure of the mental mechanism and seeks to attain permanent results and lasting changes as its objects.

The hypnotic suggestion treatment, in its time, very soon passed the bounds of medical application and established itself in the service of education of young persons. If we may believe the reports, it has proven itself an effective means of overcoming the faults of children, disturbing physical habits and traits of character otherwise incorrigible. No one raised objections at that time or expressed surprise over this extension of its field of usefulness which has become fully intelligible to us only by the aid of psychoanalytic investigation. For, today, we know that the pathological symptoms are often nothing else than substitute formations for bad, i. e. unsuitable, tendencies, and that the conditions of the symptoms are established in the years of childhood and adolescence—at the same time in which the individual is the object of education—whether the maladies actually appear in youth or only in a later period of life. Education and therapy now appear in a reciprocal relation to each other. Education will take care that from certain dispositions and tendencies of the child, nothing harmful to the individual or society shall proceed. Therapy will come into play if these same dispositions have already caused the unwished-for result of a pathological symptom. The other outcome, namely, that the unsuitable dispositions of the child have led, not to substitute formations in symptoms, but to direct character perversions, is almost inaccessible to therapy and most withdrawn from the influence of the educator. Education is a prophylaxis which should prevent both results, the neurosis and the perversion; psychotherapy will render the more labile of the two results retroactive and institute a kind of re-education.

In view of these facts, the question presents itself whether one may not utilize psychoanalysis for the purposes of education as the hypnotic suggestion has been utilized in its time. The advantages of this use of psychoanalysis would be obvious. The educator is prepared on the one hand, through his knowledge of the general human dispositions of childhood, to guess which of the childish dispositions threaten to attain an undesired outlet and if psychoanalysis is of influence in such errors of development, he can bring it into use before the signs of an unfavorable development are established. Thus, he can influence children who are still healthy, prophylactically, by means of the analysis. On the other hand, he can detect the first signs of a development toward a neurosis or perversion and guard the child against such further development, at a time when, for a number of reasons, it would never be taken to a physician. One could conceive that such a psychoanalytic activity on the part of the educator—and the pastor in Protestant countries who occupies a similar position

—might afford invaluable assistance and often render the intervention of the physician superfluous.

It may be asked whether the practice of psychoanalysis does not presuppose a medical education which must remain lacking to the educator and pastor, or whether other relations are not antagonistic to the purpose of placing the psychoanalytic technique in other than medical hands. I confess that I see no such obstacles. The practice of psychoanalysis demands much less medical education than psychological preparation and free human insight; the majority of physicians, however, are not fitted for the practice of psychoanalysis and have completely failed in placing a correct valuation on this method of treatment. The educator and pastor are bound by the demands of their vocations to exercise the same consideration, forbearance and restraint which the physician is accustomed to observe and their being habitually associated with youth makes them perhaps better suited to have a sympathetic insight into the mental life of this class of persons. The guarantee for a harmless application of the psychoanalytic method can, however, only be afforded in both cases by the personality of the analyst.

The approach to the field of mental abnormalities will compel the analyzing educator to make himself familiar with the most exact psychiatric knowledge and to take the physician into consultation where the diagnosis and outcome of the disturbance may appear doubtful. In a number of cases, results will only come from mutual co-operation of educator and physician.

In a single point, the responsibility of the educator may perhaps exceed that of the physician. The physician, as a rule, has to deal with mental formations already fixed and will find in the already developed individuality of the patient a boundary already established for his activity, but also a security for the patient's independence. The educator, however, works on plastic material which is sensitive to every impression and he must observe the duty of not molding the young mental life according to his own personal ideals but rather according to the dispositions and possibilities inherent in the object.

May the application of psychoanalysis in the service of education soon fulfill the hopes which educators and physicians attach to it! A book like this of Pfister's, which will make the analysis known to educators, will then be assured of the gratitude of future generations.

Vienna, February, 1913.

INTRODUCTION

By G. STANLEY HALL, President of Clark University

THIS volume upon its appearance in German in 1913 at once took its place in the literature on the subject as the most adequate of several earlier compends that had appeared, both in German and English. I immediately adopted it as a reference text for my own classes and even went so far as to make a rather lengthy epitome of it myself for the use of those members of my classes that were not familiar with German. The author has been intimately and personally associated with the psychoanalytic movement from the first, and has practical acquaintance with its technique, but is not a physician and approaches the subject in a way which, without being less serviceable to practitioners, makes the theme on the whole more accessible to laymen. He has the still greater advantage of having held sufficiently aloof from not only the controversies between Freud and Adler but those between what might be called the Vienna and the Zurich schools. The author's method here is to present each topic in a clear and concise way and then to illustrate it by cases. The translation is not only at once the most timely and will be welcome to all English-readers interested in the subject, but it is made by a thoroughly competent and experienced hand whose earlier translation of Hitschmann's "Freud's Theory of the Neuroses" has been widely commended and widely used. Pfister certainly has rare ability to condense, elucidate and take us to the heart of problems, as may be seen in his pithy article lately printed in the American Journal of Psychology (January, 1915) on "Psychoanalysis and the Study of Children and Youth."

G. STANLEY HALL.

Clark University,
Worcester, Mass., May, 1915.

PREFACE

When I had proceeded some ways on a special work on psychoanalysis for psychologists, pedagogues and theologians, the "Herausgeber" of "Pädagogium" (Prof. Dr. Messmer) surprised me with the advice to write a book on the same subject designed especially for the professional educator. Reluctantly I gave up the former alluring plan. The eloquence of Prof. Dr. Messmer and still more his own keen and understanding penetration into the spirit of pedanalysis, as well as other pleasing observations among our mutual colleagues, convinced me that the pedagogues, because of their mental equipment and their longing for the great thing here represented, were especially well prepared in advance. I was also compelled to see that an impartial attention to the interests of three professional circles would have too greatly expanded my book.

Futhermore, there is only one theory and technique of psychoanalysis. Therefore, psychologists and theologians, as well as my brother educators, for whom my book is intended, can use it as an introduction to the investigation of the unconscious submerged forces in their fields. Indeed, if certain medical leaders of psychoanalysis are right, even physicians will gain in the following work an explanation of the fundamental presuppositions of their analytic labors since the book marks the first attempt at a systematic presentation of pyschoanalysis derived by induction.

As a book of one seeker of truth intended for other seekers, the following investigations are intended. I wished, not so much to show what splendid things we have accomplished, as rather by the proof of indisputable results of greater range to awaken a desire for new and perhaps still greater conquests.

Therefore, I have presented pyschoanalysis as a growing method, struggling toward knowledge, constantly broadening its field of influence by sturdy efforts.

Many critics and laity will reproach me for not giving a confident answer to important questions. Certain psychoanalysts will insist that where they themselves have attained certainty, it should be demanded of me, and certain inquisitive ones who prefer to have their mental food served well-done, will receive my conservatism ungraciously. In defence, I can only present the shield of my scientific conscience and hope for the support of those for whom co-operation in the solution of great problems, the exploration of the virgin land of great promise but also of great difficulties, affords a greater attraction than the visiting of well-mapped lands.

Expressions of criticism, I look upon as sincere desire for knowledge. I know that my first pedanalytic attempt goes forth into the world with not a few defects and am therefore very susceptible to expert instruction. Thus far, criticism hostile to analysis suffers throughout from a fatal disease which I would call "ontophobia," fear of the facts. It will be sad for me if my work also falls into ontophobic hands, for it is intended only for those who test for themselves, those who are hungry for facts.

With a few insignificant exceptions, I am not going into polemics. He who does not understand that holy "tolle, lege," "take, read!" which points to the book of reality as the instrument of delivery from error and bondage, is not to be won by ever so striking dialectic means.

Not because of the opponents but out of love for the truth, I have laid great stress on the proof that the much calumniated and more than once misused psychoanalysis, is not only compatible with the highest ethical and religious demands but absolutely presupposes them, something which the very malicious and ignorant ones may laugh at. The analysis has strengthened me in the conviction that the human being is in no way merely a sexual being of the highest order (which no psychoanalyst has ever asserted) but that the varied mental wealth and noble characteristics which the idealistic philosophy has found in him, really belong to him. To be sure, I could not avoid the insight that the sexual life possesses a far higher significance in our mental household than the traditional psychology—in contrast to many poets and other students of humanity—is willing to admit. The closer investigation immediately showed, however, that the sexual life may be most intimately bound up with the affairs of the mind so that the purely animal in it, being the less important, is forcibly crowded into the background. We are also not shocked by the fact that in art, poetry, morality and even religion, love plays a predominant rôle and that Jesus makes a definite love, a primary commandment. Gounod says beautifully: "The law of life, like the law of art, is described in the saying of St. Augustine: 'Love is all.' " Why should anyone become excited when also in disease of the mind, in the dream, in apparently accidental acts, in short, in all performances in which mind has a part, the influence of love comes to light?

In conclusion, I wish to thank most heartily those who have contributed in the preparation of this book, first of all, Prof. Dr. Freud who aided me with excellent advice and active interest; further, Dr. Jung, who, after the completion of the manuscript, most kindly called my attention to a number of improvements. Finally, I thank most sincerely Prof. Dr. Messmer who placed most freely at my disposal his psychological library and his intimate knowledge of the most recent psychology and in addition had the kindness to prepare the index.

Now may the work, in spite of its imperfection, prove a blessing to the noble work of education and help the pedagogues to an acquirement of that which psychoanalysis brought me: an immeasurable enrichment of scientific investigation and practical knowledge!

OSKAR PFISTER.

Zurich, May, 1913.

TRANSLATOR'S NOTE

Those who have read the original German edition of this book will notice several changes in the translation. The author entirely revised the book in 1915 and sent me these revisions and changes to be incorporated in my translation. This revision has been carried out exactly as ordered. The only other change from the original edition is the omission of chapter two which deals with the philosophical aspects of the subject.

C. R. PAYNE.

TABLE OF CONTENTS

TABLE OF CONTENTS

LIST OF ILLUSTRATIONS

CHAPTER I

DEFINITION AND HISTORY OF PSYCHOANALYSIS

PSYCHOANALYSIS, as its name denotes, concerns itself with the separation of mental processes into their constituent elements. We might, indeed, conjure up all kinds of harm if we did not at once warn against considering this provisional statement as an exact definition.

There has been analysis of psychic phenomena since prehistoric times. The psychologist who separates the contents of consciousness into its constituent parts and traces them back to their causes, the historian of art who seeks the origin of an important creation, the biographer who is engrossed in the development of his hero, the physician who attempts to elucidate the compelling motives of a melancholia, the educator who endeavors to understand the mental condition of his pupil, in short, everyone who is intent upon penetrating the mental life of others would be, according to the statement heading our train of thought, a psychoanalyst. In reality, not a few representatives of ancient traditions, in view of the results of the successfully advancing movement which bears the distinctive name, pride themselves that they have already done psychoanalysis for decades.

They would be quite right if the meaning of the word was derived by merely splitting it into its parts. The name has, however, gained its content by an historical process, to overlook which would create a fatal confusion. In order to escape the annoying cobwebs and arrive at the correct definition, we have to present in detail how the originator of the name and the very special procedure connoted by the same, reached his theory and technique. We shall see that the criterion of psychoanalysis lies in a special kind of inquiry into the uncon-

1

scious mental processes which powerfully influence the conscious life.

In the year 1893, Sigmund Freud * published, in collaboration with his colleague, Josef Breuer, an epoch-making article entitled "Concerning the Psychic Mechanism of Hysterical Phenomena" ("Über den psychischen Mechanismus hysterischer Phänomene").

In order to understand the fundamental ideas of this short but important work, it is advisable to investigate its connection with the father of the hysteria investigation, J. M. Charcot of Paris (1893). The celebrated director of the Sâlpetrière was the first person to free hysterical individuals from the stigma of ridiculousness, earnestly to study and systematically to arrange their symptoms, in doing which, he was also able to demonstrate hysteria in the male sex. Especially important was his discovery, made by researchers on hypnotized patients, that the hysterical paralyses which appear after severe emotional shock, the socalled traumatic † paralyses, arise from ideas which control the persons in moments of special dispositions. The motor disturbances may be produced ‡ in hypnosis and even in suggestion.

These results at first exercised no effect on therapeutic methods. Charcot remained true to physical and chemical procedures. He advised pressing on the ovarian region at short intervals, under certain circumstances for hours, in order to lessen the severity of the convulsive attacks or indeed to dissipate ‖ them. To overcome an hysterical epileptical condition, he ordered ether or amyl nitrite.¶

One of his pupils, Pierre Janet, cured a case of complicated traumatic hysteria by taking the patient in the hypnotic state back to the time when the shock was received and suggesting

---

* Sigmund Freud, born May 6, 1856, in Freiberg, Moravia, Austria, is to-day Professor of Neurology in the University of Vienna.

† From "trauma," wound, thus about: caused by injury.

‡ Sigmund Freud, Sammlung kleiner Schriften zur Neurosenlehre I, p. 12.

‖ J. M. Charcot, Leçons sur les maladies du système nerveux, 5th ed., Paris, Vol. I (1884), pp. 339, 400.

¶ P. 401 f.

that the shock was harmless. We will quote the account of this instructive process for the reader's perusal:

Marie, a girl of nineteen years, suffered upon her admission to the institution from periodic convulsions and deliria. Before the beginning of her menstrual periods, her character changed, she became gloomy and violent and had pains in all her limbs together with nervous disturbances. Barely twenty hours after the onset of the flow, the menstruation would suddenly cease, a severe chill would shake her whole body and a severe pain slowly ascend from body to throat and the great hysterical crises begin. The violent convulsions were soon succeeded by deliria. Now, the patient uttered cries of terror, meanwhile talking constantly of blood and fire and fleeing to escape the flames, now she played like a child, spoke with her mother and climbed on the stove or furniture. Delirium and convulsions alternated with short intermissions for forty-eight hours. After repeated vomiting of blood, the normal condition gradually returned. Between these major monthly attacks, Marie had minor muscular contractures, various changing anesthesias (entire loss of sensation) and in particular, complete and constant blindness of the left eye.

For seven months the disease resisted all medical procedures. Especially did suggestive measures regarding the menstruation have only bad effects and increased the deliria.

The hypnotic investigation yielded the following: At the age of thirteen, about twenty hours after the onset of the first menstruation, Marie, impelled by false shame, secretly took a cold bath, by which the flow was suddenly interrupted. At the same time there appeared severe chills and delirium lasting for days. When, after five years, the menstrual periods returned, they brought the above described condition with them. Thus, the patient repeated the bath scene monthly without knowing it.

The cure did not succeed by the mere hypnotic removal of the fixed idea. Only when the patient in hypnosis had been taken back to the age of thirteen, could the conviction be awakened that the menstrual period would normally come to an end in a course of three days. Immediately, no further periodic disturbances were to be seen in the patient.

The cries of terror were explained by the circumstance that Marie, when sixteen years old, saw an old woman killed by a fall from the stairs. With considerable trouble, the girl was shown in artificial sleep that the old woman only stumbled and had not died. The cries ceased from that moment.

Most difficult was the explanation of the hysterical blindness. Finally, it was discovered that Marie, when six years old, had been compelled one day in spite of her outcries, to sleep with a child of similar age which had scrofula on the whole left side of its face. Soon after, Marie developed the same trouble on the same place. When the scrofula disappeared, it left behind anesthesia of the left half of the face and blindness of the left eye. Again the girl was taken back to the time of the first shock. The physician pictured the pretty comrade entirely free from scrofula. At the second repetition of the scene, the now convinced patient caressed the imaginary child and upon awakening could see perfectly normally.*

The method applied by Pierre Janet, although recognized † by Delboeuf and Binet as an effective means of treatment, was not considered a regular method nor established theoretically.

An accidental discovery, the enormous importance of which its fortunate discoverer himself did not sufficiently appreciate, opened up new paths. In the years 1880–82 the Vienna physician, Dr. Josef Breuer, was engaged with a famous patient.‡ The girl, aged twenty-one, suffered from severe hysteria, the most important symptom of which consisted of paralysis and anesthesia of the limbs on the right (less often left) side of the body, of squinting, cough and other physical troubles. The walls seemed to be falling on the patient. Two sharply differentiated mental conditions could be noted:

---

* Pierre Janet, L'automatisme psychologique, Paris, 1889, pp. 436–440.

† Freud, Sammlung kleiner Schriften I, p. 18, 1909.

‡ Breuer & Freud, Studien über Hysterie. Leipzig & Vienna, Deuticke, 1895, 2d ed., 1909.

One, almost normal, which was distinguished only by sadness and another, abnormal condition of extreme excitement which was often accompanied by hallucinations. The power of speech disappeared and for two weeks the patient was dumb. One day when she was sitting on her father's bed, she saw a snake which would bite her. In the attempt to ward off the reptile, she noticed that the fingers of her hand changed into snakes with death's heads. From fear, she attempted to pray but could recall only an English child's prayer. From that hour, without noticing it, she spoke only English and no longer understood her mother tongue. In unconsciousness, she murmured some words. When one of these words was kept before her, she phantasied an episode from which she received a certain ease of mind. A year after the death of her father, the two conditions changed so that the patient lived as a normal person in the present but repeated from day to day, in the abnormal state, the events of the preceding year, as the mother could substantiate from a diary she kept.

Though this clinical history already affords enough of striking nature, another particularly important circumstance was added. When Breuer had dictated to the hysterical patient in hypnosis what she had whispered in her unconscious state (absence), she gave an account of the whole phantasy from which those words came. It showed that the scattered words were like the flag appearing above a wall, behind which was marching a body of troops bearing it. If the events which had caused the symptom could be successfully drawn out, then the cessation of the pathological phenomenon followed the oral description. For example, the fear of water, the girl traced back to the impression that a dirty little dog had drunk from a glass without her being able to raise any objection. After this memory, the aversion to the drinking of water disappeared. The squint and exaggeration of visual objects went back to the circumstance that the girl with tears in her eyes, had brought the clock close to her face in order to tell the time. When the whole story of suffering had been traced back to its causes, her health had also completely and permanently returned.

From these and similar phenomena, Breuer and Freud, who urged his colleague to publish the material which he had been gathering for more than a decade, drew the following conclusions: Very many of the hysterical symptoms are occasioned by an idea which occurs to the patient with strong affect at a time of sleepiness (166). In case the latter is not conducted along normal mental association paths and, as you might say, distributed, it jumps to abnormal physical and mental paths and produces the hysterical phenomenon. Thus, the hysterical individual suffers, as we may say, in great part, from reminiscences. The cure is effected by bringing that reminiscence accompanied by its suitable excitement into consciousness and then allowing it to fade away normally. To put it differently, the pent-up affect is brought into consciousness and carried out in speech or removed by medical suggestion; it "is abreacted." Since Breuer's intelligent patient gave the name of "chimney-sweeping" ("Kaminfegen") to the talking treatment, which had been tried on her, her fortunate discoverer called the method the "cathartic method" (from καθαίρειν to purify). Its differentiation from that of Janet's lies in the fact that a bit of the patient's past, which is lost to his memory, namely the occasion of the disease, is rendered conscious, and on the other hand, the intentional bringing at the same time of a suggested idea standing in contradiction to the pathological idea, is given up. We again call attention to the fact that hypnosis and abreaction, the speaking out of a forgotten but affectful traumatic happening which has hurt the mind, now brought back to consciousness, constitute the essential features of the cathartic method.

Breuer and Freud presented the views thus gained in a short preliminary publication * and again in the book, "Studies in Hysteria" ("Studien über Hysterie" †) which

* Breuer & Freud, Über den psychischen Mechanismus hysterischer Phänomene. Neurolog. Zentralblatt, 1893, Nos. 1 & 2.

† Leipzig and Vienna, Deuticke, 2d ed., 1909. (The citations refer to the latter edition.)

appeared in 1895. This important work contains in Freud's contributions the fundamental ideas which led to the psychoanalytic method. We will mention the most important: Many hysterical symptoms, for example visions, express symbolically ideas which may be found below the threshold of consciousness (51, 157ff.). This idea was once conscious but on account of its painful character, was repressed (99, 145, 235); some of its parts, however, still break through into ordinary consciousness (57). All hysteria rests on such repression (250). The content of the repressed idea is of sexual nature (224) and various analogous causes must be present to produce the symptom (63, 229). Hypnosis * can be dispensed with (92f.) but the resistance which the patient presents against the repressed ideas being brought into consciousness must be overcome by strong pressure (234f.). Already, Freud ventures on the interpretation of dreams, without, however, recognizing the importance of these in the treatment of hysterical troubles (57). Impressions of earliest childhood are already given attention (115). Also that phenomenon to which Freud later, when he had lost faith in the omnipotence of abreaction, ascribed the determining influence in the healing process, the socalled "transference," is in good part outlined. Of this, Freud knew that the patient transferred upon the physician some of the painful ideas emerging from the unconscious during the analysis (266f.), thus, for example, the wish cherished for a kiss from another man would be changed to a similar wish toward the physician. Mittenzwey is greatly in error when he believes that Freud's progress beyond Breuer's ideas at this epoch consists merely in the extension of the method to all the neuroses, in the introduction of the term "defence" ("Abwehr") and the exclusively sexual causation of the neuroses.†

One peculiarity of the Freudian method may now be

---

* Authors like Forel and Frank (Die Psychanalyse (1909), Munich, Reinhardt) who speak well of psychoanalysis but cling to hypnosis, are adherents of the "cathartic" but not of the psychoanalytic conception.

† K. Mittenzwey, Versuch zu einer Darstellung und Kritik der Freudschen Neurosenlehre. Zeitschrift für Pathopsychologie I (1912), p. 413.

pointed out: Freud allows his patient to tell without criticism everything which comes into his head while in the physician's presence. Where he observes gaps or striking discrepancies, he directs the apperception directly to these points and has the patient give associations to them. The associations thus collected, he submits to a method of interpretation which he has developed from many years of experience; the independent substantiation of this method, no regular analyst can or will avoid. The essential features of Freud's psychoanalysis are, in addition to the abandonment of hypnosis, an association and interpretation method. In these sentences, we have given the characteristics of the psychoanalytic method.

It is now high time to give the reader an answer to a question which must have gradually aroused his impatience. How does all this concern the educator? Professionally, he has nothing to do with hysterical individuals. I cannot better answer the justifiable interpolation than by continuing with my sketch of the history of the development of psychoanalysis.

Freud recognized ever more clearly that the processes which produced nervous disturbances are also of highest influence on the mental life of normal individuals and can be equally well studied in them. Without being unfaithful to the medical interest, the Vienna neurologist developed a new kind of psychology which penetrated to the unconscious causes of mental performances. He once defined psychoanalysis as "the investigation of the unconscious part of the individual mental life."* For a long time astute judges of human nature had asserted that many of the highest performances of the mind were created, not in the laboratory of conscious thinking, feeling and willing, but in the subterranean chambers which had often been denominated as the unconscious. Schiller describes this conception in the familiar lines:

> "As in the air the storm wind blows,
> One knows not whence it comes or goes,
> As the spring gushes forth from hidden depths,

* Freud, Das Tabu und die Ambivalenz, Imago I (1912), p. 220.

So comes the poet's song from within
And awakes the power of dim emotions
Which wonderfully slumber in the heart." *

Again Schiller says: "The unconscious united with discretion makes the poetic artist." †

Also, artistic inspiration, religious experience (James, "Religious Experience," 443f., 461–467), indeed even philosophical speculation (Nietzsche) have long ago been traced back to mental processes lying under the threshold of consciousness.

Freud's investigations not only substantiate these surmises but also afford the proof that the whole conscious mental life, especially on its affective side, is ruled and directed by such subconscious ("subliminal" from limen, threshold) motives. Freud and his pupils are interested, first of all, in the neuroses (popularly, nervous diseases) and mental diseases in which anatomical anomalies are not demonstrable, the socalled functional psychoses, then further, in numerous affairs of normal mental functions which had been partly treated cursorily as mysterious, partly left unobserved. In 1900, appeared Freud's "Traumdeutung"‡ ("Interpretation of Dreams"‡), the most comprehensive, perhaps also the most important work of the author. He who would judge it, must certainly overcome his aversion to the mysterious title and his resistance to a not unimportant mental product. Further, he cannot avoid the trouble of working over a number of his own or another's dreams according to Freud's formulæ. Otherwise, it is obvious that an acceptable scientific judgment cannot be formed.

In 1901, appeared Freud's book, "Psychopathology of Everyday Life" ("Zur Psychopathologie des Alltags" ||) on forgetting, errors in speech, superstition and mistakes. In

* Compare my article: Anwendungen der Psychanalyse in der Pädagogik und Seelsorge, Imago I (1912), pp. 55–82.
† From O. Rank, Das Inzestmotiv in Dichtung und Sage, p. 1.
‡ Leipzig and Vienna, Deuticke, 2d ed., 1909, 3rd ed., 1911. Also English translation by Brill of New York.
|| Berlin, Karger, 2d ed., 1907.

this work, the writer seeks to prove that the actions mentioned in the subtitle, as well as many other accidental or apparently meaningless acts, frequently come from unconscious motives and owe their origin to the same mechanism which prevails in the dream, neurosis and functional psychosis. In 1905, followed an extensive investigation of wit and its relation to the unconscious.* In 1907, Freud considered the foundation of religious psychology in his article, "Obsessional Acts and Religious Practices" ("Zwangshandlungen und Religionsübung" †). The same year, pedagogy received its first attention from a psychoanalyst in the open letter on the "Sexual Enlightenment of Children" ("Zur sexuellen Aufklärung der Kinder" ‡). These works were followed in 1908 by the first psychoanalytic treatment of a literary work, entitled, "The Delusion and Dreams in W. Jensen's 'Gradiva'" ("Der Wahn und die Träume in W. Jensen's Gradiva" ||). Psychology of children which had already been taken as a field for analytic investigation as early as 1905, in "Three Contributions to the Sexual Theory" ("Drei Abhandlungen zur Sexualtheorie") received in 1908 the first work specially devoted to the subject in the article "Concerning Infantile Sexual Theories" ("Über infantile Sexualtheorien" ¶). The views set forth there were substantiated in the "Analysis of the Phobia of a Five Year Old Boy" ("Analyse der Phobie eines fünfjahrigen Knaben" §). Into the domain of ethics, Freud entered in 1908 with the essay, "Cultural Sexual Morality and Modern Nervousness" ("Die kulturelle Sexualmoral und die moderne Nervosität" **). The psychology of poetry and art received new elucidation in the article, "Poet and Phantasy"

---

* Leipzig and Vienna, Deuticke.
† Kleiner Schriften II, 122–131. (Originally in the Zeitschrift für Religionspsychologie, I, Part 1.)
‡ Same, pp. 151–158.
|| 1910.
¶ Pp. 159–174.
§ Jahrbuch für psychoanalytische und psychopathologische Forschungen, I (1910), pp. 1–109.
** Kleine Schriften, II, pp. 175–196.

("Der Dichter und das Phantasieren" (1908) * and in the monograph "A Childhood Reminiscence of Leonardo da Vinci" ("Eine Kindheitserinnerung des Leonardo da Vinci") (1910).† Finally, in 1910, Freud published glimpses into philology in his short article, "Concerning the Contradictory Meanings of Primitive Words" ("Über den Gegensinn der Urworte").‡ For a long time no attention was paid to psychoanalysis. Its results called forth some respectful bows but mostly only a shaking of heads. The first persons to second Freud in scientific publications were C. G. Jung,‖ psychiatrist in Zurich and his chief, E. Bleuler,¶ Professor of Psychiatry and Director of the Cantonal Institute for the Insane. After these two investigators, in spite of the fiercest hostility, recognized the correctness of Freud's assertions, the movement which had previously been received in dead silence, soon became discussed in the farthest circles. In the spring of 1908, the adherents of the new psychology assembled in Salzburg and arranged for the publication of a periodical journal as an organ for the propagation of their ideas. As a result there has appeared annually in two impressive half-volumes, the "Jahrbuch für psychoanalytische und psychopathologische Forschungen" (Vol. I, Part I, 1909) (Yearbook for Psychoanalytic and Psychopathological Investigations). The series of pamphlets devoted to applied psychology ("Schriften zur angewandten

* Kleine Schriften, II, pp. 197–206.
† Schriften zur angewandten Seelenkunde, Part 7.
‡ Jahrbuch, Vol. II, pp. 179–184.
‖ Jung, Ein Fall von hysterischem Stupor bei einer Untersuchungsgefangenen. Journal f. Psychologie und Neurologie, Vol. I, 1902. Die psychologische Bedeutung des Assoziationsexperimentes, Archiv f. Kriminalanthrop. Vol. 22, p. 145. Exper. Beobachtungen über d. Erinnerungsvermögen. Zbl. f. Nervenheilk. und Psychiatrie, Year XXVIII (1905), etc. See the index to the literature in the Jahrbuch, Vol. II, pp. 363–375.
¶ Freudsche Mechanismen in der Symptomatologie von Psychosen. Psychiatr.-neurolog. Wochenschrift 1906. Affektivität, Suggestibilität, Paranoia. Halle, 1906, contributions in the "Diagnostischen Assoziationsstudien" edited by Jung.

Seelenkunde"*) edited by Freud is constantly growing. The Congress sitting at Nürmberg in 1909 concluded the formation of the International Psychoanalytic Association which soon had sections in Vienna, Zurich, Berlin, New York and Munich. For the U. S. and Canada, a general American association was founded. Since the "Yearbook" could not contain the wealth of scientific material,† two new periodicals appeared: In 1910, the "Zentralblatt für Psychoanalyse," a medical monthly for mental problems ‡ and in 1912, the bimonthly *Imago*, a journal for the application of psychoanalysis to the mental sciences.‖ Since January, 1913, there has appeared the "Internationale Zeitschrift für ärztliche Psychoanalyse" (published by Heller, Vienna, 18 marks a year; edited by Ferenczi and Rank).

In November, 1913, appeared the first number of an American quarterly devoted to psychoanalysis. This is the *Psychoanalytic Review*, edited by Drs. William A. White of Washington and Smith Ely Jelliffe of New York City.

In the first number of *Imago*, we find a list of all articles in the field of mental sciences published up to the end of 1911. It names almost two hundred articles from the fields of psychology, sexual-, dream-, everyday-, and child-psychology, pedagogy and theory of morals, characterology, biography,

* Up to the end of 1912, thirteen parts: 1. Freud, "Gradiva." 2. Riklin, Wunscherfüllung und Symbolik in Märchen. 3. Jung, Der Inhalt der Psychose. 4. Abraham, Traum und Mythus. 5. Rank, Der Mythus von der Geburt des Helden. 6. Sadger, Aus d. Liebesleben Nikolaus Lenaus. 7. Freud, Eine Kindheitserinnerung des Leonardo da Vinci. 8. Pfister, Die Frömmigkeit des Grafen L. v. Zinzendorf. 9. Graf, Rich. Wagner im "Fliegenden Holländer." 10. Jones, Das Problem des Hamlet un der Ödipus-Komplex. 11. Abraham, Giovanni Segantini. 12. Storfer, Zur Sonderstellung des Vatermordes. 13. Rank, Die Lohengrinsage. 14. Jones, Der Alptraum in s. Beziehung zu gew. Formen d. mittelalterl. Aberglaubens.

† Vol. I, 594 pp., Vol. II, 747 pp., Vol. III, 857 pp., Vol. IV, Part 1, 606 pp.

‡ Published by Bergmann, Wiesbaden. 18 Marks per year. Edited by W. Stekel. Suspended publication in 1914.

‖ Hugo Heller, Vienna. 15 Marks per year. Edited by H. Sachs and O. Rank.

esthetics, mythology, religious-, speech-, social- and criminal-psychology.

Among pedagogic journals, two have entered the service of psychoanalysis: at the beginning of 1912, the *Berner Seminarblätter*, journal for school reform, organ of the Swiss Pedagogic Association, issued under the auspices of Dr. Ernst Schneider, Director of the Higher Seminary in Bern, in conjunction with Prof. Dr. Oskar Messmer in Rorschach, Dr. Otto von Greyerz in Glarisegg and the author of this book. Some months later, the "Monatshefte für Pädagogik und Schulreform" (Vienna) was won by Alfred Adler for psychoanalysis.

The first pedagogues who publicly recognized the importance of psychoanalysis were Prof. Adolf Lüthi, who in 1910 in the yearbook of the "Unterrichtswesens in der Sweiz" (page 197) reviewed in most friendly manner my first pedagogic articles of psychoanalytic nature, further Prof. Dr. E. Meumann,* Prof. Dr. O. Messmer,† and Dr. P. Häberlin,‡ Privatdozent of Philosophy in Basel, who had previously, while Seminary Director of the Thurganischen Lehrerbildungsanstalt in Kreuzlingen, extensively practiced the new pedagogic method. Pastors who have entered the literary field in favor of psychoanalysis are A. Waldburger ‖ in Ragaz, the Calvinist, Th. Johner,¶ a conservative theologian, and Adolf Keller in Zurich.

Two or three years ago the reproach was hurled at the psychoanalyst that aside from Freud and Bleuler, whose importance no one disputed, no university teacher had joined the

---

* Meumann, Pädag. Jahresber. 1910, 63rd Year, Leipzig, p. 134.

† Messmer, Die Psychoanalyse u. i. päd. Bedeutung. Berner Seminarblätter, V, Part 9 (1911).

‡ Häberlin, Sexualgespenster. Sexualprobleme, Vol. VIII, pp. 96–106 (1912).

‖ Waldburger, Psychanalyt. Seelsorge u. Moralpädagogik. (Prot. Monatshefte, XIII (1909), pp. 110–114. A defence of my article which appeared in the same journal.)

¶ Johner, Die Psychoanalyse im bernischen Kant. Pfarrverein. Der Kirchenfreund (Basel), XLIV (1910) No. 24.

new school. To-day this criticism, which many consider unendurable, has already disappeared. A constantly increasing number of high school teachers, in spite of a threatened boycott and much derision, have joined the outlawed psychoanalytic association. The following are analysts: the psychiatrist of Bern University, Prof. von Speyr, the neurologist of Harvard University, Prof. James J. Putnam, a man of wide experience and great philosophical attainments, further, the professors of psychiatry, Ernest Jones (Toronto), Adolf Meyer (Baltimore), August Hoch (New York), Davidson (Toronto), Jelliffe (New York), White (Washington). Among the psychologists is the first college president to acknowledge Freud, the influential founder of experimental religious psychology, G. Stanley Hall; among investigators of speech, P. C. Prescott, Professor of the History of English Literature in New York and H. Sperber in Upsala; among the representatives of internal medicine, Prof. R. Morichau-Beauchant in Poitiers. A large number of other investigators, especially in Germany and Switzerland, accept psychoanalysis in its important points. This rapid spread of a theory which had such a tremendous resistance against it, within a very few years, is nothing short of marvelous.

In spite of the large number of publications, it is to be regretted that the literary work has not kept pace with the practical and theoretical advance. Very many results especially important for pedagogy are scarcely touched upon in psychoanalytic journals. Of the analytic educational work with pupils, who, without being really ill, still because of inner inhibitions, make themselves and their families unhappy, there is almost no mention anywhere. How the hitherto unobserved impressions of childhood control the whole later development of the normal individual, even to the peculiarity of his style, his choice of a vocation and of a wife, as well as the most insignificant subordinate affairs, finds too little discussion. The enormous loss of love for fellowmen and of power for work which many individuals suffer, mostly without knowing it, as a result of unfavorable educational influences, have not, up to

the present time, been given their proper weight in the literature. I gave a few examples of this in my article, ''Applica-
tions of Psychoanalysis in Pedagogy and Pastoral Care''
(''Anwendungen der Psychoanalyse in der Pädagogik und
Seelsorge''*). I described cases of untruthfulness, kleptomania, tormenting of animals, destructive rage, aversion to
work, dislike of certain foods, meaningless gestures, portentous
corporal punishment, withholding of sexual enlightenment,
eccentric gaits, pathological hate, hysterical physical defects as
a pedagogic problem, creation of hobgoblins out of the unconscious in choice of a husband or wife, unhappy marriages as
result of psychic traumata of youth, religious abnormalities
from similar causes. From these experiences chosen at random, I drew the conclusion: Countless numbers of persons who
bring heart-breaking grief to their parents and other people
and cannot help bringing it because they are under neurotic
obsessions, can by the aid of analysis be changed into agreeable
useful individuals.† The proof for the correctness of this assertion which ought to have emphasized the difficulty of the
analytic work more strongly, I hope to afford in the present
book.

Corresponding to the external modifications in the psychoanalytic movement, there are internal changes which are much
too little noticed by those not intimately associated with it.
Many a justifiable reproach from the side of its opponents applies to the analysis as once practiced but not to the present
method. It is obvious that so new and penetrating a method of
investigation was and is subject to errors. That which once
appeared to the astonished gaze of the discoverer as evident
certainty, discloses here and there to closer observation other
causal connections. Where from a number of coincident results, a comprehensive principle was derived, later, contradictory observations, setting the earlier formula against a new one,
may compel a hypothesis embracing both the old and the newest
knowledge. This transition is common to all sciences and it

* Imago, I, pp. 56–82 (1912).
† P. 77.

would not be just to forge weapons against the method from
this adaptation to the progress of experience.   I am not at all
averse to voicing the opinion that psychoanalytic science has
very much to learn and will learn from the observation of
earnest pedagogues and any critical co-worker who discloses
errors and ambiguities will be most welcome.

I shall name some of the most important transformations
which the analytic theory and technique has undergone since
its inception: The theory that the repression of an affectful
idea into the unconscious was always accomplished by a painful, shocking experience.   The shock or trauma theory was
given up in favor of the conception that everything is of importance, the repression of ideas or phantasies.   Where once
the emphasis lay on the sexual trauma, the unconscious attachment to the parents was found to be the chief cause of the
neuroses and of other conditions of dependence on the unconscious which influenced life.   The sexual theory, previously the
greatest stumbling block, underwent a radical change, since,
not only the assertion of the causation of every neurosis in a
sexual irritation in the ordinary sense, was abandoned, but also,
the term sexuality received a great amplification, so that the
poorly oriented reader scarcely understands any longer what
the analyst means by the word and strikes wrong interpretations.   Where at that time, one considered the ''abreaction,''
the affectful ''speaking out,'' as the healing agent, to-day we
know that the transference of repressed wishes upon the
analyst, forms, at least in severe cases, an indispensable condition of the cure.   Where in the first period, the analytic
attack was directed at the symptom, now, it is, in a certain
sense, neglected, in order to turn all attention to the resistance
against analyst and analysis.   If at first, one aims only at the
elimination of the internal conflict, he presently strives for
independent adaptation to reality which comes from the overcoming of the internal two-sidedness, the turning of the
patient's mental forces toward reality in accordance with the
limitations of his personal peculiarities, and thus rounds out
the analytic educational work by assisting conservatively self-

education. Freud's fight against the scientifically and ethically reprehensible "wild psychoanalysis," * which expects cure from promiscuous sexual gratification without regard to scruples or love, has also raised the moral standing of the analysis.

By all these modifications, which are due in only the slightest measure to hostile criticism, almost entirely to psychoanalytic experience, the agreement with traditional views and especially with prevailing pedagogic ideas, has been essentially increased. In 1907, Isserlin explained: "If we emphasize the disposition somewhat more and deprive the trauma † of the decisive rôle which it would play in the causation of hysteria, the contending opinions would have come closely together." ‡ We have seen that the original historical and psychological chasm which seemed unabridgable in the beginning, became narrowed also at other points. He who travels in an unknown land, at first notices the new and strange; only gradually does the "partout comme chez nous" come into its rights.

It would now be my task to describe how the critics met and accompanied the forward march of psychoanalysis. To my satisfaction, Bleuler has performed this necessary task in his discerning article, "Die Psychoanalyse Freuds." The battle raged in the most diverse affective states; from perfect neutrality to furious insult, to boycott, indeed in one instance, even to denunciation before the public, in which scarcely an insinuation was omitted. As a strange cultural curiosity, one example may be mentioned without anger or intent to complain or apply for the martyr's crown. I can mention it with all the greater equanimity since it only reacted in favor of psychoanalysis. On the 15th of December, 1911, a neurologist in Zurich, specialist in electrotherapy, gave a public lecture in

* Freud has from the beginning fought against this with all possible vigor, for example, Kl. Schriften I, p. 109 (1895), pp. 137 ff., 199, 230; II, pp. 14, 34.

† M. Isserlin über Jungs "Psychologie der Dementia praecox und die Anwendung Freudscher Forschungsmaximen in der Psychopathologie." Zentralblatt für Nervenheilkunde u. Psychiatrie. 1907, p. 341.

‡ Jahrbuch II, pp. 623–730.

which he pictured the objectionableness and perversity of psychoanalysis. To this end, he drew a caricature which estranged even non-analysts. In order to show what kind of a business an analysis was, he picked out of Freud's "Fragment of Hysteria-Analysis," that is, from an article intended only for the medical profession, one of the most delicate portions and described to the public, among which were many young boys and girls, how Freud discussed coitus in os. One can imagine the indignation of some, the joy of others. What would that speaker have said if one had pictured orally to a totally unprepared audience containing many very young individuals, in a voice of moral indignation, the things which that physician did to women and girls in his gynecological practice? And in this, it would not be a question of perversions which would be exposed to the phantasy of persons half-developed sexually. The refusal of a public debate by the analytic side led to a violent contest in the daily press, the end result of which was favorable to psychoanalysis in that the denounced literature was really devoured and the rush to the analysts increased wherever possible.

Since Bleuler's article in defence of psychoanalysis, there has appeared only one important criticism of psychoanalysis: that of Arthur Kronfeld.* In its depth of thought, neutral reserve and repeatedly, indeed, in its honest admiration of Freud, it places all other discussions in the shade. Still, it is one with its predecessors in that it does not trouble itself in the least about the fundamental facts underlying psychoanalysis and avoids a priori empiric tests. The hypotheses and theories which Freud and his pupils have been compelled to believe from the phenomena observed, it puts under the head of "general psychological foundations" and thus stands the whole system on its head. How would a representation of the Wundtian psychology work, which began, say with the principle of the

* Über die psychologischen Theorien Freuds und verwandte Anschauungen," Archiv für die gesamte Psychologie, Vol. XXII (1911), pp. 130–248. While this book was in press, an excellent anticriticism against Kronfeld by Gaston Rosenstein appeared (Jahrbuch IV (1913), pp. 741–798).

aim of heterogony, and from there went backwards but was promptly silent every time Wundt disclosed a psychological fact determined empirically or proposed an experiment? The effect would plainly be similar to that in a cinematographic production if a dramatic scene was produced backwards by reversing the film. All causal connections would be destroyed, the whole would be incomprehensible. So proceeds Kronfeld with the analysis. Also the most everyday observations, for example, the transposition of an affect from one idea to another, he denies without going to the trouble of a test. Like all the hostile critics, Kronfeld seems to suffer from a strange fear of the facts, an "ontophobia." Hence his industry, his learning and his sharpsightedness serve no purpose, the discussion is hopeless though one would gladly meet so chivalrous an opponent.

In the following statements, I shall give careful attention to the voices of the critics. Especially shall I consider the expressions of Alt, Aschaffenburg, O. Binswanger, Dubois, O. Fischer, F. W. Foerster, Friedländer, Heilbronner, Hoche, Janet, Isserlin, Klien, Kraepelin, Kronfeld, Lehmann, Mendel, Moll, Näcke, Oppenheim, Morton Prince, Siemerling, Skliar, Vogt, Wiegandt, Ziehen. I hope that no important argument of these opponents will escape me. The mockers among the opponents, I would ask to recall that old saying which Goethe gives in his "Faust": "We are accustomed to men jeering at that which they do not understand."

The many other authors who, after proving for themselves, have broken lances in favor of the violently opposed theory, should be considered with the same precision.

If the objection be raised that pedagogy ought to wait in silence until the physicians have solved the problem of psychoanalysis, two facts should be remembered: psychoanalysis is also important for normal individuals; these are of no concern to the physician but of much concern to the educator. Further, this professional quarrel of the physicians may not be settled for decades; meanwhile, however, the great new educational problems are waiting and can no longer be put off. The scientifically trained pedagogue is just as good an expert in regard to the child's mind and the influencing of this function as the physician is for the sick child. Therefore, the teacher has a right to his own judgment and the stimulating encouragement of Freud as well as all other competent analysts can only strengthen him in his undertaking.

From our historical sketch, we may now derive the definition: Psychoanalysis is a scientifically grounded method devoted to neurotic and mentally deranged persons, as well as to normal individuals, which seeks by the collection and interpretation of associations, with the avoidance of suggestion and hypnosis, to investigate and influence the instinctive forces and content of mental life lying below the threshold of consciousness.

Whether or not the claims expressed in this definition are justified, we have now to determine.

PART I

THE THEORY OF PSYCHOANALYSIS

CHAPTER II

THE PSYCHOANALYTIC CONCEPTION OF AN UNCONSCIOUS

WE may now approach the question: what are we to think of subliminal mental processes? Are there in general subconscious psychic facts? Does an unconscious exist and is it scientifically conceivable?

The prevailing psychology is not very kindly disposed toward the unconscious. True, its existence is seldom disputed. At the most, some representatives of the psychophysical materialism, as for example, Ziehen, deny its existence. The psychiatrist named considers it in all seriousness as doubtful whether all the very complicated acts of hypnotised persons are not without parallel psychical processes and thereby readily leads us to the standpoint of old Cartesius who denied animals all mental experiences and considered them "creaking machines."* It cannot surprise us that this hypothesis of psychoanalysis receives little favor and is explained without trial as "nonsense." † The other psychologists allow the validity of the unconscious. Indeed, Th. Lipps considers consciousness as such, as a passive, indifferent, in itself unimportant by-product of unconscious processes.‡ This appreciation, how-

* Th. Ziehen, Leitfaden der physiolog. Psychologie (9th ed., Jena, 1911, p. 259).

† Ziehen, in a psychiatric meeting, flatly explained the Freudian theories as nonsense. The printed report to which we owe this communication, neglected to say whether Ziehen gave reasons for his opinion.

‡ E. v. Hartmann, Die moderne Psychologie, Leipzig, 1901, p. 99.

ever, is made of less value by the fact that Lipps does not know
how to render the unconscious accessible to scientific observation.
We poor psychologists stand before the screen of unconsciousness
without any hope of learning to know the picture-making machinery.
Wundt uses us a little less roughly. He
does not lift the subliminal, at least at first, to so high a rank
before establishing our helplessness in comprehending it.
"Our knowledge of the elements which have become unconscious
has to do with nothing more than the possibility of
memory." *

Besides denying the existence of the unconscious or scientific
recognition of it, psychology presents a considerable confusion
of terms which we must consider in order not to increase it.

In order to fix the concept of the unconscious, we proceed
from that of the conscious and consciousness. But does not the
same confusion prevail here?

The psychologists make it easy by explaining: one can only
experience consciousness, not describe † or define it.‡ Against
these opinions, Dürr maintains with justice that everything
which science discusses must permit of a definition.‖ Wundt
also saw himself forced later to the formulation of a definition.

"Consciousness" is derived from "conscious" which word
is used in reference to an object or to the objectivated subject,
for example: the "conscious" matter; "an idea becomes clearly
conscious," "I am conscious."

Both meanings occur in derivatives. Whoever is "conscious"
exercises a function, for example, a perception, an idea.
In reference to the subject, the expression "conscious" always
has an active meaning, to an object, a passive one.

In the mental experience, as also in "knowing," we are accustomed
to distinguish subject, object and function. The

---

* Wundt, Grundriss der Psychologie, p. 243.
† Kirchner, Katechismus der Psychologie, Leipzig, 1883, p. 52.
‡ Wundt, Grundzüge der phys. Psychologie. 2 (1881) II, p. 195.
‖ Dürr, Bewusstsein u. Unbewusstes in der "Tiefenpsychologie."
Grundfragen der Psychologie u. Pädagogik II, p. 37.

psychologic reflection has elaborated the concept of consciousness in each of these three directions:

1. As subject concept, it denotes the subject of the mental life.* As, for example, in the phrase, "the man or the mind is consciousness." † This latter can therefore appear as acting. I mention the expression which has become old-style, because from it, in the expression "the unconscious" or "the unconsciousness," important counterparts have developed.

2. As function concept, the term "consciousness" has very many meanings. Some of these meanings are: (a) as "connection of the mental images." According to Wundt, the meaning of the term would be that it expressed that general union of mental processes from which the individual images arise as narrower combinations.‡ According to this definition there prevails in deep sleep or in a fainting spell, a state of unconsciousness, something which Wundt admits. Nevertheless, an isolated sensation in sleep, for example thirst, or a simple dream-picture not connected with other psychic images, would be unconscious, while a dream scene would be conscious. This use of language will therefore not enlighten us.

(b) Consciousness = "the totality of mental affairs belonging to an individual" (Witasek).‖

(c) Consciousness = the inner outcropping of our sensations, ideas and emotions (Höffding).¶

(d) Consciousness = "All actual ideas" (Herbart) § or "the comprehension of objects" (Dürr).**

(e) Consciousness = "the knowledge concerning the existence of all or a part of psychic affairs belonging to an individual; in general, the knowledge about all the psychic and also physical

* Same, p. 39.
† Rehmke, Die Seele des Menschen, Leipzig, 1902, p. 43.
‡ Wundt, Grundriss, p. 238.
‖ S. Witasek, Grundlinien der Psychologie, p. 60.
¶ H. Höffding, Psychologie, 2d ed., Leipzig, 1893, p. 95.
§ Herbart, Psychologie als Wiss. Sämtl. W. W. (Kehrbach). Vol. V (Langensalza 1890), p. 193.
** Dürr, Bewusstsein u. Unbewusstes in der "Tiefenpsychologie." Grundfragen der Psychologie u. Pädagogik II, p. 39.

objects of which the individual thinks, of which he is accordingly conscious."* According to this condition, a knowledge about mental experiences or content would be necessary, a self-observation, an "inner sense."

We add the description of Lotze:

(f) Consciousness = Waking state.† Therewith all dreams would be unconscious, no matter how vividly I may experience them in myself nor how exactly I know them, nor how powerfully the selfconsciousness appeared in them. In favor of Lotze's statement speaks the fact that one is not accustomed to attribute consciousness to persons overcome with sleep.

In contradiction to this, one speaks of a lowering of consciousness, indeed of a suspension of consciousness, where a passionate excitement prevents our knowing what we are doing (Ulrici).‡ From this, follows,

(g) Consciousness = Waking state in every relation free from extreme passion.

(h) Consciousness = Waking state in normal mental activity. The last description leads us already to the third kind of elaboration of concept.

3. As object concept, consciousness is differentiated from the process of knowing in the following expressions:

(a) Consciousness = Content of knowledge or what is known. In this sense, we speak of a moral or religious consciousness, in which of course, we think not of a mere fund of knowledge but of an affectful experience and inner reaction.

(b) Consciousness = Existence in the selfperception or in the selfconsciousness. (Similarly Leibniz).‖ Against this limitation, Dürr justly remarks: "A child which sees houses, trees, animals and people, also has consciousness, although it cannot yet state psychological considerations concerning his perceptions and his other mental life."¶

---

* Witasek, p. 61.

† H. Lotze, Grundzüge der Psychologie, Leipzig, 1894, p. 81.

‡ H. Ulrici, Leib u. Seele. Leipzig, 1866, p. 277.

‖ Wundt, Grundz. d. ph. Psych. II, p. 348.

¶ Dürr, p. 39.

Thus the terminologies intersect one another in a confusing whirl. For etymological and practical reasons, I define consciousness as the existence of any kind of psychic phenomena. Thus I assign the dream and the delirium in which there is often so strong selfconsciousness and perception to the conscious activities as well as incoherent dream fragments.

It is now not hard for us to mark off the different concepts of the unconscious against those of the conscious.

For our purpose, we distinguish the philosophical definitions, thus the metaphysical of a Schelling, Schopenhauer, v. Hartmann, the theological of an I. H. Fichte and Ulrici, the epistemological construction of an Ed. v. Hartmann.*

Here, we have only to deal with the unconscious as a psychological concept, that is, such an one as results from a scientific elaboration of psychic phenomena. Its logical foundations are to be sought in psychophysics and pure psychology.

The psychophysical parallelism assumes that psychic processes correspond to excitations of the central nervous system. It denies the view "that the phenomena of consciousness may be derived from objective events or inversely, the objective results from states of consciousness." † Since among conscious phenomena, connections are missing, that principle can be carried through only under the presupposition of unconscious phenomena. This is especially strikingly the case in the recollection of memories. What has become of the conscious content in the moment of forgetting? Does it remain in existence as Herbart ‡ assumes or does it only leave behind a disposition to its recurrence? ‖ In any case, however, there existed a complex of conditions beyond consciousness to recall a conscious content.

Or when a minimal stimulus in the central nervous system slowly increases, goes beyond the threshold of consciousness,

* v. Hartmann, Die moderne Psychologie, p. 79.
† G. F. Lipps, Grundriss der Psychophysik. Leipzig, 1909, p. 25 f.
‡ Herbart, Vol. V, p. 338 ff.
‖ Witasek, p. 54 f.

grows strong and slowly diminishes, should then only the strongest stimuli produce a psychic accompaniment?

Unconscious processes or those which have become unconscious accompany all perception and cognition, thought and volition. We do not know, for example, without psychological instruction why and in what way we have attained to an idea of space and location in space. We think in concepts, the full extent of which is not present with us.* We decide according to values, the foundation and coacting motives of which in great part escape us. The same is the case with instinct, time, many habits, actions which have become mechanical, mysterious feelings, dreams, etc.†

Experimentally, an unconscious was first proven by the hypnotic investigation. Forel, for example, argued: "Often we are unable to recall a familiar name and just so much the less, the more we seek it. . . . In hypnosis, such interpolations and omissions are intentionally brought about by suggestion and the conscious part of the brain activity is constantly displaced by the temporary results of suggestion executed in unconscious ways." ‡ By well conceived hypnotic procedure, the first psychologist outside the Freudian school to demonstrate unconscious functions in normal mental life was Narziss Ach and this in reaction experiments. He formulated the statement: "It is the rule that the effective goal-idea, upon the appearance of the concrete idea of reference, does not appear in consciousness as such but nevertheless exercises a determining influence. . . . These peculiar activities proceeding from the goal-idea, related to the idea of reference, we designate as the determining tendencies." || Perhaps many will take ex-

* Th. Lipps, Leitf. d. Psycholog. Leipzig, 1903, p. 40.
† Höffding, pp. 94–112.
‡ A. Forel, Der Hypnotismus, seine Bedeutung und seine Handhabung, Stuttgart, 1889, p. 55.
|| Narziss Ach, Über die Willenstätigkeit und das Denken. Göttingen, 1905, p. 224 f. Ach lays great stress on his priority in the discovery of this "determination" (Über den Willensakt und das Temperament, Leipzig, 1912, p. 286), but he does not perceive the immense import of his find.

ception to calling an activity, a tendency. Then he will prefer the definition: "These mental attitudes acting in the unconscious (=non-conscious), proceeding from the significance of the goal-ideas, directed toward the approaching idea of reference, which actuate a spontaneous appearance of the determining idea, we designate as determining tendencies."* Another pupil of Külpe, K. Koffka, speaks of non-conscious reproduction, and determining tendencies which have an influence on the course of ideas.† Concerning the latter, he remarks: "On one side, determining tendencies may call forth conscious ideas, on the other side, thoughts liberated termining tendencies. If we think of the existence of a tendency before its realization: it is then a thought and this would have to occasion the like tendency to which it owed its origin. This becoming conscious of the tendency thus retroacts on its force, the tendency is thereby strengthened."‡ Max Offner, who collects in his study of the memory the results of the experimental psychology, arrives at the same conclusion: "The assumption of these subliminal psychic processes, this unconscious but similar to conscious mental activity, is not to be avoided if we would not consider the conscious psychic events as a mere succession and juxtaposition of experiences but would bring them into an inner relationship as we inwardly associate the strokes of the clock with the hours by the knowledge that they are caused by the action of a mechanism built and acting according to fixed laws which is separated from our perception. Liebmann points out an excellent analogy: "There are dramas," he says, "which would remain absolutely unintelligible without what goes on behind the scenes. To these dramas, belongs the human mental life. What takes place on the stage of clear consciousness are only broken fragments and shreds of the personal mental life. It would be incomprehensible, indeed impossible, without what

* P. 228.

† K. Koffka, Zur Analyse der Vorstellungen und ihrer Gesetze, Leipzig, 1912, p. 299 ff. Still nearer comes Freud: G. F. Lipps, Weltanschauung u. Bildungsideal, Leipzig u. Berlin, 1911, page 155.

‡ P. 316.

transpires behind the curtain, that is, without unconscious processes.'' ''For considering these unconscious processes as something not really unconscious but only as conscious in a limited degree, as carrying a 'differential' from consciousness, observation affords us no justification. Only the unjustified presupposition that psychic and conscious are interchangeable terms is the occasion of that empirically unsubstantiated assertion.'' * Thus with Ach, the unconscious has obtained entrance to the experimental psychology, and indeed not only as a general explanatory principle but as an empirically demonstrated fact. To this state of affairs, I expressly call the attention of those who still continue to deny the unconscious as an unscientific concept.

The concept of the unconscious limited to the causal relationship of psychic phenomena now receives different interpretations. Many conceive of it as purely physiological (Jodl, Külpe). Proceeding from the supposition that sensations, ideas and emotions are conceivable only as having happened, thus as consciously experienced, they explain the condition of the unconsciousness of these phenomena as a contradiction and consider ''conscious'' and ''psychic'' simply as identical. So far then as they admit that this physiological unconscious influences the conscious, they destroy the psychophysical parallelism and thereby saw off the bough on which they are sitting. They deliver themselves over to materialism which they consider as long abandoned and no longer tenable.   Moreover, they do not explain the pretended difference between brain processes with and without consciousness and likewise leave the constant interaction between conscious and unconscious incomprehensible (Höffding).†

Again, many consider the unconscious as a ''psychic disposition of unknown kind.''   This is especially true of Wundt who considers it probable ''that the psychological condition of the ideas in the unconscious stand in a similar relation to their conscious purpose as the accompanying physiological processes or

* M. Offner, Das Gedächtnis, 2d ed. Berlin, 1911, p. 135.
† Höffding, p. 107.

conditions hold to one another.'' * Höffding speaks cautiously
and conservatively of psychic analogues which constitute the
unconscious, the nature of which he leaves entirely undeter-
mined, and of which he demands only that they render possible
both the origin of conscious phenomena and the relationship
between conscious and unconscious activity. He leaves it undecided whether one may speak of an unconscious mental life.†
Theodor Lipps, who has broken so many lances in defence of the
reality of the unconscious, says: ''Since unconscious sensations and ideas are the same regarding real processes as the
conscious, so they are subject to the same rule of law. They
use a similar mode of action. On the other hand, we may only
speak of unconscious sensations and ideas, where psychic activities, that is ultimately where purpose, coming and going of
conscious experiences and the constitution of the same, force us
to it. Or rather, the maintaining of unconscious sensations
and ideas ultimately proves nothing else than that in the psychic life-connection, activities may be encountered and formulated which are similar to the activities of conscious sensations
and ideas, without possessing the corresponding conscious content.'' ‡ The unconscious, in itself, is an entirely undefined affair; by an overstepping of the threshold of consciousness and a
lowering of the same, a process is not changed from an unconscious into a conscious one, as it were, inverted, but to it, the
conscious content comes or from it, disappears (38). There
are no unconscious or unnoticed contents. Thus, unconscious
sensations and ideas are psychic realities without content (37).
Who can conceive of such a thing? Is not something psychic
without content as inconceivable as color without extent?

Only a few philosophical authors of to-day speak of a psychic
existence of the unconscious elements of the mental life which
carry and determine all conscious processes. To this number,
belong, besides Th. Lipps, Friedrich Paulsen || and Max Offner.

* Wundt, Phys. Psych. II, p. 204.
† Höffding, pp. 108, 110.
‡ Lipps, Leitfaden, p. 39 f.
|| Paulsen, Einleitung in die Philosophie, Berlin, 1898, p. 126 ff.

The former explains unconscious ideas as "potential inner perceptions" or better, as not absolutely non-conscious but rather a less-conscious, a conscious perhaps lowered to complete imperceptibility.* In these statements, I miss definitive clearness. Less conscious and completely imperceptibly conscious are as different concepts as conscious and unconscious, for to consciousness belongs, as one may also comprehend the term, perceptibility, existence. Less conscious is no longer purely potential. Thus this defender of unconscious psychic phenomena loses himself in unfathomable contradictions. Only Max Offner, so far as I know, speaks candidly of unconscious psychic phenomena.

Thus, we arrive at this result: modern psychology cannot get along without an unconscious. It frequently attributes to this function the greatest significance for the conscious mental life but it can develop nothing systematic out of it. Beyond vague surmises which contribute nothing to the scientific explanation of psychic phenomena, it does not proceed. For psychology, the unconscious is an important but entirely unknown make-shift. If Wundt is right in his statement that we must give up forever the hope of learning the nature and thus also the laws of the unconscious, then psychology is in a bad way. Every knowledge-seeking investigator of mental phenomena must feel indebted to him who furnishes information concerning the subliminal processes.

Is the psychoanalyst this man? In order to decide this question, let us proceed from the facts which led him to an assumption of an unconscious. That the analysis proceeds from facts and only then formulates laws, is in opposition to the views of those who assert that the analysts have derived laws arbitrarily and by the help of these laws, constructed facts which should then afterwards again prove the laws.

Breuer and Freud came to their conception of unconscious ideas without any special kind of interpretation method. The former obtained from his famous patient while he kept before

* P. 129.

her a word whispered by her during an "'absence,'" * information which could be checked up accurately by external means.
I, too, came, by a method which differs in nothing from the
usual, customary scientific stipulation, to the assumption of unconscious psychic phenomena by an examination which hardly
deserves to be called an analysis.†

A pupil of about sixteen years is one morning dumb, sees
his surroundings in late forenoon still veiled in darkness, as
if it were not yet day; as he rises, his legs refuse to work,
while over his chest, a strange tension makes itself felt. Urged
to confide in me the secret which is troubling him, he tells me
the previous history of his illness up to the afternoon in which
he was prevented by a feeling of shame from following his intention of confessing to his mother that he practiced onanism
and had stolen from her. In this moment, appeared the painful thoughts: "I can no longer speak as I would! Now all
is dark before me! I hang only by a thread!" ‡ This mono-
logue the patient had completely forgotten during his hysterical
disturbance.

I state emphatically that this memory caused me great surprise and was in no way influenced by me as to content. Following our analytic or qualitative criterion of causality, we are
inclined to connect the hysterical symptoms of dumbness, disturbances of vision and gait, as well as the feeling of a closely
defined zone of considerable extent on the chest, which is difficult to understand psychologically, with the complaint expressed the day before, which corresponds exactly in content.

* Under "absence" is understood what is usually called unconsciousness.

† All the examples in this book come, when not otherwise specified,
from my pedagogic and pastoral practice. All refer to persons with
ethical or religious defects. All afford only fragments of analyses. It
has not been possible to avoid giving the impression that the analytic
work is simpler than is really the case. The overcoming of the resistance (see Chapter XIX), the avoidance of the so-called collateral paths,
the interweaving with other symptoms, and the like, could not be
demonstrated.

‡ The details are in my article: "Psychanalyt. Seelsorge u. experi-
mentelle Moralpädagogik." Prot. Monatshefte, 1909, pp. 3–42.

How the causal connection is to be conceived, is as little clear to us as that between the idea and the execution of a voluntary movement of the arm. It would indeed be too remarkable if the otherwise absolutely enigmatical, affectful thoughts and the hysterical inhibitions should have happened accidentally at the same time. No one will believe this.

In order to proceed with entire certainty, let us look around for similar cases. - They are very easy to find for everyone who has opportunity and ability to observe. I do not see at all that the facts asserted by Freud cannot be tested, as Kronfeld asserts.* Analogous examples in great numbers meet every educator, pastor and physician who is willing to see, hence the second causal criterion, that of constant result, is also fulfilled. A few simple examples may follow:

A girl of fifteen and one-half years suddenly exhibits during the analysis swollen lips. I seek to learn whether this phenomenon has appeared before and discover that this actually occurred, one morning, five years before. [What happened at that time?] † "A student had wanted to kiss me the day before and I successfully defended myself against him." Since that time, the girl has hated the students until the pastoral treatment. Before the recrudescence of the hysterical phenomenon, the girl had once more refused the kisses of a young admirer.

A girl of twelve and a half years frequently suffers from severe migraine and pelvic pains which confine her to her bed. She has the feeling that all her hairs are being pulled out. [!] (After longer hesitation:) "One day, my brother took the liberty when we were alone, to do improper things to me. As I struggled, he seized me violently by the hair." [The pains in the pelvis.] "It seems to me as if a cogwheel were revolving in me. My brother was in the habit of biting off his fingernails

---

* P. 68 (see foot-note on page 18).

† Throughout the whole book, square brackets contain my words addressed to the subject of analysis, round parentheses, my notes intended for the reader. An exclamation point represents the question: "What comes into your mind?"

so that the edges were uneven." From that hour, the symptoms ceased. Of a possible sexual cause for hysteria, the girl knew nothing.

The same highly talented patient, whose hysteria, unfortunately, formed only the superstructure of an epilepsy, presented a very striking series of symptoms. Some months before I made her acquaintance, she was seized, after the midday meal, with a spell of clucking. In spite of the application of various household remedies, the tormenting trouble continued until after the evening meal, when the little one went to the bookcase and read some passages from Scheffel's "Ekkehard." Henceforth, as often as the clucking became disturbing, nothing helped but the book named. Suddenly, this remarkable, hitherto prompt and unfailing remedy also lost its power, when my help was sought.

It is perhaps somewhat presumptuous to present this example at this time, since it is complicated. But it shows certain peculiarities of the unconscious and the analytic method so prettily that I cannot bring myself to suppress it. According to my stenographic notes, the exploration ran the following course: [The clucking.] "With us at home, that is called 'Schnackerl.' I call it foolishly 'Goschnill,' in which, I emphasize the last syllable. This word seems to me very significant: 'Cochenille' means the purple snail. My brother has a specimen in his collection. I have the strange impression that the 'Goschnill' could hop. This seems to apply more to the word than to the object. I do not know at all why I find it so significant. [Goschnill.] Gosche, one calls the mouth vulgarly. 'Schnill' might refer to schnellen (to jerk), oh yes! Clucking is a jerking with the mouth. The hopping 'Goschnill' reminds me of hopping crabs in the dune sand. I enjoy having one of these animals hop on me while I lay there dreaming. My brother gave me countless lectures on them. My brother, when he is eating or is alone with me, makes his hands jump constantly. (We shall discuss this obsessional neurotic individual on page 73). He jerks them into the air."

It is plain that many hysterical symptoms, externally considered, are simple imitations. The suspicion is at once awakened in everyone who knows this fact, that the mouth jerking of the sister is connected with that of the brother, and at the same time that the purple snail and the hopping crabs also refer to him. The further investigation of the case affords us confirmation of this surmise.

"Ekkehard" is our youth's favorite book. The girl could not read it to the end, however, and is anxious concerning the conclusion. Her favorite is Frau Hadwig. She loves an "educated, awkward, intolerant monk whom she can never marry and a handsome servant, Praxedis." [Ekkehard.] "My brother is also educated, awkward and would gladly live as a hermit in a little church in the wilderness." [Praxedis.] "She reminds me of my English teacher whom I love very much."

It was directly ascertained that shortly before the failure of the reading as a defence against the clucking, the news of the departure of the beloved lady had been announced. Now, is the conclusion too strained that our patient was freed from her automatism by the fact that without noticing it, she compared herself to the duchess, nevertheless, contrary to her expectation, was left in the lurch by the story when the comparison no longer tallied? We shall later meet numbers of such comparisons. He who finds incredible our supposition of unconscious trains of thought as the connecting member between the facts of the clucking and that of the relation to the brother, as well as to the romantic ideas, can turn to the course of the hysterical process of our patient.

About two weeks after the subsidence of the clucking, a tormenting itching of the scalp broke out. A moderate rash as result of use of bromide did not explain the sensorial irritation. By questioning, I found, at the same time carefully avoiding all falsification from suggestion: the young girl scratched herself till blood came ("as if I would scalp myself") and tore out whole wisps of hair. The itching, in spite of its painfulness, was a pleasure. In more striking manner, during the intense feeling, she had to fix her eyes on her brother constantly. Previously, she had noticed that the latter, who had formerly also had a nervous skin eruption, had a dirty scalp.* "Itching" can signify a motor function and is then synonymous with jerking and also a sensory affair. This symptom also disappeared immediately after the analysis.

We shall frequently see how, in place of a prohibited neurotic manifestation, another makes its appearance. As our patient had previously imitated the brother's itching by a motor symptom, the clucking, so now she does it by a sensory one. Therefore she looked at him constantly while she was having her hysterical symptoms. It becomes quite evident here that below the threshold of consciousness, an elaboration of the symptom, in the sense of choice and automatic realization of a new symbol, takes place. Some further compensations appeared after the quickly attained cure. For the sake of brevity, we must pass over them.

In order to accustom the reader to the thought that we are really dealing with laws derived from facts, I will give a few apt examples out of many dozens of such.

A lady of twenty-five years has suffered for nine years from severe migraine in the temples. [Do you recall the first attack of the trouble?] "No." [Press on the temples and think of the first attack.] "It was in the pension. I had just received a letter. From my father. He is a drunkard. On his departure, he had said: 'Do not be surprised if you receive a letter telling you that I have shot myself.' As a child, I had often received a blow there, especially during quarrels. The migraine became far worse after I had seen in a print the corpse of a man who had shot himself in the temples."

These communications were interrupted by digressive (or apparently digressive) remarks. They sufficed to banish the suffering from those places. The same hysterical patient, one day during the course of the analysis, created a crown of painful points of pressure on her head. By the observation of this phenomena, she awoke the memory that, as a girl of sixteen, after her pastor had described the innocent One, persecuted

---

* Jung calls my attention to the fact that Goethe's sister also had an eczema on neck and breast when she would appear decolleté.

and crowned with thorns, she plaited a crown out of thorn branches and placed it on her head. At present, she feels herself likewise innocent but persecuted. May we venture the surmise that she consoles herself by identification with the Savior? At all events, we will not dispute an unconscious connection after the analogy of conscious trains of thought. The crown of thorns disappeared at once after the autoanalysis.

He who hesitates to give his assent or thinks to escape with mere psychic dispositions should give his attention to the following example: A boy of sixteen years suffers from many points of pressure on his head which go back to falls, beatings, etc. The father, a teacher, was in the habit of boxing his son on the ear during piano instruction, until the painful places called a halt to the practice. Immediately after the discovery of these facts, the trouble disappeared but after a little while, re-· appeared as an hysterical crown of thorns. This time also, the apperception of the symptom led to the Savior, crowned with thorns, whose passion the patient had viewed with pity in the primary school. This identification, too, would console for undeserved persecutions. In the next consultation, the boy surprised me with a line of pressure which, when more closely examined, brought forth the associated memory: "Often, my parents said to me: 'You are an odd saint!'" The unmasked pseudo-messiah thus satisfied himself with a somewhat more modest rôle. Who would now assume that the brain centers which allowed the imaginary thorns to be felt, have, without psychic intervention, yielded their function to quite different ones which have brought forth the feeling of an aureole?

An unintelligent person of forty-eight years, whose superstition long bothered me, asked me on occasion of a visit: "Do you not think, Pastor, that people who were born on special days can see wonderful things which are hidden from ordinary people? [Did you come into the world on a special day?] "Certainly, on the birthday of the Confederation." [What secret thing have you seen?] "Thirty years ago, one evening at nine o'clock, on the steps, I saw a white figure with piercing black eyes, long black hair and long fingers. It looked at me without moving. I was at first rigid from fright but then ran into the room and shouted that someone was standing out there. My parents, however, saw no one. Some days later, the angel appeared to me in my sleeping room." [Good! Put yourself back with strained attention to the moment of the vision. Consider the piercing black eyes. What comes into your mind?] "Our neighbor had such eyes." [The hair of the angel.] "This too corresponded with that of the neighbor." [The angel had long fingers which is not usually related of the messengers of God.] "Marvelous! The neighbor also had long fingers." (Later addition: "On that afternoon, a saleswoman had said to me: 'Your neighbor will find no rest in the grave for she has obtained her house through legacy-hunting.' " Hence the long fingers.) "She liked to scare children. We couldn't endure her!" (By chance, I had just analyzed two dreams of the funerals of living people and had found confirmation of Freud's assertion (Traumdeutung, 3rd ed. p. 179) that behind these dreams, lurks the repressed wish for the death of the person in question. Therefore, I continued:) [The neighbor was hostile to you but you wished her not simply death but made her in your vision into an angel of God. What better could you wish for a person if you would put him aside?] "I see that you are right; now I have rejoiced over my angel for some thirty years."

(One recalls that professional murderers of children were called "angel-makers," in which title, likewise, the base motive is hidden by one outwardly sublime.)

I will not suppose that the reader will believe my interpretation. Provisionally, we have only to deal with the question whether between the neighbor and the angel, a causal connection existed and whether the change seen in the hallucination may be traced back to unconscious mental work. Only from a series of observations of such connections will we look for the laws according to which the subliminal mental activity occurs.

From the large number of religious hallucinations which I

have explored, I add a further example.* A youth of seventeen and one-half years had the following experience: "Six and one-half years ago, I was approaching my home after coming from a neighboring village. Suddenly, I was attracted to look at a mighty oak. There appeared from behind the tree and coming toward me, a great black figure as if it had sprung out of the ground. It rubbed its hands toward me as if it would wash them. At the same time, there was a sound like thunder. For some minutes, I was as if paralyzed. I would gladly have run away but could not. Finally, I ran home in great excitement." [Describe the figure accurately and tell what comes into your mind.] "The figure had black curly hair. Otherwise nothing. Yes! It was naked. A terrible enemy whom I had, also had such hair. He spread the rumor concerning me that a certain girl had been impregnated by me. Strangely enough, this girl came from the village which I had left shortly before the vision. The physician examined the girl and declared her pure. My father complained for me of injury to my honor. Before the justice of the peace, I said to my calumniator: 'You are a regular devil!' I received an indemnity of thirty francs which I gave to the poor. The bad fellow also had black curly hair just like the devil. Otherwise, I know nothing." [The devil was naked.] "Because it was an impure thing. Because he stood there in his nakedness." [Rubbing the hands.] "Perhaps in rage. When my enemy was in a rage, he rubbed his hands."

[That you did not recognize your enemy in the devil for seven years shows that not all the traits correspond. Name the most important difference.] "The nose. My enemy's was considerably larger." [The nose of the devil.] (Simon laughs.) "It is very interesting! That girl had a strikingly small nose like the devil in my apparition."

Since I already knew the laws of unconscious processes to be considered in this connection, I drew a conclusion which I do not expect the reader to accept unconditionally as yet: "The

* Pfister, Die psycholog. Enträtselung der rel. Glossolalie u. autom. Kryptographie, Leipzig und Vienna, 1912, p. 15 f.

hallucination probably expressed the wish that the hated enemy might be changed into the devil, standing there in his nakedness in helpless rage (like Lady Macbeth after the king's murder in Shakespeare's drama) and seeking to cleanse his hands by washing and bearing, in addition, the visible sign of his calumniation, the nose of the injured girl." I am going still a little deeper into the interpretation. Nevertheless, at the present status of our investigation, I do not once expect the reader to accept even the repeated interpretation. I hope only to show here that a connection exists between the devil and the enemy as well as the girl, perhaps even a purposeful connection, concerning the formation of which, every psychologist is curious.

In order to increase the expectation somewhat more, I add a third hallucination which, like the foregoing, may also show by the way, how the psychoanalytic method leads the apperception of the object and the entirely uncritical association to facts which bring nearer to our understanding the relations of origin of the product of unconscious activity. A physician of forty-seven years told me that twenty-five years before, during a walk in the forest, he suddenly saw most distinctly in front of him at some distance, the plaster bust of Schleiermacher. He went up to it. Just as he was about to grasp it, it disappeared. I went from there gladdened in spirit. [!] "My father, a pastor, possessed such a bust." [!] "Once the maid broke the glass bell mounted over it. I was still a child. My father made an awful fuss about it. The affair did not concern me. I thought the insignificant damage was not worth so much excitement on father's side. I always regarded the bust with awful fear. That the figure stood there, I took as a sign that it was well with father." [In what state of mind were you before the vision?] "I was much troubled because an important letter from home did not come in spite of pressing requests. My brother had developed delusions of grandeur, bought horses and was always telegraphing for money. In order not to spoil his career, father was unwilling to have him committed to an asylum. As I had received no recent information, I thought father might again be beside himself with excitement.''

The reader may now test for himself whether my questions, which certainly did not suggest their own answers, afford material which may lead us to an understanding of the vision. Has the memory of Schleiermacher in the critical moment a real meaning? I think so. The identification of the two worthy theologians, the father and Schleiermacher, rendered it possible that the perception of the latter might also afford assurance of the safety of the former. The memory of the blind rage on account of the onetime endangering of the statue brought the consolation that now too the father's excitement may be greatly exaggerated. For the rest, the person who had the hallucination is innocent of the affair and only indirectly concerned.* Thus, we now understand also the cheerful mood which would otherwise be difficult to comprehend. A candidate in medicine, just before the state examination, must have known that an hallucination is to be considered as pathological.

I leave to the reader to seek a simpler interpretation of the vision. But he cannot well dispute the following: Between the vision and the facts gained by psychoanalysis, just as in the examples previously mentioned, there must exist a connection. He who does not deny every causal relation on the ground of a prejudice similar to that which caused Descartes to consider all animals as creaking machines, must assume a purposeful work below the threshold of consciousness similar to that of conscious deliberation. In the three last described analysis, the apperception of the hallucination (angel, devil, Schleiermacher) led us to facts which have a very intimate relation to a present, easily ascertained wish. Thus, the hallucination expresses a really purposeful thought, which, because of grounds provisionally withheld from our understanding, forms below the

---

* If the reader does my book the honor of a second reading, he will find in this parallel the allaying of the evil wish which must have been repressed and thereby occasioned the hallucination.

threshold of consciousness and manifests itself psychically or physically in disguised form.

That, even in old age, such processes occur, a lady of sixty-nine years shows. One day there occurred an automatic twitching of the upper lip toward the left ear, accompanied by a ringing and buzzing which seemed to come from a mosquito. [Mosquito.] "The mosquito is a sucker of blood. My son wrote me before the outbreak of twitching and buzzing that his lady friend, for whom he had made pecuniary sacrifices, and who had promised to marry him, has turned him down. I find this customary with her. She too was a blood-sucker." [The twitching.] "I find nothing." I knew that the son mentioned had a scar on the same place. As he returned from the mensur (duel), his mother, in her first awful fright, thought someone had tried to murder him. The ringing in the ear reminded her also of that of a rapier. The lady probably connected the present (financial) loss of blood with that which had once actually occurred and which, at that time, had such a harmless outcome. Of this logical operation also, there was not the slightest trace in consciousness.

Finally, I mention an observation which shows us the unconscious at work in a normal individual. A gentleman of thirty-six years told me that for some days he had been tormented by a word, the meaning of which was entirely unknown to him. He only knew dimly that while in the preparatory school, some twenty-two years before, he might possibly have heard it in Greek history but could not remember to have heard it again since. The word was called "Pentakosiomedimne." He asked me to give him the meaning of it or help him to seek it. Fortunately, my memory also failed so that I turned to analysis and began: [Think of the word intently and tell me what comes into your mind.] After a long pause, I received the following: "The word 'Medimne' reminds me of 'Medusa.'" [Keep it sharply in view.] "Now I see clearly the distorted face of a near relative whom, on account of incurable insanity, I was compelled to take to a sanitarium some days ago.

I have to put up for the cost of his care which goes hard with me.''

Here the conversation was interrupted by lack of time. The next time I directed his attention to the beginning of the word. After some hesitation, the association came out: ''Pente must mean five. I think of a chemical agent which is composed of five ingredients. Ah so! On the morning when the obsessing word appeared for the first time, I was lying down with a pain in my stomach and took a narcotic. I thought of my relative. Then the thought came to me: If one could only give the poor paralytic a powerful narcotic too, and indeed so much that—.'' Later, it showed further that under the suffering of the patient, five persons nearly related to the one being analyzed, were strongly concerned.

Is it so entirely unreasonable if we now seek a purposeful connection between the associations and the facts indicated by them with the obsessing word? A priori, an inner relation between obsession and worry is probable. Further, the associations point to it. If, however, there is a psychic connection, then nothing prevents asking for the meaning of an obsessional idea. It is quite easily found, for ''Pentakosiomedimne'' signifies, as the person under analysis certainly knew in his time, the members of the highest class of citizens under Solon. Our subject has suffered long from pecuniary embarrassment since he has previously had to care for many relatives. For some time, he has experienced an essential bettering of his income. The obsessional idea acquired, as in so many of the foregoing cases, the good meaning of a consolation: The economic care occasioned by the mental disease is offset by the financial improvement.

If we do not dogmatically deny an unconscious mental life, we observe in this example various subliminal performances: A group of ideas, which confers the full logical meaning on the technical expression (''Pentakosiomedimne'') belonging to it, has disappeared from memory and yet, the expression suits the situation surpassingly well. Likewise, in the final result, different ideas which have become acute, are intelligently joined

together, ("medimne"—medusa, distorted face, pental—soothing, sleeping-potion, pente—five persons concerned).
. I have put forward for the reader's consideration a collection
of cases intentionally left unarranged. It would be as easy as
it would be aimless and tiring to fill a portly volume with similar observations, for similar facts and processes come to the
view of the analyst in great numbers, both in his practice and
in his daily life. Generally, one will not and cannot see them.
It is now our task to draw conclusions necessarily resulting
from our material.

The unconscious is not easier and also not harder to demonstrate than the conscious of another person. As Cartesius, on
the ground of his conception of thinking, denied animals all
psychic impulses, so one can consider all other people as mere
creaking machines without the possibility of being contradicted. The immanent philosophy which allows the whole
world to exist only in my idea, has produced something quite
different. Animal psychology, under the circumstances, could
never have convinced a Cartesius redivivus if it had spent fifty
years on this one task. Only a conclusion from analogy assures
us of the existence of an animal mind and of mental life in other
persons, and conclusions from analogy can always be disputed.
But what reasonable man would go so far in scepticism? He
who would deny that psychic motives lie at the bottom of individual acts of other people, would be ready for the madhouse.

In assuming an unconscious mental life in the cases observed,
we do nothing different than when we presuppose a consciousness outside ourselves in this or that psychical or physical performance. We hold ourselves to the criteria of relationship of
content and constant results. We saw automatic dumbness,
visual disturbance and feeling of tension with paralysis, in
temporal conjunction with the affectful complaint, forgotten at
that time: "I cannot speak and see, I hang only by a thread."
In numerous cases, we see physical and psychical phenomena,
which would otherwise remain entirely unexplained, arranged
as to causality or brought nearer to our scientific understanding
when we fall back on the hypothesis of a subliminal mental life.

Thus it is incorrect when Kronfeld asserts that psychoanalysis is not founded on facts but constructs such with the help of a theory.* We saw the unconscious, never as a mere disposition, but always as a molding, creative force. Even where there seems to be a mere reproduction in an automatism, upon closer consideration, a more complicated thought process is unmistakable, as for example in the following case: A youth of seventeen years has felt for some days, a strange sensation in his left arm. The occasion and meaning of the symptom are entirely inexplicable to him. When his attention is concentrated upon the symptom, he recalls that as a child, he was about to be vaccinated but struggled so violently that the hated procedure had to be given up. At the present also, there is something unpleasant in view: the father wishes to transfer his son to another institute which is displeasing to the son. Thus, the hysterical innervation expresses the wish that this time too, the father's plan may be frustrated by obstinacy. This logical connection is entirely lacking in consciousness. Not once does the scene with the physician become conscious without analytic assistance. If the scheme of refractory conduct had been clearly conceived, then that picture from youth could quite well appear. Now, however, at the moment of the appearance of the symptom, an unconscious thought presents a merely suggestive expression which selects from an experience an especially characteristic agency and brings it to automatic expression.

We recognize many more complicated unconscious performances in the more complicated phenomena, for example, in the clucking and itching, in the crown of thorns and the halo, in the long fingered and short nosed angel, the devil with the features of two familiar persons, etc. Later, we shall meet very many more elaborate productions of subliminal activity, even to the most sublime structures of art and religion. Since below the threshold of consciousness, the most imposing trans-

* Kronfeld, über d. psych. Anschauungen Freuds, p. 64.

formations and new creations take place systematically, it is incorrect to call the unconscious a mere "disposition" or to consider it as a purely physical affair.

This unconscious productivity, in which, emotion, will and intellect have a share, thus unconscious sensations, ideas, emotions and inclinations, is the first fact which we emphasize. The other fact is: It has been possible for us with the help of our attitude toward the manifestations of the unconscious and the collection of the ideas associated with these, to gain a meaning for the phenomena to be explained, often with surprisingly little trouble. Often, the associations gained from the apperception, at first run in all directions, somewhat like the slapdash lines of a rapidly sketching cartoonist. Suddenly, however, one perceives in the apparently meaningless and haphazard mass of ideas, a purposeful whole which agrees very well with the situation of the subject.

Here, a word may be interpolated in reply to the objection that the analyst allows himself to be deceived by the subject of the analysis or is selfdeceived by giving suggestion and thereby causing the results. One prevents suggestion so far as it may falsify the answers by the tone and manner and the same stereotyped question: "What comes into your mind?" The subject of the analysis will certainly often seek to lie. Still he can only lie about what comes into his mind and that is the important material. He cannot invent the structure of a neurosis. External substantiation of the replies is often possible. Especially in dreams and the reaction experiment, the liar is often drolly unmasked, since he betrays himself without noticing it. Finally, the patient perceives that he injures only himself and not the analyst by untruthfulness. In a case published from the semianalytic side, the physician may be duped by an invented tale. The difficult patient who had been nourished for years by the probe, experienced a relapse and now confessed repentantly to the physician who applied the real analysis, her deceit, whereupon the treatment could be continued and permanent recovery obtained.

Without the psychoanalytic method, we would absolutely

never have attained an insight into the structure and cause of the symptoms of the majority of our simplest cases, concerning some of which very sharp-sighted people had racked their brains. I do not say that psychoanalysis is the only method by which the unconscious may be ascertained. One can also afford the proof synthetically by giving an order in hypnosis and commanding at the same time to forget the occasion of the order. For example, a teacher may be commanded to put a little paper hat on the top of the stove in his room the next day, nevertheless, to forget that this was expected of him. The man will do it after he has invented some kind of a plausible motive, perhaps a very clever one, perhaps the desirability of greater practice in triangulation. The real motive remains unconscious.*

We are now in a position to characterize descriptively the unconscious with which psychoanalysis has to deal. "Unconscious," "subconscious" or "subliminal," we call the intellectual processes taking place outside of consciousness, which processes, we infer according to the principles of causal connection derived from physical and psychical phenomena. These subconscious mental phenomena, we conceive to be exactly analogous to the conscious, only the characteristic of being known is lacking to them. The hypothesis of localization in certain nerve centers is denied to no one, but because of the intellectual importance of the subliminal mental products and of the material utilized, these phenomena cannot be made subordinate, as Janet and Grasset believe.†

According to Freud, the distinction between conscious and unconscious ideas is not merely a dynamic one, somewhat of the kind that the unconscious idea lacks the power to become conscious as in the case of a weak sensory stimulus. An unconscious idea, to which an instinct is attached, can rule the

---

* Beautiful examples are given by Narziss Ach, über die Willenstätigkeit u. d. Denken, Göttingen, 1902, p. 188 ff.

† J. Grasset, Le spiritisme devant la science, Paris, 1904, pp. 99, 110 ff.

whole life, devastate it and cripple it in its development.* Hence, Freud distinguishes foreconscious ideas which lack only the conscious investment of energy, from the real unconscious, but attributes to this distinction more practical than theoretical value.† Both kinds, the foreconscious and the unconscious, come under the term subliminal. I see no occasion to fix sharply the distinction between the two, as something like Kant's distinction between the world of phenomena and the thing in itself.

As the mental life is divested by many psychologists of its own causality and traced. back to purely physical causality without the psychological investigation falling along with it, so also can the unconscious be reduced to physiological processes without psychoanalysis coming to naught thereby. Some analysts incline to this hypothesis of psychophysical materialism.‡ Why I do not do this, I have previously explained. But the representatives of the purely physiological unconscious must take to psychological formulations, for the knowledge of the brain processes affirmed also by the adherents of the psychological unconscious is entirely denied to us.

Similarly to the expression, "consciousness," that of the unconscious has different meanings. Now, it denotes the totality of what is non-conscious, now, the unconscious mental life including its own activity. In this significance, Freud denotes it by the abbreviation "Ubw." (Unc.).‖

* Freud, A note on the Unconscious in Psycho-Analysis. Proceedings of the Society for Psychical Research, Part LXVI, Vol. XXVI (1912), p. 314.

† P. 316.

‡ Freud also formerly expressed himself in this sense, for example, Kleine Schriften, I, p. 52.

‖ Traumdeutung, p. 318.

SECTION I

REPRESSION AND FIXATION

CHAPTER III

THE UNCONSCIOUS AS PRODUCT OF REPRESSION AND AS ENTITY FREE FROM REPRESSION

ALTHOUGH we have attained a clear definition of our object and a general description of the method of investigation to be employed and elaborated, there still floats before us a rather nebulous conception of our field of work. In order to lift the veil, we will attempt a genetic consideration of the unconscious.

Janet thought he could explain the phenomena of hysteria as degenerative phenomena. Because of a degeneration of the nervous system, there appeared a mental splitting of the personality so that the mental processes which belonged together could no longer be synthetized to a unity, but remained dissociated.* Degenerative? There, we have again a horrible word, under which, anything can be comprehended because no one sees anything clearly intelligible and obvious in it, or if he does, someone else comes along and explains that this is not degenerative.† Of a degeneration of the nerves as a foundation for dissociation, we know nothing; further, the astounding performances of many hysterical individuals in perception, memory, phantasy and other functions, do not speak for degeneration.

Instead of trusting ourselves to the cheap vessel of the

* Freud, Über Psychoanalyse, p. 16 f.
† I have discussed the conclusions of Bär, Kurella, Näcke, Bleuler and Lombroso in my book, "Die Willensfreiheit" (p. 106 f.).

physiological hypothesis, we will seek to attain our goal by psychological analysis.

First, we must get clear some fundamental concepts of psychology. In the following pages, there will be much mention of sensations, perceptions and ideas, of emotions, instincts, acts of the will and similar mental phenomena; the scientific determination of these terms is a bone of contention among the various psychological schools and parties. It is right to ask ourselves in what sense we understand these words.

For our immediate experience, there are only psychic events, in which we distinguish an intellectual and an emotional side.* We distinguish what is related to objects outside of consciousness, all sensations, ideas and thoughts, as intellectual content, from that which depends on the behavior of the subject, thus from emotions and inclinations. Pure sensations, ideas and thoughts are as scarce in conscious mental life as pure emotional reactions, volitional reactions and actions. The expression, "emotionally toned idea," if it did not suggest strong emotional emphasis, would be a pleonasm.

Psychology, like psychoanalysis, has the greatest interest in the question whether both sides of the mental phenomenon may be traced back to one fundamental form. One group of authors believe they can separate the emotional into intellectual elements. Herbart would explain all mental processes as statics and mechanics of ideas, Spencer and Steinthal consider the will as a mere idea, Münsterberg, Lehmann and Wahle conceive it to be a complex of ideas and sensation.† Ziehen and Ebbinghaus lay special stress on the idea of activity, without which idea, according to their conclusions, attention cannot once appear.‡ Of the intellectualistic theories, I can illustrate only one, at the same time, however, indicating the errors of its sisters, namely, that of Meumann.‖ This theory con-

---

* Wundt, Grundzüge der phys. Psych., 6th ed. Vol. I, 1908, p. 404.
† O. Külpe, Die Lehre vom Willen in der neueren Psychologie, Leipzig, 1888.
‡ Ziehen, Leitfaden der physiol. Psychologie, p. 173. Ebbinghaus, Abriss d. Psychologie (Dürr), Leipzig, 1910, p. 81.
‖ E. Meumann, Intelligenz und Wille, Leipzig, 1908, p. 192.

siders as indispensable attributes of every voluntary act: (1) the goal idea; (2) the judgment corresponding to it; (3) the bringing about of the action to be performed by these two elements and at the same time the causative action itself and our consciousness of this action (188). According to Meumann, the consciousness of activity in the volition is "nothing else than a consciousness of this personal preparation for the act" (188f.). "In a volitional act, we notice how nothing else appears in our consciousness except causative energy, except the goal fixed by us, the approved motive corresponding to the aim and our appropriate act. In general, where this selection brought about by us among psychic processes, appears, we know ourselves to be voluntarily active. The nucleus of the will process is accordingly this selection phenomenon and its causation by suitable goal ideas which we ourselves have fixed and to which we have imparted an inner acquiescence. It is not every selection among our ideas but this active selection which constitutes the will" (191). In this presentation, an emotion does not come into consideration. "It contradicts the nature of emotions, which are always objects of pleasure and displeasure, to impose on them thoughts of an activity" (191).

I do not see that Meumann could explain the emotional element as purely intellectual. It lies hidden already in the goal idea, as well as in the judgment corresponding to it and in the causation of the act to be performed. If Meumann had analyzed these phenomena, it would have been plain to him. The same applies to the amplifying and explanatory formulations of the same psychologist: In consciousness of "personal causation of the action" lies the knowledge of the activity reposing in the will. Further, the selection is derived from the tendency inferred in the goal idea. Meumann did not analyze the volitional process itself as it is experienced but as it is looked at from without. Hence, he made a fatal mistake right at the decisive point: out of the experienced activity, this center of the volitional act, he makes a mere knowing of the personal activity. The latter, he changed from a constituent factor of the volitional performance into a mere object of knowledge, the content of which, the personal, that is, mental activity, is not raised beyond all doubt. Thus, Meumann can assert the primacy of the intellect, cast doubt on the spontaneity of the subject in a volitional experience, deny psychic causality and allow credence only to the physical in the sense of psychophysical materialism.

Concerning the psychology of emotion, not much more need be said. One widespread theory attempts to reduce the emotions like the will to sensations and indeed to sensations in organs. Lange supports the standpoint that emotion may be the sensory reaction to vasomotor stimuli (excitation of the arteries), while James lays more stress on sensations associated with physical movements of expression.* In the sense of Lange, we would say: "We feel because our vessels expand"; James says outright: "We are sad because we weep and angry because we tremble." Meumann considers the emotions as blendings of organic sensations.†

The expression, "feeling," is used in various senses. Its application to tactile sensations is to be rejected for only confusion results from this speech usage. On the other hand, for scientific language, a terminology is justified which designates as feelings, states of consciousness which, although composite and including intellectual factors, nevertheless, are essentially determined in their characteristics by the predominance of the joyous or painful, the pleasant or unpleasant, of pleasure or pain.‡ Thus, one may speak of a feeling of pity, love or hate. Only, one must make himself clear that here too, no pure feeling exists, that rather, the whole is named according to a predominating subjective attribute. Where strict, sharp observation is necessary, we limit the expression

---

* W. James, Psychologie. German by Marie Dürr, Leipzig, 1909, 376 ff. P. Fischer, Darstellung und Kritik der Hauptansichten über die Natur des Gefühls in der neuesten Psychologie, Breslau, 1897, p. 13 f. An excellent presentation of the investigation of the psychology of emotion from 1900–1909 is given by Mathilde Kelchner in the Archiv f. d. ges. Psychologie (Lit.) Vol. XVIII, pp. 97–164.

† Meumann, Int. u. Wille., p. 290.

‡ Witasek, p. 317.

"feeling" to the perceptible factors of pleasure and displeasure in a mental experience.

In criticism of the physiological theories of emotion, may be advanced: the asserted organic sensations are admitted. Ebbinghaus alone rightly recalls in this connection that the emotional theory of James and Lange cannot explain why emotions can never appear in consciousness without content to which they are connected and why sensations like those of pain, hunger, etc., are inseparable from the emotions belonging to them.* Further, sadness is something different from perception of weeping and its accompanying innervation sensations plus the idea of a state of affairs. "I am glad" says something different from "I have intestinal sensations, brain innervations and more of the same." For psychoanalytic work, however, the deciding of this debated point is not necessary.

Many psychologists assign feeling, with Wundt, to the volitional acts, so far as in every pleasure, an inclination exists, in every displeasure, a disinclination, and every emotion prepares or can prepare for a volitional act.† The transition to the volitional act is formed by the affect, this "coherent flow of emotion of unified character." ‡

As simplest form of volition, one usually considers the volitional act which, under the influence of an affect, proceeds toward the goal of setting aside this affect. "The affects which arise from sensual emotions, as well as the omnipresent social affects, such as love, hate, anger, vengeance, are the original sources of the will, both with man and the lower animals." ||
The affect, with its accompanying idea, forms the motive for the act and indeed, the former is the impulse and the latter, the motive. In the decision, the emotions mutually inhibit one another and thereby always lose more and more in intensity.¶
The will seems then (falsely) determined by purely intellectual

* H. Ebbinghaus, Grundzüge der Psychologie, 3rd ed. (Dürr), Leipzig, 1911, Vol. I, p. 543 f.
† Wundt, Grundriss, p. 217.
‡ P. 214.
|| Grundriss, p. 216.
¶ P. 223.

motives. In similar repeated external or internal decisions of the will, the previously subordinated motives appear weaker and finally disappear * altogether, the victorious motive also retreats, the volitional act is set free by the external stimulus without appearing in consciousness, it becomes mechanical, automatic.†

In this whole development, I find no occasion and no opportunity to separate causality of will and assign it to physiology, to the psychophysical materialism. Even if one traces the will back to an act of judgment, the formula of Fouillée holds: "La volition est la détermination par un jugement qui prononce que la réalisation de telle fin dépend de notre causalité propre." ‡ "Aucune combinaison de passivités n'expliquerait d'une mainére intelligible le sentiment d'activité, et le vouloir-vivre est aussi clair en nous que la sensation même." ||

All volitional impulses may be comprised in groups according to their aims and traced back to some few purposeful efforts of the volitional subject. Such simple tendencies of definite aim, to speak with Höffding,¶ such pressure of activity directed by the goal idea, the development of which tendencies is seen in the varied extent of mental processes, we call, from the psychological side, instincts. In every-day life, one speaks of hunger-, self-preservation-, sexual-, knowledge-instinct, etc. In general, one traces them back to two fundamental instincts: the instincts for preservation of self and the race,§ hunger and love (Schiller) or to the ego instinct and the sexual instinct (Freud).** I do not think that one can be satisfied with this division, so far as one understands with Freud under the ego instincts, only the strivings toward preservation of the in-

* P. 226.
† P. 227.
‡ Fouillée, La psychologie des idées-motrices, Paris, 1893, 2d. Ed. II, p. 263.
|| P. 232.
¶ Höffding, p. 119.
§ Witasek, p. 364.
** Freud, Psychoanalytische Bemerkungen ü. e. autobiographisch beschriebenen Fall von Paranoia, Jahrbuch III, p. 65.

dividual being. It seems to me that it is quite as good to speak of an instinct for individual and racial improvement, continuation or enrichment. If we express the instincts in these definitions according to their motive impulses, then we can denote them according to their sources as life impulse, pleasure hunger or libido. It is really arbitrary to limit the latter name entirely or principally to the sexual instinct.

The psychological derivations gained, do not necessarily belong to the presuppositions of psychoanalysis, to which fact I call especial attention. Freud himself is close to psychophysical materialism when he sees, for example, in instinct, "the psychic representative of organic forces." * At all events, however, psychoanalysis favors, as we shall see, the voluntaristic psychology which considers the instincts as the determining factors, the ideas more as only the organs of these.

Let us proceed now, after having gained the very necessary and valuable connection to the earlier psychology,† to an investigation of the unconscious.

Can a common attribute be shown in the examples cited by us, from which we may succeed according to our formulæ of hypothesis and law to a scientific comprehension of unconscious mental forces?

As a matter of fact, one characteristic predominates in our collected cases: throughout, as we followed the causes of striking phenomena, we encountered painful ideas which had once been conscious, then however, and just at the time of those phenomena, disappeared from consciousness. The idea itself was painful because it corresponded to a very strong wish which was prohibited by a higher demand. The phenomena we have presented, which we recognized as offshoots of unconscious mental impulses, turn out to be compromise products, in which two opposed currents of high intensity effect a compromise.

* Same.

† The psychoanalyst is very glad and ready to learn from the experimental psychologists since he in general does not pose as having the only proper method.

We will show this in our examples. On account of the simplicity, I will choose the schematic form on page 56.

The unconscious motives which are reflected in the symptoms, were unconscious, in part only at the moment of the symptom, in part in general foreign to consciousness until the analysis raised them above the threshold.*

The conflicting ideas, as well as the nature of the conflict of these ideas, will be discussed in the following chapters. Likewise, we shall have to investigate why not every conflict of two emotionally toned ideas furnishes a subconscious motive for phenomena such as we found in the previous examples.

So far as the collision of two ideas occasions a subliminal motive influencing the mental or physical life, we speak of a **repression**. Accordingly, an idea is repressed when it comes into conflict with one or more other ideas of higher value to the individual in question and, as a result of this conflict, is forced out of consciousness.

That there may be such a repression of conscious content by opposing content, was not first discovered by Freud. Herbart has already originated a theory of repression. He says: "We all notice within ourselves that of our total knowing, thinking and wishing, in any particular moment, an incomparably smaller amount actually occupies our attention than that which might appear upon proper occasion. In what condition does this absent but not dissipated knowledge, which remains and persists in our possession, exist in us? . . . What can prevent our firmest convictions, our best intentions, our cultivated emotions, often over long periods, from becoming effective? What can produce the unfortunate sluggishness in them, which so often exposes us to vain regret? Other thoughts have busied us too completely! This we all know already from experience. And yet we have preferred to lose ourselves in the heresies of transcendental freedom and radical evil, which destroy all healthy metaphysics, to making exact investigations of the psychological mechanism on which plainly

---

* From later experiences, it is shown that also behind the conscious motives, powerful unconscious ones lurked.

Symptom	Unconscious Motive	Affectladen Idea (a)	Affectladen Idea (b)
1. Dumbness, dimness of vision, astasia, tactile sensation on breast.	"I cannot speak, now all is dark, I hang only by a thread."	Need for confession of sexual and property offences.	Feeling of shame.
2. Swollen lips.	"I have been kissed excessively."	Wish to be kissed.	Ditto.
3. Migraine with pulling out of hair, clucking, itching of skin, migraine, allaying of clucking.	"I wished it were again as at that time the brother did improper things to me." "I answered the itching of my brother by a similar performance." "I am in the position of the woman Hadwig."	Incestuous relation to brother.	Ditto.
4. Migraine of temples.	"I have been hit in the temples in place of the father."	"May the father shoot himself."	Self-punishment.
5. Crown of thorns.	"I am persecuted like the innocent, thorn-crowned Savior."	Wish to be this.	Audacity of this wish.

Symptom	Unconscious Motive	Affectladen Idea (a)	Affectladen Idea (b)
6. Vision of angel.	Elimination of neighbor.	Death wish.	Remorse, hence distortion.
7. Vision of devil.	Elimination of enemy.	Wish that he might be a real devil.	Ditto.
8. Vision of Schleiermacher.	"The alarm is false as at that time when there was a fuss over Schleiermacher."	Wrath of father and hate against him.	Wish not to think of this love of father.
9. Tic nerveux, hallucination of buzzing bug.	"The son misused by a bloodsucker suffered harmless bleeding."	Memory of suffering son.	Wish to forget him. Love to son.
10. "Pentakosiomedimne"	"I am rich enough to bear the burden."	Death wish against insane relative.	Remorse.
11. Innervation in arm.	"I will behave again as stubbornly as at the vaccination."	Removal from school.	Wish to forget and abandon school.

the blame must lie. ... Two ideas suffice to repress a third completely out of consciousness and to occasion a totally independent condition. One idea alone cannot do this against the two. ..." *

"As we speak of the rise and fall of ideas, so I would call an idea 'under the threshold' when it lacks the power to fulfill those conditions under which it is perceived. Just the condition in which it then exists is always the same as complete inhibition; still, it may be more or less completely 'under the threshold' according as more or less strength is lacking to it, and must be added in order to pass the threshold." †

We find these important thoughts entirely substantiated. To-day, too, one usually prefers to flee into metaphysics, especially into psychophysical materialism, rather than trace out the conditions of the repression. The psychoanalytic investigation confirms in surprising degree, as we shall see later, the observation that one idea alone is never sufficient to repress another. Behind the ideas given in our table, there lurk, without exception, further submerged, related ideas ("overdeterminants"). We shall also find Herbart's sharp-sighted theory of the degrees of repression to be correct.

It is not necessary to enumerate the whole list of psychologists who, since Herbart, have recognized the repression as existing. I mention only one especially keen student of humanity, Nietzsche, who says: " 'That have I done,' says my memory. 'That have I not done,' says my pride and remains inexorable. Finally, memory yields." ‡

Also, psychiatrists like Pick and Hellpach already recognized before Freud that repression plays a rôle in certain "nervous" diseases.‖

It is to be emphasized that by no means all the unconscious

* Herbart, Psychologie als Wissenschaft, neu gegründet auf Erfahrung, Metaphysik und Mathematik, Part I, Section 47. (Werke, herausg. v. Kehrbach, Vol. V, Langensalza 1890); p. 292.

† P. 293.

‡ Nietzsche, Jenseits von Gut und Böse, IV, p. 68.

‖ Bleuler, Die Psychoanalyse Freuds, Jahrbuch, II, p. 692. Schultz, Psychoanalyse, Zeitschrift f. angewandte Psychologie, 1909, p. 486.

is brought about by repression. Freud lays stress on this statement.* That which is commanded in hypnosis or that which is forgotten without the pressure of antagonistic ideas, to reappear again sometime, is not repressed and yet unconscious. Also, according to Wundt, the underlying, ultimately absent, motives in similar decisions of will, are repressed.† Further, we can assert with Dürr "that every disconnected content, appearing beside other psychic processes, brings with itself an encroachment upon the consciousness of those processes." ‡ Pedagogy, and that of the intellect as well as that of the will, has to do in great part with this unrepressed unconscious and has exact knowledge of its existence.

Psychoanalysis also deals with this matter. One should not be deceived by the plan of this book concerning this condition of affairs! But to-day, the analytic movement founded by Freud stands in a stage which is devoted almost exclusively to the repressed unconscious. With the other subliminal components, the traditional psychology and pedagogy is already busying itself more than it knows. Pedagogy has always proceeded toward the origin of ideational and emotional dispositions. Psychoanalysis gained entirely new ground and wholly new pedagogic possibilities for work from the investigation of the repressed phenomena below the threshold. Further, the knowledge of repression-free subliminal components, as it has thus far been attained by the help of the Freudian investigation, proceeded from the repressed material and can best be shown in connection with those investigations. Perhaps, in a few years, the presentation here sketched, which proceeds from the repression, will no longer suffice.

* Freud, Gradiva, p. 40.
† Wundt, Grundriss, p. 226.
‡ E. Dürr, Die Lehre von der Aufmerksamkeit, Leipzig, 1907, p. 149.

CHAPTER IV

THE INDIVIDUAL REPRESSED MATERIAL

HAVING traced the unconscious by the aid of analysis to its subterranean lair, we will now with true sportsman's zeal, examine the valuable savage at closer range. In this, we should not allow ourselves to be influenced by any preconceived opinion. He is a miserable hunter who would allow his quarry to be run to earth by a forester, beforehand, and afterward complain that he should have come skillfully to his object! Fortunately, not only has Freud constantly and fundamentally changed his views concerning our object, but there prevails among his followers a multitude of different opinions. This occasions the lively opposition of the critics. Hence, one cannot avoid the tedious developing of one's own judgment.

I. FREUD'S THEORY.

I shall not take back with the left hand what the right gave, if I, nevertheless, present some theories in which Freud and others have formulated their insight into the nature of the repressed material. By my procedure, the reader will see on what things to depend and he will be protected from all kinds of errors into which so many critics, in manners conceivable and inconceivable, have fallen. Thus I ask, not for rude Frau Fama faith which, according to Friedlander's complaint, has brought the reproach of "pansexualism" against psychoanalysis, but to test in unprejudiced manner what Freud has said and then to investigate in truly objective manner in how far his view is correct.

Nothing has so injured the estimation of Freud's work as his thesis that the cause of every hysteria, anxiety and obsessional neurosis is to be sought in the sexual life. This statement has its previous history. In the beginning (1894), the founder of psychoanalysis asserted only that he had found as cause in all cases of obsessional neurosis investigated by him, a painful affect from the sexual sphere, but nevertheless, he did not exclude affects from other fields.* In the "Studies in Hysteria" (1895), he said, however: "The observation forced itself upon my attention that in so far as one may speak of a cause by which neuroses are brought about, the etiology is to be sought in the sexual agencies." † That he came to this insight against his will, he declares ‡ by saying that it was long enough before he was "converted" to this view; this he mentions three years later.‖

The original thesis was soon (1896) made more explicit by Freud's assertion that the sexual traumas of early childhood were the cause of hysteria; these traumas consisted of actual irritation of the genitals, coitus-like procedures, sexual passivity in presexual periods.¶ At the same time, Freud believed he could establish § the origin of the obsessional neurosis in sexual activity, namely in "aggressions carried out with pleasure and participation in sexual acts associated with pleasure." In spite of the violent opposition which arose against him, he saw in every case the ultimate foundation of an hysteria in a sexual experience in early childhood and indeed in sexual intercourse (in broadest sense).** In addition, according to a communication in 1898, the thought prevailed that the sexual cause of the neuroses might not be the exclusive one, but that it "only added one more to all the known and probably rightly recognized etiological agencies of the authors." ††

Later (1906), Freud went beyond these hypotheses. In a

* Freud, Die Abwehr-Neuropsychosen. Kl. Schriften I, p. 51.
† Studien über Hysterie, p. 224.
‡ P. 226.
‖ Kl. Schriften I, p. 158.
¶ P. 113.
§ P. 118.
** P. 160, 162.
†† P. 189.

personal article, he partially retracted his previously expressed
views regarding the rôle of sexuality in the causation of the
neuroses.* A mass of later observations made him certain, in
the course of a decade, that a traumatic experience did not
necessarily lie at the bottom of the malady but often only a
phantasy ("memory fancy").† As the outer activities lost
in importance, the inborn tendencies, now however, as "sexual
disposition," gained the upper hand.‡

It remained, however, in the statement that the psychoneurotic suffers ‖ from a repressed sexual complex, the word taken in
its broadest sense. More recently, it has been announced that
the sexual instinct affords the only constant condition and the
most important source of energy in the neurosis, "so that the
sexual life of the person in question expresses itself, either
exclusively or predominantly or only partially, in these symptoms." ¶ The hysterical individual bears within himself a
bit of abnormally strong sexual repression alongside an excessive elaboration of the sexual instinct. "The occasion for
the malady develops for the hysterically disposed person, when,
because of the progressive maturing processes or external relations of life, real sexual demands make their appearance in
earnest." § This statement has likewise proved to be unten-
able since hysterical children have been analyzed.

Freud's sexual theory underwent a sharp elaboration in the
formulations of the year 1908: "The hysterical symptom
corresponds to the return to a manner of sexual gratification
which was real in infantile life and which has since been repressed." ** "The hysterical symptom can assume the representation of various unconscious non-sexual impulses but cannot dispense with a sexual significance."††

* Kl. Schriften I, pp. 225-234.
† P. 229.
‡ P. 230.
‖ Kl. Schriften II, p. 119 (1906).
¶ Drei Abhandlungen zur Sexualtheorie 1905, p. 8; 2d Part 1910,
p. 25 f. Kl. Schriften II, p. 180.
§ P. 27.
** Kl. Schriften II, pp. 142, 150.
†† P. 143.

Only in the last few years did Freud see himself compelled to revise the definition of sexuality. He did it in 1910 in the following important words: "It cannot have remained unperceived by the physician that psychoanalysis is accustomed to suffer the reproach that it extends the term, sexual, far beyond the customary extent. The complaint is just; whether it may be applied as reproach, may not be discussed here. The term sexual includes far more in psychoanalysis; it goes both below and above the popular sense. This extension is justified genetically; we reckon to the 'sexual life' also all play of tender emotions, which have sprung from the source of primitive sexual impulses, both when these impulses experience an inhibition of their original sexual goal or have exchanged this goal for another one, no longer sexual. We speak, therefore, preferably, of psychosexuality, putting emphasis on the fact that one should not overlook nor undervalue the mental factor of the sexual life. We use the word sexuality in the same comprehensive sense as the German language does the word 'love.'"*

How much indignation and animosity would have been avoided if this explanation had been given earlier! But a long struggle was necessary before this stage of knowledge could be reached. That we are in no way dealing with an entirely new theory, Freud pointed out, later still, when he asserted that "all our valuable emotional relations in life, those of sympathy, friendship, faith, etc., are genetically joined to sexuality and have developed by the decline of the sexual goal from purely sexual desires, however pure and non-sensuous they may seem to our conscious selfperception. Originally, we have known only sexual objects; psychoanalysis shows us that the merely esteemed and revered persons of our reality may still always be sexual objects for the unconscious in us." †

If one adds these statements to Freud's previous expositions, they contain no very startling thoughts. Insert for "sexuality" the word "love" and no one will deny that sympathy

* Freud, über "wilde" Psychoanalyse. Zentralblatt f. Pse. I, p. 92.
† Freud, Zur Dynamik der Übertragung, Zbl. II, p. 171.

and friendship and faith have something to do with sexuality. For who can conceive of those ethical functions without love? Further, that they are based on sensual experiences of childhood is obvious. It is only questionable whether for the latter, the predicate of sexual is to be recommended. We shall speak of this later (Chapter VIII) after our data is more complete.

We see on the one side, the term sexuality constantly more generalized until it is finally withdrawn from speech usage to the most extreme unintelligibility, and on the other side, the range of activity of sexuality extended ever further and further. In 1900, Freud said that the majority of the dreams of adults deal with sexual material and bring erotic wishes to expression, even when one does not see it in the content of the dream.* Of late (1911), he has traced back the day-dreams, which are so important for pedagogy, and indeed religion, art and education, in great part, to sexual processes of development.† To the capability of the sexual instinct to exchange the immediate sexual goal for more remote and socially more valuable ones, or to yield contributions of energy to the latter, Freud ascribes a decisive importance for the attainment of the highest cultural achievements.‡ The idealistic characteristic of his sexual theory here comes beautifully to expression.

The criticism of this theory did not long remain absent. From the side of opponents as well as from that of adherents, besides high admiration, there were presented weighty considerations. We understand the opposition right well. Freud's original assertions and the later terminology were very challenging. But it was unfair to accuse the analysts of trying to spy out sexual motives. The emphasizing of that kind of causes is founded rather in the force of circumstances, which is felt as very troublesome. Thus, Ferenczi says: "At the Third Hungarian Psychiatric Congress in Budapest, I committed an error in my paper, several years ago, which is difficult

---

* Traumdeutung, 2d ed. p. 197, 3rd. ed. p. 205.

† Formulierungen über die zwei Prinzipien des psych. Geschehens. Jahrbuch III, p. 5 f.

‡ Freud, Über Psychoanalyse, p. 61.

to make good: I left out of consideration the investigation of neuroses by the Vienna University, Professor Freud. This omission was all the more culpable since I had knowledge of the works of Freud. Already in 1893, I had read his article. To-day, when I have been convinced in so many cases of the correctness of the Freudian theories, I must ask myself why I so rashly reproached them at that time, why they seemed to me at that time a priori improbable and artificial and especially: why the assumption of a purely sexual pathogenesis of the neuroses called forth in me such a violent resistance that I did not once accord them a closer study. In palliation of my attitude, I must at all events state that the vast majority of my colleagues still to-day maintain toward Freud an entirely negative attitude. The few, however, who later tested it, usually became enthusiastic adherents of the hitherto entirely unconsidered movement.''* Bleuler and Jung also could not believe in Freud's emphasis of the sexual causes of the neuroses until they turned to the authority against which the opponents of psychoanalysis cherish an insurmountable aversion, the personal observation.† Bleuler emphasizes that he guarded more than enough against leading his patients by his questions to sexual matters.‡ I have already said that I had exactly the same experience.‖ And so it has gone with many others who, like the experienced neurologist, Prof. James J. Putnam,¶ felt themselves at first repelled by certain assertions of Freud, then recognized the duty of testing and changed into ardent adherents of psychoanalysis.

II. Personal Observations

We shall first present the facts in the case. In this, we shall carefully consider whether we come upon sexual causes and

* Ferenczi, Wiener Klin. Rundschau, 1908, No. 48.
† Bleuler, Die Psychoanalyse Freuds. Jahrb. II, p. 642 f.
‡ Bleuler, Dementia præcox oder Gruppe der Schizophrenie, Leipzig and Vienna, 1911.
‖ Psychoanalyt. Seelsorge u. exper. Moralpäd. Prot. Monatsh., 1909, p. 34 f. Ev. Freiheit, 1910, p. 19 f.
¶ Putnam, Persönliche Erfahrungen mit Freuds psa. Methode. Zbl I, 533.

promise now, as we are standing before important decisions, that we will neither deny sexual facts because of prudery or fear of men nor will assert such from preference for a clever doctrine.

I begin with a few cases chosen at random, the sexual motivation of which lies on the surface.

1. EDUCATIONAL PROBLEMS PLAINLY DEPENDENT ON SEXUAL MATTERS

A young woman of twenty-three years is suddenly pursued by tormenting hallucinations. On the street, snakes glide over her feet; snakes hang from the ceiling of her sleeping-room to her bed, the stove-pipe, the telephone cord, a stick in the cellar a finger long, change into snakes, so that she can no longer visit certain places because of anxiety. In bed, she cannot stretch out lest she touch a snake; further, eating is prevented since she is afraid of biting the same animal.

Some days before the outbreak of the trouble, a woman had warned the girl in a religious conversation. The latter had confessed that she often yielded to sexual impulses and asked if this were sinful. The answer was so disquieting that immediately a fervent vow against the evil habit came into the field. The analysis quickly disclosed the meaning of the hallucination. Previously, the girl had been afraid that there might be a man under her bed, now she believes that there is a snake lying there. He who knows that in Greece at certain feasts, a serpent was likewise laid in a chest like a phallus, sees through the meaning of the anxiety symptom already. A quieting explanation, which afforded the excited instincts opportunity to adapt themselves to idealistic goals, eliminated the visions in a few conversations. Whether complete sublimation * at once occurred, I do not know, since I have no information on this point. Some weeks after the hallucinations had disappeared, this victim of anxiety-hysteria visited a pietistic preacher who gravely warned against sins. The girl remembered the ideas of her counsellor and renewed her vow. Some days later, the snakes

* Transposition into activities of higher ethical value.

were promptly in their places, to be likewise promptly banished by renewed and deeper analysis; this time probably forever.

A girl of sixteen, who fairly hates all men, suffers from severe anxiety upon going to sleep. All men except Jesus can be imagined only with erect penises. Often, she hallucinates a man who disappears behind her bed. In dreams, she sees herself naked, pursued and whipped by her father. The man whom she hallucinates evenings, plainly resembles a boy who misused the little girl sexually in her eighth year, in company with her brother and another boy. The girl says she has a burning desire to give herself to the first man or boy she may meet. Life is repugnant to her. In an analysis lasting eight or nine months, often tedious, the important hysterical symptoms were eliminated but the anxiety still remained, although in much less intensity and this only completely disappeared when the girl left her parents' house and removed to another city. Since then, the girl, in whom the physician had diagnosed beginning dementia praecox, has been cheerful and genial and her ethical conduct is most commendable. The parents whom she hated bitterly in past years, she loves tenderly.

The woman of forty-eight years mentioned on page 36, who had hallucinations of an angel vision, reported in the same quarter hour, an attack of anxiety which seized her every evening as dusk was coming on. [Have you experienced previous to the beginning of the anxiety attacks, something very painful in the hours of dusk?] "My father caused hateful scenes." [Did you not also experience something which would still more excite an eighteen year old girl?] "Yes, a friend of my brother once made improper demands in the hours of dusk but I resisted him. In the beginning, I feared the young man would come again. This thought soon disappeared but the anxiety remained." [When you are in this condition today or to-morrow, recall exactly the experience with the young man.] For two or three months, this person, who was of limited mentality, was free from anxiety. When this returned, I found that the memory of the content of our conversation was entirely absent. When I simply impressed it again, definite recovery occurred, at least no relapse has occurred up to to-day (three years). Even if superstitious suggestions, which I could not prevent, aided, still the easily performed analysis of a condition of thirty years standing, which analysis had not taken a half hour altogether, was well recompensed.

A student, aged twenty-two, has been subject since his thirteenth year to a severe case of obsessional washing. In spite of all ridicule on the part of his associates, he washes his hands countless times. The obsession broke out after his father had treated him for masturbation by boxing his ears and whipping him. In some other cases of obsessional washing, I found a similar cause.

The same patient has suffered for seventeen years from severe asthma, because of which, he has had to leave the preparatory school repeatedly, losing in all one and a half years. The infirmity would overtake him on the open street so that he would drop down; it frequently caused a loud whistling during his speech and most grievously disturbed his rest at night. One day, I found that the patient, when five years of age, had suffered from pathological fear of steam rollers and fires and had slept constantly under the covers. The apperception of the idea "steam roller" immediately called forth associations which the patient recognized as descriptive of a marital embrace. The steam roller proved to be a symbol for the puffing father. (Somewhat later, a fear of horses which this patient had had when two years old, was traced back by himself, by means of the associated words, to an exchange of the horse with the begetting father so that the case agreed completely with Freud's later published case of phobia in a five year old boy.*) Two days after the interpretation of the machine-phobia, it was noticed that the asthma had ceased coincidently with the latter. The suspicion of hysteria was strengthened by the fact that in his eleventh year, when the boy had shared the sleeping room with an asthmatic patient, the whistling sound in breathing had appeared as difficulty in breathing. I therefore advised the patient with complete avoidance of suggestive pres-

* Jahrbuch, I, pp. 1-109.

sure, to throw away the smoking powder and upon the outbreak of oppression in the chest, to recall exactly what kind of thoughts were running through his mind at that particular time. The energetically applied autoanalysis revealed every time a sexual scene in which the patient practiced that puffing which he had already recognized as the cause of the fear of the steam roller. As the connection of the asthma with the sexual idea was made clear, the anxiety disappeared in a twinkling. After one or two weeks, the last remnant of a tormenting affliction of seventeen years' duration had disappeared without leaving a trace. The cure has since lasted some years as the patient assures me. It is to be noted that practically simultaneously an immense network of hysterical symptoms, phobias and obsessions was overcome, so that the youth, at one time of apparently superior religious and moral nature, who for many years had been unbelievably depraved and been treated in various psychiatric institutes without result, may be considered cured in two or three months. A quarter of a year later, several psychiatrists pronounced him completely restored to health. In autumn, there appeared a relapse into disorderly habits, since the Don Juanism, which was still unknown to me at the time, had not been analyzed and probably ethical feeblemindedness was also present. The youth left me in anger and resumed many pathological symptoms including the asthma. A short written communication, in which I expressed my indifference toward such puerility, again restored health.

The elimination of the asthma came about, as the reader sees, by the autoanalysis, almost without interpretation by the educator, a case, which unfortunately does not always occur.

To illustrate the elimination of a very painful, and for the moral development, dangerous phobia, I submit the following case. The hysterical and obsessional neurotic patient just described, underwent, while in the preparatory school, every forenoon about nine o'clock, an anxiety condition which drove him out of school. Trusted comrades, he begged imploringly to hold him fast. Father or mother acompanied him daily to the school building which he nevertheless often left by a side door. When, after wild adventures, he had been enabled by analysis to resume his studies, the phobia appeared again. Therefore, one day, I directed the patient's most concentrated attention to the symptom, requested any association, even though it should be beside the point and received the following: when the patient, years before, suffered severely from pollutions, forenoons at nine o'clock, an inspection of his body-linen was made, at which time, sharp rebukes for his masturbation were given. The teacher, who read at nine o'clock, reminded him of his father, as the strict teacher at that time had done. The former, like the father, had remarked: ''Nervous people must sleep long!'' The phobia left at once when the patient, upon my instruction, kept the scenes with the father before his eyes when the anxiety condition appeared. Here too, the phobia is explained by the splitting off of the idea and the appearance of the affect belonging to it alone. Results which entreaties, tears, threats, punishments and rewards had not brought to pass, the analytic religious instruction attained with ease.

In all observations of anxiety, not organically conditioned, on closer examination, a sexual inhibition became evident. This happened also with the obsessional acts and ideas, which, as is known, also punish with anxiety those disobedient to their demands. I give only two examples which may claim pedagogic interest.

The first was an obsessional neurotic patient, a single man of forty-seven years, who has had, since his twelfth year, an unbelievably obstinate struggle against the number thirteen. His suffering compelled him to leave the preparatory school and has muddled his whole life. He must constantly take the number into consideration: every thirteen minutes before and after an hour brings an attack of anxiety, likewise, every position of the hands of the clock which yields thirteen, for example, 8:23 (sum). Other situations which call forth anxiety are—to select a few from hundreds of cases: it strikes eleven o'clock, two persons are in the room, or the clock points to eight, five persons are sitting at table. He cannot stay away from home thirteen hours. The whole month of March, 1910, is an unlucky month in which he can undertake nothing important, likewise February, 1911, etc. The hours from five to eight o'clock are dismal because of their sum, 26 = 2 x 13. Every thirteen lines of a letter, every number thirteen in additions, brings torment. Not only the houses numbered 13, but also all persons dwelling in these, he must avoid. Many times, the anxiety is traced back to the fateful number by very artificial connections.

Further, the highly intensive religious life of the patient is influenced by the number 13. Every thirteenth verse of a chapter is unlucky. A section which begins with verse 13 affords no consolation. Because a song of Gellert stands in the song-book as No. 13, he can read no other of the same poet.

Most noteworthy is the prohibition to go to bed at ten o'clock. Every evening, he must say three prayers, which makes with the hour again thirteen. The prayers are:

1. "Now I go again in God's power
   In Christ's strength
   In Jesus' blood
   That no evil one may do me harm.
   In the name of the Father, the Son and the Holy Ghost, of the Father (sic)."

2. "Guard me and protect me, my God, my soul and my body, my honor and my property, guard me, God, my dear father, guard me, God, my dear mother, guard me God, ... brother, sister, acquaintance and relative, that I beg of you, my God in Heaven! Amen." The father had died twelve years before, the mother fifteen.)

3. "Great God, forgive me my grievous sins! Amen."

The following things serve for defence: avoidance of critical situations, selection of favorable times, in particular, however, consideration of a church clock.

The connection with sexuality was easily seen: Before the outbreak of the illness, the boy tormented himself, even to melancholia, with reproaches and vain struggles against onanism, to which two men had misled him. All his lifetime, he was tremendously afraid of pollutions and considered sexual intercourse a cause of weakness and insanity. Besides, the question troubled him whether abstinence might not also be injurious. Countless times, the very wealthy and handsome man attempted to become engaged but found himself every time forced to back out. Strong was his constantly suppressed desire to compare his sexual member with that of others.

Without doubt, the disease is nevertheless determined in its form mostly by the parents. With the austere, superstitious father, who chastised him sharply, he always got along badly. So much the more fervently, did he love the mother, who suffered from anxiety and obsessional washing. Both parents feared the number 13. But also, in relation to the parents, sexuality played a rôle: from the sight of the parents with few clothes on, the child felt himself powerfully repelled and cried out in anxiety if the mother had to rise in the night and went to the bed of his brother.

The analysis was not completed, for my visitor wished only a cure by prayer from me and would not submit to the demands of an analytic treatment. The therapeutic result was a priori doubtful.

The other case is that of a sixteen year old boy of good endowment, who for ten years had been compelled to hold his hands out of the water when in a warm bath and got into the greatest excitement if he was prevented from this. At the beginning of the trouble, three years ago, the physician prescribed carbonic acid baths for him with slight results. The reaction experiment ("Water-Snake") immediately aroused the suspicion that something had happened to him in the bath which had some connection with the virile member. As a matter of fact, it turned out that the baths in common with his father had left behind the impression that there was something horrible in the water. Without the slightest suggestion from my side, the memory recalled by the patient himself in this connection sufficed to banish the obsession.

The continuation presupposes previous knowledge of symbolism. I therefore beg the reader to leave the psychological means out of consideration and to pay attention only to whether, without suggestive illusion, sexual roots of the neurosis were found. The youth, in whom we recognize the brother of the clucking Princess Hadwig (see above page 33), for years tossed plates, glasses and food into the air, to put them down again at once. This, he did, however, only when one of the sisters, especially the younger one, who is known to us, was present. The sight of the restless boy is painful. If the boorish acting fellow is refused the evening greeting by his sister, he walks up and down his room weeping for a long time. The analysis of this symptom took the following course: the boy cannot describe for me with certainty the action practiced countless times daily for years (with few exceptions). I had it demonstrated by the other members of the family. Then I called the youth himself to produce the motion with closed eyes and sharp apperception and received this: "It reminds me always of the leaping-bugs, crabs and fleas." [Leaping-bugs!] "Little insects which jump very often. These I found once in X." [X!] "There, I found for the first time 'impatiens noli me tangere.' (The mother afterwards substantiated that the fruit of this plant had made a great impression upon the boy at that time six years old; the boy knew the meaning of the name.) They jump just like little leaping crabs." [Crabs.] "At the time when I would eat no fish I would also eat no crabs. Before, I had eaten a fish, a flounder, the member of which had struck me unpleasantly." (A sterotyped dream in which a dragon and indeed a composite figure of flounder and flying dragon had given the boy anxiety some six years before, likewise went back to that experience.) [Fleas.] "And cicadas, they all jump alike. I think that my habit arose still earlier from the crabs because these always excited me." [Did a sexual organ in the crabs impress you?] "No indeed—still, the hind parts of the crabs in question, from which one drew the shell, was wormshaped like the member of the flounder." (He showed me in his collection the different animals, the similarity of which was important to him.) [The fear of crabs and the impression of the "leaping bugs" are thus sexually conditioned. The latter led you before to "noli me tangere!"] "That is probably also sexually conditioned: it is called: do not touch the snake (!) (Hence the gestures in the bath.) The fruits of the 'noli me tangere' are worm shaped; upon being cracked open, they roll up. My movement only occurs when the family is present, never in my room." [Thus, when the sister, with whom you were morbidly in love, or are now, somewhat, was also near you. Her presence makes you lustful, you wish to repress this instinct. From this conflict, proceeds the action.] "That is possible."

It is seen that the patient, on account of my interpretation, given in the end by himself, which, by exercising greater patience, I could quite well have let him find himself, was not yet completely convinced. Nevertheless, the somewhat summary method was sufficient: From that same evening, the painful habit has disappeared for good.

Of other obsessional acts, only one may be mentioned: The patient could endure no open drawers, especially, when napkins rolled-up lay therein. The latter, in general, he gladly let alone. [Think of the drawer in imagination!] "I see the napkins rolled up in it. My napkin-ring suddenly disappeared. It bore a picture of X" (the place where you found the 'noli me tangere'). [Go on.] "Plants and crabs. . . . The rolled up napkins had much the same form as the fruit of the noli me tangere. Accordingly, napkins entirely open, make no impression on me, rather only closed ones. You see here a representation of the noli me tangere. When the fruits are opened, they roll up like the napkins."

From this hour, the obsessional impulse was definitely eliminated, still the napkins ("Noli me tangere = touch me not") were left lying open for some weeks longer until I called the boy's attention to the reason for the omission. The attitude toward the sister also became normal.

Also in hysterical symptoms, the sexual basis is often in plain view. An eighteen year old pupil has suffered for three weeks from severe blinking of the eyelids (tic nerveux). The under lid of one eye is automatically drawn sideways. Asked concerning the way it originated, he says, that at that time, he rubbed a bit of coal dust out of his eye. Having his attention sharply fixed on this occurrence, he remembered that he had formerly seen a girl who winked in this way and thought at that time she might have injured her nerves by bad habits. He himself struggled in vain against masturbation which he considered a disgrace. So far the associations. If we have understood the metaphorical meaning of many symptoms, then we shall not consider it farfetched if we consider the automatism as a representation of the unconscious motive. ''The sexual misdeed is removed like the soot from my eye.'' The tic disappeared from that moment.*

Some examples among healthy individuals which are instructive for educators, may follow:

Untruthfulness. A member of my parish asked me to give him the name of an educational institution to which he could take his untruthful foster-daughter. The sixteen year old girl spread the rumor that she was attacked with obscene and vulgar expressions by him, the foster-father, and a certain pastor. Also in other matters, she lies with unbelievable impudence and obstinacy. I explained to the man that first the mental status of the delinquent should be determined before the question of institutional care could be decided. The conversation with the young sinner revealed the following particulars, almost all of which I could substantiate as authentic:

The girl spoke to the pastor she accused only once and was kindly treated by him. She loves him because the youth who has gone abroad, on whom she has cast her eye, is strongly attached to the man. The little liar maligns, in the manner described, only men with whom she is in love. From the untruthfulness, which came over her in her twelfth year, she gets no advantage. Sobbing, she reports that she often has to weep in bed because she lies so terribly, and seems unworthy of

---

* Such brief analyses afford the beginner a certain satisfaction, but not the psychologist and thorough worker. I would not present them as models to be copied, but wish rather that the reader consider the analysis as a really tedious, slow and difficult educational work. (See Chapter XXIV).

instruction for confirmation. Often, she prays to God for freedom from her faults but the next day, everything goes just so much the worse. In the house of the pastor who gave her religious instruction, she suffered, while climbing the stairs, such violent anxiety that she could scarcely leave the spot.

The latter occurrence, as well as the violent trembling of the guilty girl during her confession and the content of the lies, show us the hysterical, obsessional character of the untruthfulness in queston. The slanders express‾ a wishfulfillment: The little girl would like to be attacked and treated as a prostitute by the passionately loved men. But she represses the wish which now comes forth as a demon from within, with irresistiblè power in the form of evil reports. The vain love changes into hate and gratifies itself in phantastic verbal violence. The untruthfulness was just as old as the masturbation and expresses the tendency to conceal and dissimulate a fault, whereby she refrained from actual delinquency.

Kindly instruction concerning these connections brought an immediate end to the lying impulse. Not a single untruth more was observed in the following months, to the astonishment of the foster-parents. That which requests and punishments, self-reproaches and prayers had not attained, was accomplished by the analytic pedagogy with ease, while a reformatory institution would perhaps only have made matters worse.

Kleptomania. A seventeen year old pupil feels an irresistible compulsion to steal a rubber ring (bicycle tire) in his store, although he possesses no bicycle and must assume that his theft will come to light. After a long struggle, he succumbs. He steals the tube, plays with it in great excitement for some minutes, and indifferently sends it to a comrade. His action was punished by dismissal. He overwhelmed himself with reproaches and believes himself a born criminal since he committed the crime against his will and involved his father in a dishonesty. Other emotional complications appeared, sleeplessness prevented peace of mind and thus there has existed for a long time severe melancholia.

The "thief against his will" had repressed masturbation and

therefore indulged his evil passions in a symbolical phantom, the tube.

The female counterpart to the male symbol just mentioned, excited another of my pupils. The eighteen year old lad, in broad daylight, in spite of the high probability of being discovered, unscrewed from a bicycle in front of a butcher-shop the clasp in which the pump should be carried. The youth, who was of an excellent and well-to-do family, was also caught. Shortly before, he had attempted to observe his mother in the bath-room.

These results confirm those of Otto Gross, Stekel,* Riklin and others. He who knows the exigency of many kleptomaniacs, will wish that a teacher, trained in analysis, may very soon meet the unfortunates. Thieves who are ethically defective, in whom, from birth, the moral consciousness is lacking, are not considered in this category.

Cruelty to Animals and Passion for Destroying Things.
A candidate for confirmation, aged sixteen years, who has become estranged from God, the world and himself, the son of a luetic, confessed to me his self-danger. One day, he sees a charming kitten sitting in the sun. At once, there awakens in him the burning desire to maltreat it. A fearful unrest seized him until he had procured a stick and struck the sleeping animal on the nose with all his strength. The young cat was half dead from pain and fright but the boy had a strong feeling of pleasure. Gratified, he made off. Another time, he felt compelled in the empty school-room, to destroy the mantle of a Welschbach burner and again experienced a kind of sexual orgasm. Flies, he maltreated to as slow death as possible.

The same boy loves games in which he is tormented. He gladly allows himself as captured Indian to be bound to the martyr's stake and urges his companions to draw the bands still tighter, to throw things at him still more recklessly. In the torture he feels the sweetest delight.

Cat and gas-mantle represent, as so often in dreams, male

* W. Stekel, "Die sexuelle Wurzel der Kleptomanie." Zeitschrift für Sexualwissenschaft, 1908, pp. 588–600.

and female sexual objects. The young sadist practiced mutual onanism with his younger brother but gave it up from considerations of health. The animal represents to him, the brother, whom his passion seeks. The rod signifies in his vulgar speech, the male organ. On the sister, the mantle-destroyer projects incestuous phantasies. The damming up of the sexual desire violently inflates the sadistic-masochistic instinctive tendency.

One sees from our example, how invertedly those pedagogues act who subject every tormentor of animals to corporal punishment. They wish to enforce sympathy with the animal's feelings of discomfort. Very many tormentors of animals are, however, sadists, consequently also, more or less masochists, and obtain from painful punishment only that which gratifies them and strengthens their cruel instincts.

Aversion to Work. A girl of eighteen, who is engaged, willingly performs all the duties of the housewife except cleaning windows which is revolting to her. The symbolism of the window so frequently demonstrable in dreams, solves the riddle. It has to do with the repression of masturbation. Freedom from the symptom resulted immediately from the analysis.

Symptomatic Acts. He who engages for a long time in the analysis of apparently meaningless gestures, which constantly recur, gradually becomes able to read intimate secrets with certainty from these stereotyped habits.

A fifteen year old pupil was accustomed to make frequently a peculiar grimace, in which he turned up his nose and finished it with the outstretched index finger under it. Often also, he drew the chin down and scratched under the right corner of the mouth. One day as I was speaking from the text: 'Sin is at the gate,' I decided to send up a little analytic exploring balloon. Glancing indifferently at the boy, I spoke of the temptation to lying, cheating, stealing and boasting. The boy's face remained unchanged. Still, as I pointed out that unfortunately, obscene, evil things were spoken and done, his finger shot under his nose and scratched according to his habit. At the end of the hour, in repetition, I repeated the experiment with the same result.

Although I knew already that a severe conflict was troubling the pupil, I did not urge my help. I knew for a certainty that the boy would tell of himself. Nine months later, he appeared and asked my aid. The turning up of the nose expressed disgust at an odor. The outstretched finger closed the one nostril to protect him and simultaneously expressed symbolically the cause of the unpleasant exhibition. The youth had masturbated. The odor of semen was repulsive to him and yet he longed for it. Hence, the one nostril was held shut, while he breathed through the other. A similar compromise was betrayed by the action of the finger which passed as female symbol, thereby refusing cohabitation. (Similar phantasies and symptomatic acts are often found in impotent individuals. By picking the nose, in spite of all commands to the contrary, or when a youth is all the time sticking his finger through his buttonhole, no matter how much the teacher admonishes against it, the analytic teacher knows that the appetite of the lustful one knows no limit in his phantasies.)

The scratching at a corner of the mouth went back to an ulcer which my pupil had long had in that place and in masochistic inordinate desire, did not allow to heal. The defect in good looks vexed the somewhat vain boy and he wishes it away. Now, as he torments himself with reproaches because of masturbation, he makes use of the earlier material: Like the earlier, so also may the present defects be banished. Also here, the same finesse as in the mimicry in the nasal zone: The scratching keeps up the defect which should still be eliminated. Thereby, the wish is expressed to practice masturbation and still be freed from the blemish. If this favorable outcome appeared in the physical defect why not in the moral? The gesture ceased from that hour.

2. REPRESSED MATERIAL FOUNDED ON EROTIC CONFLICTS

Frequently, the educator, while investigating a disturbance of moral conduct, a psychogenic (= mentally caused) physical symptom or some other repression symptom, comes upon emotional conflicts. Many times, upon deep investigation, he finds behind the disturbance of the relation to the parents, brothers or sisters, comrades or other companions, still another complication which we designate as sexual in the sense of the ordinary narrow speech usage. It is, however, not always the case, so that we shall speak of a sexual etiology only when we trace back the eroticism in general, especially the love to the parents and other people, exclusively or predominantly to sexual experiences.

According to my view, love toward other people, even at the very first, is dependent on the instinct for the preservation of the race; as I do not make the latter synonymous with sexuality, however, (compare Chapter VIII, 1) so I cannot designate that love as sexual. Further, the eroticism is established, in good part, on the cultivation of the ego emotions. That, also in the eroticism, energies which once belonged to sensuality, are constantly utilized, is in no way denied by this statement.

A girl of about eighteen years, who was sent to me because of antipathy against all people, with the exception of one girl comrade, and distaste for life, showed, soon after entrance into the school (age of 7 to 8 years), strong dislike towards parents and companions. The latter she avoided and at about twelve years of age, displayed an aggressive scornful behavior toward them. In the first period, she frequently had a stereotyped anxiety dream: "On a straight road, she goes between two swamps, from which many hands are extended toward her to pull her down." The analysis easily revealed: The other pupils laughed at the child who still believed in the Christ child and the angels who bring children and informed her that the mother carries the baby in her body and if she could not quiet her child, they cut off her breasts. Still other hateful ideas, they brought to the terrified child. In the dream, there is indicated the wish to allow herself to be pulled down by her companions of same age into the swamp of obscene ideas and probably also of acts, but at the same time, the still stronger desire to escape from them. From her twelfth year, after reading a book about

Buffalo Bill, the girl often dreamed she was an Indian chieftain and killed a crowd of Pale Faces. The masochism is alternated by sadism. In her homosexual phantasy, the outlaw knows how to avenge herself grimly, which corresponds to her conduct in reality, only that life imposes limits on the hate. Would the whole attitude toward humanity and life not have taken another direction if a sensible enlightenment on the part of the mother had been given at the proper moment? The well-meaning woman spared no sacrifice for her daughter whom she educated affectionately and intelligently regarding other things. But her endeavors went to pieces on the repression. Since symptoms of dementia præcox were present, the girl was taken by me to an analytic psychiatrist and apparently cured by him, at least she has remained perfectly normal for more than a year.

A girl pupil of fifteen years complained of peculiar sensations in the hands and feet, which cause her to seek her bed immediately. Upon the report of sudden illness or unexpected death, she got into violent excitement and trembled in her whole body. I commanded her to concentrate her attention on the prickling places and give her next association. "My friend. I am so fond of her." [And she of you?] "Just as fond." [Press the places on the hands which have the crawling sensation.] "Again this friend." Somewhat later she related the dream of the night before. "I was going along the street. Someone embraced me." [Think of the place in the street.] "I know it. I met the friend there yesterday." It turned out that the little hysteric in the presence of her friend, felt an uncontrollable desire to embrace her. The girl is going away soon, my pupil fears she will be forgotten and left entirely alone. The tactile hallucination gratifies the need for affection (Moll's Kontrektation). Now it was explained also why the girl had felt the phenomenon so vividly the second day previously when the mother remained away so long and a longing for her broke out. With the mother, the child does not get along well but eagerly wishes for her affection.

Further, the excitement upon the news of sudden illness and death, brings forth the memory of a friend. Two years before, she played one day in the bed of a little sick companion whose father had accidentally left his finger-ring. Our patient put the ring on her own finger in play. The comrade died unexpectedly that same night. From that time, the excitement began. Three years before, her own luetic father had died of a disease which was localized in the same organ as that of the friend. I forgot to ask whether the death of this man, even if also long expected, had occurred suddenly. Probably that was the case.

Now when a shocking report of illness is heard, the memory of the analogous previous experience is not awakened, but merely the accompanying affect, the anxiety. The idea belonging to this affect, as is often observed in similar cases, remains repressed.

In this description of the occasions for anxiety, sexuality exercises a decisive rôle. The inhibition of the emotional forces seems to turn the scale. Now, however, the girl relates an anxiety dream which she had immediately after the death of her father, in which dream, the latter plays a rôle. The analysis was not possible since unfortunately, after the one conversation, the symptoms disappeared without leaving a trace, unfortunately, since a real unraveling of the conflicts still present would have been necessary. Still, it is probable,— we will later show the origin of the anxiety—that behind the dream, unsatisfied sexual desires existed. After another half year of complete health, slight distaste for life appeared and the well known hysterical jealousy toward a sister had in the meantime planted a grudge against me so that I was shunned. The earlier symptoms remained absent.

This sister, aged twenty, suffered, besides from many easily removed hysterical obsessions (mild squinting, turning of the head, twitching of the corner of the mouth and melancholia) from a very unpleasant phenomenon, an obsessional love. In her pastor, who had confirmed her, she was, in spite of his earnest remonstrances, immoderately in love, so much the more as she struggled against it. It is worthy of note that in solemn moments, especially in church, she had to laugh, for which, in the pension, she was repeatedly punished in vain.

The girl related that from her childhood, she was greatly slighted by her father and hence disliked him. She also disliked her mother. When something was to be shared, she never seemed to get her rights. Toward her numerous sisters, she was envious.

The first obsessional laughing occurred during the funeral sermon which the pastor preached at her father's bier and indeed following the remark, how sad it was that the father had to be separated from so large a family. The instruction for confirmation, the girl sought gladly, only she hated the teacher since he praised her too little, but she rejoiced greatly over every word of recognition. The ceremony of confirmation excited her to laughter when the speaker said: ''And you, Father, and you, Mother, do you not rejoice at the sight of your daughter?''

Removed to a distance, our pupil fell passionately in love with a woman teacher who showed her kindness, kissed her every evening and, especially on days of illness, overwhelmed her with attentions. Much speaks in favor of the illness itself representing an extortion of tenderness. The previously strong religion suddenly disappeared at that time, to reappear again as quickly after the separation from the passionately loved one.

After the return home, she acted coldly toward the pastor until he, one evening (probably accidentally), pressed her hand in friendly fashion, but on the other hand, overlooked her sister and friend who were standing close by. From that hour, she loved him passionately. Plainly, she found in him again the longed-for father as she had before hated him as such. The obsessional laughing, the beginning of which was expressed by the twitching of the corner of the mouth, betrayed the gratification over the father's death and especially the malicious joy toward the sisters.

In this report, there is lacking the proof of sexual factors.

But we see that this patient also leaves us in the lurch since she lost her obsessional love after the second session and in a base attack captured the lover of her elder favored sister. If one finds a scientific explanation among cured patients of this class, still, upon closer investigation, one discovers a number of other conditions, since every neurosis possesses a very complicated bundle of roots. That also in our case, a sexual cause was decisively at work, we could only assert if we were sure that the decidedly sexually colored love toward the pastor was an unchanged new edition of that toward the father. But we have not yet discussed the transposition of emotion.

The following case of stuttering seems to be conditioned on asexual eroticism. A boy of sixteen, candidate for confirmation, could not get beyond the beginning of his speech. After violent effort, he produced a sobbing tone, spoke a few words normally and again stuck fast. His father is a drinker. His sister, ten years his elder, educated him harshly and as it seems, without love. She often struck him and if he broke out crying, she increased the punishment. For years, the youngster has had no one in whom he could confide and felt himself unfortunate in life. Only at night in bed, could he give way to weeping, by day, he throttled his suffering. We understand well that the boy expresses his suffering in his speech disturbance and comes automatically to his weeping. But we suspect further that other material is hidden deeper. Unfortunately, after the conversation, the inhibition remained absent and the boy likewise. After about a year, the evil returned, but not bad enough to send the deserter to me. At that first time, he had told of improper acts of his comrades and played the dear innocent. Probably he feared to tell the whole truth. I cannot definitely assert this, however.

It is in no ways to be wondered at, if many observers quickly assert that no sexual motive was present calling for careful reticence. I myself plead guilty of having originally lightly denied the sexual etiology in cases which I thought I could see through, until to my confusion, I was taught better. I know also how uncommonly difficult it often is to penetrate to the foundation of a neurosis * and cannot therefore, admire the diagnostician who, after two or three or even after one consultation, asserts that a sexual etiology is not present. From the fact that in some sputum examinations, no bacilli are found, it does not follow that the patient in question has none. Every profound shock to the individual—and only such an one occasions a neurosis—also implicates the sexual sphere and is also reflected in sexual phantasies, for the psychic life constitutes an organism, in which the suffering of one part causes suffering in other functional fields. From the existence of sexual inhibitions, therefore, we may not yet decide that these have exclusive etiological significance.

3. The Asexual and Anerotic Repressed Material

(a) the traumatic neurosis

Something which is often urged against Freud's sexual theory is the occurrence of traumatic hysteria. From ancient times, it has been believed that merely a terrific shock was sufficient to occasion a nervous malady. The father of psychoanalysis found in such cases without exception, however, that the disease was prepared for by a sexual difficulty. A man of forty-five years who became ill from anxiety upon the report of the death of his father, lived, for example, eleven years with his wife in coitus interruptus. This same habit which, according to the consensus of opinion of all psychoanalysts,† is very injurious, prevailed in some other examples.

I, too, could find such connections in spite of my limited experience. A young merchant complained to me that, as a result of a railroad acident, he was suffering from nervous trouble. When the accident happened, a train which he saw coming, ran into his wagon. Since then, he repeatedly hallucinates this scene on the road with great anxiety. Upon being questioned, he said that he was engaged and only gets an

* Wherever in this book, neurosis ("nervous trouble") is mentioned, I always mean psychoneurosis, that is, one based on mental complications, not the neurosis organically conditioned.

† Compare Freud, Kl. Schriften I, p. 71.

attack when, after a visit to his fiancée, he is seized on his return trip. The man had a suit pending against the railroad company for immense damages for injury from this accident. He did not seem enraptured with my advice to have himself cured by a physician skilled in psychoanalysis. The physician would not be one to be envied as I know from a second, similar case, the analysis of which went to pieces on the money-hunger of the victim.

Nevertheless, I also know traumatic neuroses which proceeded smoothly to health without sexual material appearing. Of course, in this case, a superficial exploration was sufficient, so that sexual material could very well have remained hidden. An example:

A teacher sent me a good-natured but poorly-gifted school girl of ten years for therapeutic pedagogic treatment. The little one came accompanied by her mother. She has suffered for five weeks from complete paralysis and twitching of the left arm, frequently falls on the left side, awakens every night at a quarter to ten with anxiety and twitching of the mouth. In the absence of the child, I asked regarding shocking experiences and learned that five years before, an adult had frightened the child by seizing a knife in sport, making a frightful grimace and threatening to kill the child. The latter rushed to the door and fled but had to stay three days in bed as a result of the fright. Since then, she has been abnormally timid. The evening before the illness, the child had been awakened at a quarter of ten by the cries of night rovers.

The further investigation, I carried on with the child, and indeed at first for some minutes in the presence of the mother, when I saw how confiding toward the mother she was in her presence. The child is also very kindly disposed toward her father and sister. [Do you remember the man who threatened you years ago?] ''Yes, he took a knife out of the drawer and would kill me.'' [No, no, he was only fooling, he was a regular 'Lappi' (foolish fellow), the dear God keeps you safely. How do you move the arm?] (The child twitched a few times, swung the arm forward and turned the hand outward, the three outer fingers being closed. The movement was so quick that I could not clearly observe it and did not at once grasp its meaning.) [You turn your hand as if you would say no.] "Yes." [Do you know how you lay in bed when you were awakened five weeks ago?] "Yes, against the wall." [On which side of the body?] "On the left." [And then?] "I wished to spring up but could not because I lay on my arm and leg." [And hence you thought you could not move the arm and leg? Pay no attention to that 'Lappi' and think that the singing boys who behaved so foolishly, would also certainly do nothing to make you suffer. Here you have three beautiful books which you may read if you can carry them yourself.] (The girl who could carry nothing that noon carried the books triumphantly away with firm step.)

Now, of course this was not a regular analysis. If the thought of critical psychologists had been in my mind, I would have refrained from the massive suggestion.

Three days later, the mother and child appeared a second time, the twitching of the arm and failure of the foot had almost disappeared, likewise, the pavor nocturnus at a quarter of ten, still the arm seemed quite weak. In the night following our conversation, a very disagreeable disturbance had broken out, in which frequent emptying of the stomach had occurred. [Do you experience something nauseating?] "Yes, a girl would push me into a nasty pile." (For two months, the eruptions remained away.)

The automatic distortion of the mouth went back to censure from the father. The latter reproached the child because spots were often visible on the pillow and said to her: "Shame on you! A big girl should no longer sleep with her mouth open!" The movement really only appeared when the little one was embarrassed, for example, when she could not answer a question.

After this consultation, the child was apparently well. In the third session, we found from the posture of the fingers, and turning of the hand that the arm gesture expressed the wish to open the door. The twitching of the mouth was still present in slight degree but disappeared after a few days without further analysis.

A month later, the little hysteric wished to visit me. The mother would not grant it on this day. Thereupon, the child vomited and obtained the mother's consent. For two years, the girl has been entirely well.

To-day, I regret that I did not proceed in more correct analytic manner and that I yielded so much to suggestion. Hence, I can give the case neither for nor against Freud's conception of the sexual root of the neuroses.*

Still, I know of a number of traumatic neuroses, as for example, two cases of stuttering resulting from fright from a glimpse of St. Nicholas. But I have received no patients of this class for the health pedagogic treatment as yet, since the parents, upon the appearance of such a phenomenon, which indeed falls less in the domain of the moral life, have with good reason turned to the physician.

(B) OTHER PSYCHONEUROSES

No single case of any other neurosis is known to me, in which the sexual or erotic disturbance of the mental equilibrium has been absent. Now and then, totally different conflicts stood in the foreground but without exception, they received a strong addition in emotional values from the erotic sphere, in which case, this fatal erotic situation was not necessarily founded on abnormally unfavorable external relations. Often, the inability to adapt to well intentioned and useful demands of the parents, created severe erotic denial. Excessive severity on the part of the father or the mother only sharpens the conflict but cannot occasion it if specific subjective conditions are not present.

This may be observed in two cases of writer's cramp. One of these was in a clerk of twenty-nine years, who, a year previous, had become ill under peculiar circumstances. An official of the same name had obtained a leave of absence on

---

* Freud also considers the utilization of intentional suggestion in such cases as proper.

account of a nervous malady; besides this, an office girl was absent. Thus, there fell to my patient for several months, an extra amount of work without his being satisfactorily rewarded therefor. After the return of his colleague, he hoped likewise to obtain a leave of absence but was refused his wish, although he represented to his chief that he, the solicitor, has a much harder post than his companion, not a single five minutes could he write undisturbed and he was therefore much more exposed to the danger of a nervous illness than his namesake. The writer's cramp, he considered a harmless disturbance which could be easily cured. The wish for a non-dangerous nervousness, he did not remember plainly, but rather considered his nerves as shattered by an unhealed venereal disease.

With this sexual trouble, an erotic one interacted. In order to escape an irregular life, he sought a wife by advertising in the newspaper and began a love correspondence which he maintained with bad conscience. Inwardly attached to another girl, he feigned in his letters a love which in reality did not exist. When, now, the hope of winning the one he really loved, awakened, the resolution to break off the unfaithful relations failed him, since he had already gone too far. The disturbance in writing came, therefore, as in another of the cases observed and cured by me,* to relieve a deep need and wish that he might release himself from the conflict between desire and duty.

That the non-erotic wish played an important part, however, is shown by the development of the disturbance. So long as the hysteric wished to put off only the burdensome work, his hand was drawn outward. Some months later, a change appeared: The pen jumped into the air every few moments. What had happened? The firm had dismissed him and paid him off. Now, the patient changed his plan so far as to say to himself, he would not return again to the earlier dependence but seek something "higher." From the beginning, he had wished as rich a wife as possible. I could not discover that a

* See p. 126.

change in the erotic relations and plans began when the cramp changed. Still, it is not excluded that unconsciously, a variation of the erotic phantasy was present. Since the patient was scarcely suitable for pastoral influence and really belonged to the domain of the physician, I discharged him before beginning the deeper analysis, with the advice to go to a neurologist. He remained refractory and two years later was still uncured.

Also in the second of the cases mentioned here, the disturbance of writing met an ardent non-erotic wish: The youth, aged twenty-four, wished to change his vocation but could not obtain the consent of his parents to this end. Soon, it became plain that the contracture formed only an insignificant symptom in a group of very important ones. Preëminent was a strong suicidal tendency. The neurologist to whom I sent the patient at once after this discovery, could not cure the severe hysteria; this patient will repeatedly engage our attention later, since the youth would not separate himself from the extreme, fanatical, orthodox father whose badly planned pedagogical treatment caused and maintained the disease.*

This much, I believe I may say in general, that a man who is capable of loving and whose compulsion toward love and agreement on the part of the parents, husband, bride or wife or some near substitute for these, is satisfied, can suffer no disease-forming repressions. Further, loss of property, lack of recognition, injuries to reputation, indeed religious or ethical considerations, scruples and the like, create only portentous deviations in the development of a youth when a severe sexual or erotic shock is joined to them.

We shall come later to Adler's important theory that all neuroses trace back to feelings of insufficiency.

* Another youth, whose unfortunate relation to his father caused writer's cramp, I sent at once to a physician. The analysis was at first without results, since the separation from the father, an orthodox bigot, had not taken place. Some weeks later, the patient took a position away from the family and immediately got well.

CHAPTER V

THE REPRESSING FORCE

A REPRESSION can only occur when an instinct is inhibited. This can happen by reality rendering the activity of the instinct impossible or by a second desire opposing the first one.

1. REALITY AS A FACTOR IN REPRESSION

A repression is created by reality when either a previously utilized instinctive activity is rendered impossible by a change in the external world or an instinctive function, which has become necessary to the further development of the individual, is denied. In the first case, there is a deprivation, in the second, an abstinence.

(A) THE DEPRIVATION

If, on account of the death or unfaithfulness of the beloved person or other processes, an erotic relation, whether a real relation or a strong hope, is destroyed, then a repression frequently appears. The person in question wishes to drive the tormenting idea from his mind, but thereby forces it under the threshold of consciousness, from whence it continues most unpleasant activities, often just at the time when it pushes forward another idea. If we are dealing with a deprivation of less painful kind or if the instinct affected can and will allow of some ideal substitution, either of equal or higher value, (compare Chapter XVII, Compensation, and Chapter XI, section 5, Sublimation) then the man bears the loss without pathological detriment. It is otherwise in the irreparable injuries of high emotional value or in refusal of later transferences. The latter condition, the refusal of a new love to other people, the refusal of a love substitute, is an indispensable condition of the neurosis.

It is known that the death of dear persons, the decline of health with its effects on the expectations of life or similar shocks can call forth severe emotional disturbances or renunciation of reality. Many psychoses break out after a death, also many withdrawals from the world. Francis of Assisi became a visionary through grave illness, Raimon Lull, upon the sight of the breast of his beloved, Armand Jean le Bouthillier de Rancé, the founder of the Trappist Order, eaten by ulcers, made the world a death-house, after he had met his bride in her coffin upon his return home.

On the basis of numerous observations, we shall also derive such processes from the repression. An example which presented itself in the analysis of a foreign lady in the climacteric, is as follows:

When a girl, eighteen years of age, she fell in love with a vivacious but somewhat brutal man who courted her sister but was refused. After his departure, the girl, in whose kindred and circle of acquaintances there was not a single pietist, devoted herself to a passionate adoration of Jesus which drew her into a congenial, world-fleeing conventicle. When twenty-two years old, she married a much older brother-in-law, wholly because she wished to be a good mother to her nephews. The older stepson, an image of the knightly father, she treated with rare consideration, though without affection; with the younger, an ungovernable hotspur, she was in continual conflict. As the youngster grew to young manhood, the conduct of the mother changed strikingly: she gained his affection and treated him tenderly. One day, he explained to her that the pietistic Savior, in whom he had thus far been taught to believe, was becoming distasteful to him, the pietistic mood, weak. To the general astonishment, the mother replied that she had felt the same way for some time. Soon after, the youth died. The shock drove the mother into stoicism and after several years, to grave hysteria. Four years of treatment according to Dubois was without result. In the meantime, the physician went over to Freud but severed the altruistic sublimations. Hence the patient remained dependent on him and got into the greatest need, since she had to hate the physician fiercely and at the same time to love him and during the conjugal act, had only him before her eyes. She was easy to cure in two consultations. When by the previously given analysis, the injurious transference had also been dissolved, an uncommonly strong piety set in, which placed God as the Father and his social commands in the center of her life.

The connections are easy to discern: The pietistic Jesus is the sublimated contrast-substitute for the loved one. The libido flows back to the stepson who resembles the lover so that Jesus must be given up. After the death of the erotic object, no new adoration of Jesus can ensue because this would have meant unfaithfulness to the dead. The stoicism shows us the involution of the libido; the hysteria, the failure of that attempt at sublimation in philosophy. The analysis eliminated the fixation on the youthful loved one and disclosed the transference upon the father, who, in the figure of husband and of God, stilled the longing of the heart and rendered possible a fruitful social activity. Also, the frigidity could be eliminated, and thus the marriage, after twenty-four years of barrenness, became a completely harmonious and happy one after the ethical conflict had also been removed.

An elderly woman, some weeks after the death of her husband, suddenly suffered from anxiety that her prayers were ineffective, that she could not pray any more. As we will show in numerous examples, anxiety is the constant result of unsatisfied sexual demands.

(B) ABSTINENCE

A repression may also occur without external changes, when, during normal processes of development, a hiatus is created between subjective demands and objective allowance.* The rise of the neuroses and of religious conversions during the period of puberty, the increase of melancholia in the climacteric with

---

* Freud, Über neurotische Erkrankungstypen. Zbl. II, p. 299 f.

its intensive sexual need, all go back to this process. "A young man who has previously gratified his libido (his 'love-impulse' [Liebesdrang]) by phantasies with an outlet in masturbation and now wishes to exchange this regime, which is closely related to autoeroticism, for the real object choice, a girl who has directed her whole affection toward father or brother and now would allow to become conscious for a man who is courting her, the hitherto unconscious, incestuous wishes of the libido, a woman who would renounce her polyga-mous tendencies and prostitution-phantasies in order to be-come a faithful wife to her husband and a blameless mother: all these persons become ill in their praiseworthy efforts if the earlier fixations of their libido are strong enough to resist a displacement." *

A single woman of thirty-three years became happily en-gaged to a virtuous man and held him very dear. When she would make the bridal visit to his home place and ascended the stairs with him, she suddenly felt tremendous anxiety and her love vanished in an instant. She was inconsolable over the loss of her emotion, especially as she was happy before and acted happy. He who is acquainted with the symbolism of stair dreams† or knows what erotic significance "mount-ing" has in the colloquial German speech, "monter, grimper" in the French, will not be surprised that this act of repression occurred on the stairs. My surmise that a dementia præcox was present was confirmed by the neurologist called in con-sultation. After the breaking of the engagement, there came states of excitement with ideas of persecution, yet after some months, health apparently returned.

If one examines such cases more closely, one sees that the external world only causes a repression when there was already present beforehand a strong internal tension which reaches back even to childhood. The lady who fell back upon stoicism had lost her father very early and suffered severe

* Same, p. 299.
† Freud, Traumdeutung, 3rd ed., p. 215 f. Robitsek, Leiter als sex.
Symbol i. d. Antike. Zbl. I, p. 586 f.

sexual traumata. The husband, whose character resembled that of the father, took the place of a man who was passionately loved and unforgotten and the bad experiences of the first years were again rendered acute by the conjugal demands. The dementia præcox patient who lost her love on the stairs, looked back to a youth devastated by the drinking of the father, and the husband of the friend she had just visited was likewise addicted to alcoholism. The revulsion against her fiancé soon clothed itself in fear of his drunkenness although there was not the slightest occasion in the life of the man for this accusation.

So in this collision with reality, we are dealing at bottom with an internal conflict. The person whose eroticism is well provided for, can endure incredibly hard blows of fortune and hardships, whether it is a question of the satisfaction of the love-need as it occurs in the relation to fellowmen or of the ideal eroticism in science, art, nature study, religion and other sublimated activities.

2. THE INNER LIFE AS A FACTOR IN REPRESSION

If we review our first consideration (page 56, col. 4) of the repressing motives, we are struck by the numerical preponderance of the ethical reactions. Besides these, we find, however, other considerations also, which offset the profit to be gained by the awakened effort, by a very appreciable detriment, hence exert a powerful retarding influence. We recall that neither of the two forces engaged in contest with each other, needs to be conscious. Often, the true motive is hidden behind a mask. Many times a real motive is known but only the most superficial one, for example, dislike of the vocation, while the deeper lying conditions (for example, erotic) are not even suspected.

(A) THE ETHICAL MOTIVES

He who has a poor opinion of the power of conscience will be taught a better one by the analytic method of consideration. Many maladies are nothing else than flight from a severe ethical conflict, many others represent expiations for past short-comings or counter-reactions to a burning feeling of shame.

1. *The Warning and Impelling Conscience*

A melancholy girl who has become estranged from humanity and God suffers from difficulty of hearing. Two aurists, by placing the tuning fork on the skull, diagnosticate beginning degeneration of the auditory nerve. The syphilis of the father is visited on the daughter. Nevertheless, the degree of the degenerative process cannot explain that of the deafness ac-cording to the view of the otologist consulted by me. At the advice of the latter, I undertook an analysis, although the re-sult could not be permanent because of progressive nerve de-struction. Even in the first consultation, the defect in hearing yielded almost entirely. While at the beginning, I had to shout loudly in order to be heard, at the end of the conver-sation, the patient understood fairly low speech and heard the ticking of her light running watch.

The causes of the hysterical deafness acting as reinforce-ment of the physiologically conditioned defect of hearing were as follows: 1. The father suffering from atrophy of the spinal cord often stormed about the whole night. The little daugh-ter, fleeing to the kitchen and weeping on the kitchen table, often sighed: "Would that I could hear nothing of the dis-turbance!" 2. The idolized mother became ill of cancer of the stomach. The daughter, sleeping in the same room, heard her groan and repeated the previous lament. 3. The good-for-nothing brother besieged her with begging letters. She wished to hear nothing. 4. Evil-intentioned persons accused her of improper relations with her fiancé and other men while she knew herself innocent. 5. Her fiancé, whom she did not love, occasionally spoke in harmless manner of his wish to have children. Since he did this the first time, she has not only suffered an anxiety attack every evening upon going to bed but she also feels herself strengthened in her wish: "May I hear nothing of the whole thing."

The result lasted only two days. Why? On the evening

of the second day, the girl met a friend of her youth whom she had loved years before, without finding her love reciprocated. Now, he met her with great friendliness, sent her his photograph and acted in such a manner that she thought she perceived real affection. Immediately, there arose a severe ethical conflict: "If he should propose marriage to me, do I belong to him whom I love or to the fiancé whom I do not love, to whom I gave the marriage promise and who will be unhappy without me?" Behind this conflict was hidden, as I could state definitely from analogy with more thorough analyses, a whole network of unconscious motives which stretched back even to earliest childhood. She did not know how to solve the conflict of duties by clear deliberation. Therefore, she fled to hysteria which plainly realized in the deafness the wish to hear nothing, though of course, only in symbolical manner. Thus, as it were, she avoided the collision, or rather, the duty of a well considered moral decision, for he who cannot hear, also need not hear.

It was easy to stop the new attempt at flight. The cure lasted a half year. Her spirits also improved splendidly, the trust in God arranged itself as consolation and encouragement. The anxiety had disappeared. But it remained for the girl to see that it was not right to continue an engagement merely to provide a means of subsistence. She fell out with her future sister-in-law and as a result, estranged herself inwardly still more from her fiancé. Once more, she withdrew into the deafness without, however, informing me. When she finally did come, she brought along insurmountable resistances so that I at once recognized that she was not in earnest in her will to be well. For she finally attained what she wished with a part of her being: the fiancé, who had been very badly treated, broke off the engagement and again the ethical difficulties were solved.* The warning conscience obtained its purpose with the help of the unconscious.

For the educator, those cases are especially important, in

* Scarcely had the previously unloved fiancé withdrawn than strong love appeared in the girl—which was naturally without vital roots.

which the anticipatory conscience attains its aims by utilization of the unconscious. Meanwhile, one can observe how an intended wrong is frustrated by this trick. A boy has a rendezvous, he forgets the hour in mysterious fashion, changes the place, misunderstands the arrangements, gets a nose bleed, leaves his pocket-book behind so that he cannot use the trolley and comes too late, etc.

2. *The Punishing Conscience*

In very many cases, we discover in the depths of the unconscious, as an obstacle to the activity of instinct, the memory of past wrong. In this, we are not to think of thoughts and acts which offend against public morality but of offenses against the inner imperative, against the command of the individual conscience. The young girl whose migraine in the temples went back to the death threat of the father spared herself by her pain the accusation of hostile wishes against her father. The hallucination of the neighbor changed into an angel, probably rested on a reproach because of unallowed sentiments. A new example may be added:

A girl of twenty-three years suffered from melancholia, anxiety, neuralgias in the face and stomach. The feeling of guilt ruled the waking life and originally the uppermost stratum of her dreams. She dreamed, for example, of a black marble wall, on which there projected a white tablet bearing the crucifix. In this vision, she found consolation for her suffering from sins. Homosexual tendency speaks plainly from many dreams. The cautiously phrased question concerning sexual experiences was twice definitely denied so that I allowed myself to be deceived by the prudery and moral indignation. Not yet acquainted with the technical means for analyses of resistance, I did not know how to help myself when communication was suddenly shut off by inner compulsion. I dismissed her with religious encouragement and the advice not to give so much love to the woman friend but to support herself with love to God. The anxiety had already disappeared. After four months, the patient returned, driven by change for the worse in her condition and confessed now, of her own free will, although in a severe struggle against the speech prohibition, a number of sexual transgressions with the woman friend and a dog. She considered the pains as punishment. Always when the pain in the right cheek was analyzed, there was a thought of the friend and repression of a sexual longing directed toward her, while behind the hysterical neuralgia of the left half of the face, there regularly came into view the mother, who has been dead three years. In dream and waking life, there floated before her, hundreds of song-book verses and Bible texts to which she clung during the unbearably severe pains. In this, she occasionally omitted parts which might awaken unpleasant sexual memories, for example:

"Glanz der Herrlichkeit,	Brightness of glory,
Du vor aller Zeit,	Thou of eternity,
Leben derer, die verloren,	Life of the lost,
Und ihr Licht dazu,	And their light as well,
Jesu, süsse Ruh'."	Jesus, sweet rest.

Here two stanzas are amalgamated. The first runs in whole:

"Glanz der Herrlichkeit,	Brightness of glory,
Du vor aller Zeit	Thou of eternity
Zum Erlöser uns geschenket	Sent to be our Savior
Und in unser Fleisch gesenket."	And degraded to our flesh.

This place which arouses sexual thoughts was repressed and in its place, a part of the previous stanza was quoted, which contains already the religious counter-reaction against the suppressed sexual stimulus. In general, the citations dreamed, or those occurring in the waking life, reflected in wonderful nicety the condition of the unconscious.

Twenty days after the session described, the patient awoke in the night to these words:

"Zum Erlöser uns geschenket	Sent to be our Savior
Und in unser Herz gesenket	And in our heart submerged
In der Füll' der Zeit,	In the fulness of time,
Glanz der Herrlichkeit,"	Brightness of glory.

In this connection, there came into her mind the thought, this place belongs to song No. 228, verse 2 of the church songbook. Here, however, we read the words:

"Keiner Gnade sind wir wert	Of no grace are we worthy
Doch hat er in seinem Wort	Still in his word
Klar und liebreich sich erklärt,	He hath clearly and kindly shown,
Sehet nur, die Gnadenpforte	Only look, the gate of mercy
Ist hier völlig aufgetan:	Is here wide open:
Jesus nimmt die Sünder an."	Jesus takes the sins upon Himself.

I must remark in advance that we are dealing with a demonstration of the transference. The patient, in the meantime, assimilated the homosexual repression in great part, revealed the most painful secrets and experienced a decided amelioration of her suffering. The heterosexual instinctive tendency comes forward, the desires, which in reality apply to the brother and originally to the father, are projected onto the analyst. The speaking of the parts suppressed in the previous dream had lifted the earlier sexual undertone ("in unser Fleisch gesenket" = "to our flesh degraded") into consciousness. Now the dreamer allows the idea as if she were purified from improper phantasies. In relation to Jesus, she is also innocent. But now, the pastor lurks behind him. Hence, a new feeling of guilt which is to be allayed by the reference to the stanza not quoted. This interpretation is not certain.

The analysis continued with many and long interruptions for one and one quarter years and ended very satisfactorily. Taken abroad, the one who had suffered so severely, enjoyed complete health for a long time although her external life-relations went badly. Two months after her departure, she wrote: "In spite of external affliction, it is well with me and my trust in God has become unshakable." Upon awakening, she heard the child's song: "For should I not be joyous?" She was thus not really cured. Two years later, after all kinds of injuries had been encountered the melancholia returned. I had to refuse the analysis and send the patient to the physician for nervous and mental diseases, who diagnosed, besides hysteria, dementia præcox; in a longer analytic treatment in a sanitarium, he improved the emotional conditions in some measure and also established the fact that there was little will to get well. The patient is incurable.

This case, like many others, showed me that the consciousness of sins represents in no way, merely an atonement for past wrong doing, but also a satisfaction of the instinct which finds no gratification in reality. The still active instinct, the unpermitted activity of which called forth the opposition of conscience, continues as best it may, in pathological neurotic symptoms, religious ideas of strong affect value or other performances which may be ethically very valuable.

It is important to recognize that the consciousness of guilt is also in every case a product of repression. One of its most frequent sources, where it appears with great force and joined to anxiety, is masturbation. Bleuler says: "I know as yet only one source of the feeling of guilt, which one might call religious or transcendental: onanism or some similar sexual transgressions. Where I could analyze such a feeling of guilt, I came upon sexual self-reproaches." * Jung says of the same phenomenon: "Fundamentally, it is probably to be considered as a partial sublimation of the infantile sexuality, that is to say, one which has miscarried. A certain amount of repressed libido (here, this word is equivalent to will or endeavor) † represented by corresponding phantasies, is left unattached and according to familiar examples, is converted into anxiety." ‡ The investigation of obsessional neurotic patients adds the information that very often, murder phantasies against the father and mother also call forth a pathological feeling of guilt, still we know that their disease never occurs without previous repressed infantile sexual activity. Whether these phantasies are the ultimate causes, as Freud assumes, or

* Bleuler, Über das relig. Schulbewusstseln. Z. f. Religions-psychologie Vol. III (1909), p. 5.

† Jung, D. Bedeutung des Vaters f. d. Schicksal d. Einzelnen. Jahrbuch I, p. 155.

‡ Jung, Z. f. Relpsych. III, p. 7.

only the superficial occasion, brought about by a struggle against an inner imperative and not at all meant in earnest, as Jung believes, we must later seek to determine.

It is interesting how the sexually conditioned feeling of guilt, now and then, creates repressions, which also lend great weight to self-accusations because of other transgressions. The boy whom we met as dumb, seeing dimly and "hanging on a thread," had stolen for six years from his mother without feeling remorse. Only the sexually conditioned feeling of guilt made the crime against property burning; thus it acted as setting free other moral reactions.* Another time, I observed that a boy of sixteen, who had masturbated for many years, made sexual reproaches against himself after he had committed a theft.

Ordinarily, the malady breaks out first when the onanism, previously practiced without hesitation, is left off because of threatening warnings.

A talented boy of seventeen years entered my room weeping, with the exclamation: "For God's sake, help me if there is still help!" He suffered from anxiety that his breasts had assumed female form, for which reason, he could no longer practice gymnastics and bathe (with others) and upon the military draft, he would be shamed to death. Not long before, he had listened to the lecture of a well-known itinerant preacher and at this, heard the foolish threat of gynacomasty. As a result of this, he stopped his bad habit. A short time later, the phobia appeared. Reassurance was easy. A year later, pathological sympathy broke out: The youth saw a poor girl fishing drift-wood from the sea. A comrade spoke harshly to her. The little girl looked up frightened and weeping, threw away the wood and hastened away over the stones with bare feet. This picture tormented my patient for many nights and kept him sleepless until morning. In explanation, it turned out that at that time, he had written a young girl a love letter but had not sent it because he considered it unfaithful to another girl. Behind the child whom he pitied, there thus

* Prot. Monatsh. Vol. XIII, p. 11.

lurked the jilted friend, behind the brutal comrade, he himself.

A pupil of sixteen years suffered from pathological fear of cockroaches: A comrade had warned him against onanism and predicted severe physical injuries to him. In one of the next nights, an accident happened to the fellow in whom the remarks of the friend had created great fear and imposed abstinence from onanism: He awoke right after midnight from having smashed a cockroach on his chest. Trembling, he sprang out of bed and could not go back again until morning. From that time, he had terrible anxiety for beetles. It happened that he thought he suddenly felt such an animal on his chest and in mortal dread, he would hasten away to undress himself. As cause, he found only the tape of his underclothing. From that time on, he suffered a severe attack of anxiety upon the slightest occasion until he was completely healed three years later by an analytic session with me. I explained to him the basis of his phobia and impressed on him to say this explanation over when another attack of anxiety occurred. In the afternoon before the next session, he read in bed from a guide-book. Just after going to sleep, so he asserted, the book fell to the floor; he was terribly frightened but nevertheless immediately followed my advice, whereupon to his astonishment, the anxiety at once disappeared. Two days later, he traveled across the ocean, where, some months later, new anxiety with hallucinations broke out. I gave him repeated counsel by letter and soon received the report that he felt quite well again. The exact conditions of the cure are not known to me.

Jung has recently abandoned his belief in the predominant sexual root of the religious feeling of guilt. Morbid feeling of sin, he finds in general, where a person transgresses an inalienable life-demand peculiar to his nature.

The sexual damming up is therewith not confirmed as cause of the feeling of guilt, it is merely put alongside other motives. Also, I believe that grievous offenses against the demands of conscience can excite anxiety phenomena, as Shakespeare, for example, shows in his Macbeth. But there, too, the statement holds that corresponding to such shocks to the personality, there are constantly disturbances in the eroticism or a specific functioning of the eroticism. In ambitious misdoing, the ef-́ fort to outdo the father may lie hidden, thus, an erotic motive, or in accordance with Freud's terminology, a sexual motive. There are also, however, feelings of guilt, which are to be understood simply as associative results of the infantile fear of punishment.

3. The Public Morality.

Not a few people allow more to be imposed upon themselves by the ridicule or contempt of others than by the inspirations of their own conscience. That which every educator has so often found in normal individuals, the analytic pedagogue finds confirmed in countless occurrences. Many a malady, many a reaction of the moral consciousness resting on repression, goes back to the circumstance that a demand of instinct comes in conflict with a demand of culture or society. Where- upon, the individual very often absorbs the imperative of his environment into the expression of his conscience. Especially in the erotic field, is the power of public opinion plainly, enormously strong. Often, however, the morality of the en- vironment is contrary to the personal moral insight. This conflict cannot yet cause a neurosis. A neurosis is certainly many times, as it were, the spark which is kindled from the friction of the individual and social morality and causes a mighty conflagration, but only in case the individual recognizes the social morality as conforming to his own nature and sees his own inability to comply with it. Thus, the conflict must be an internal one, even though the voice of conscience is con- ditioned by the environment. To this extent, the social morality is also of importance. The existence of devastations resulting from such internal collisions precipitated from the outside, no keen observer can deny. In this regard, psycho- analysis must open the eyes of humanity and offer sword and trowel to the universally approaching longing for a higher and deeper, freer and purer, cultural morality. Not that psychoanalysis can create the new values and landmarks! But it can and will provide a mass of facts in the case which will put the emotional and intellectual forces in mighty agitation. And further, social ethics cannot do without respect for the forces of reality. Only a few sketches may be outlined here: The neurosis, frightful as it can be, is not the greatest evil. If the highest ethical values were to be purchased only at this price, then the neurosis would have to be endured. As a matter of fact, however, corresponding to the devastation of the healthy life, there is very often a reduction of the moral value and corresponding to the pseudomoralistic commands, a loss in mental and physical health. Against this state of affairs, the analytically trained educator and people's adviser must and will take the field. In no way is this a question of licentious self-indulgence. The analysis will show us more and more that the deeper claims of the spirit are of greater importance than the peripheral discharge of erotic tensions. Many a libertine, whom the repressions of his love-demands drives with pathological compulsion into foolish efforts, can be guided by the analysis to a socially useful life. Further, where sexual denial causes great disturbance, the analysis helps to find the true ground of the trouble in soluble internal conflicts and in persons, ethically normal, to bring about that healthful direction of instinct to higher ends which we will discuss under the title of sublimation.

(B) THE REPRESSING MOTIVES WITH EXCLUSION OF THE
QUESTION OF THEIR ETHICAL DIGNITY

Very often, the neurosis bears witness to a moral refinement which struggles against the actual relations but cannot openly attain its purpose and therefore seeks its goal, wholly or in part at least, symbolically or indirectly, through some secret channel. Often, however, the repression simply goes toward sparing of pain and thus serves the pure pleasure-hunger. The repressed desire is then often of high moral tone, while the repressing desire corresponds to egoism or convenience, which takes refuge in the neurosis instead of energetically continuing the moral combat in the reality. Many an hysterical malady is a renunciation of moral deeds, a capitulation of the ethical consciousness in the face of the immoral forces of effortless pleasure-seeking, a cheap solution of serious ethical problems according to the principle of the least expenditure of effort.

Many hysterical individuals and other victims of a refractory unconscious spare themselves the great sacrifice of renunciation of certain conveniences and pleasures of life, those harsh denials and efforts which would be necessary to gain a free self-control, a healthy life conduct.

A sufferer from anxiety neurosis was thrown into the water by an enemy and during the period of his ill health, drew a high indemnity which would be discontinued with the return of health or the ability to earn his living. He must therefore perform a great moral feat in order to escape the mastery of the repressed material. His satisfaction with indolence, free from work, interposed a powerful resistance to the analysis and maintained the repression as it existed when the malady began. Obviously, there lurk behind such repressions, still other, more powerful ones. In what direction, these are to be sought, will become evident later.

Experience teaches that the repression becomes only so much the stronger when one would save himself a necessary decision, industriously drive out of mind a painful conflict or transform it into vain phantasies of which we will speak in another place. "He who observes himself attentively and without prejudice, knows that there dwells within him a being which would gladly conceal and gloss over everything difficult and questionable in life, in order to create for itself a free and easy path." * That which we would gladly diminish in conscious thought and volition, we must carry out in the unconscious with just so much the greater pains. It is the old story of the boy who will not pick up the horse-shoe but stoops for every cherry, but with this difference, that both the neurotic and the normal

* Jung, Der Inhalt der Psychose. Leipzig & Vienna 1908, p. 25.

individual must stoop and does not see the connection between cherry and money because of the repression.

No strong emotion is conceivable which may not be repressed. Ambition, desire for money, lust and cruelty are absent as little as magnanimity, generosity and selfsacrifice in the catalogue of repressing factors. Vicious tendencies are active in the unconscious as well as the virtuous ones. Those impulses which have absorbed emotional energies from other sources, especially the erotic (see Chapter VII), exert most repressing force. The conflict betwéen moral and immoral tendencies causes the greatest distraction. The moral man, like the immoral man, is strong, while the strongest intelligence and will-power with a feeling of guilt or mistrust of self may easily fall to a state of weakness.

Ethical and non-ethical motives for repression act in the sense of striving toward avoidance of discomfort.

Recently, Jung lays great stress on the point that the conflict leading to illness lies in the present (Jahrbuch V, 382) and proceeds chiefly from the circumstance that the person shrinks from a necessary task. "When the libido (the will) shrinks from a necessary task, this happens from those general human reasons of convenience, which are developed to very high degree not only in the child but also in primitive man and in animals. The primitive indolence and convenience is the first opposing influence against efforts at adaptation" (Jahrbuch V, 422). Even earlier, Freud had emphasized that the illness occurs when there is denied to the individual, as result of external obstacles or internal deficiency in adaptation, the gratification of his erotic needs. (Über Psychoanalyse, page 54). Therein, Freud has also properly estimated the present (= actual) conflict, at the same time, however, avoiding a one-sidedness of which Jung is guilty. It will not do to explain all neuroses on a basis of convenience, and only arbitrarily can one make deficiency in capacity for adaptation answerable for them. We have already mentioned under appeal to Freud a number of maladies which arose from the circumstance that a person gave up his primitive or immoral conduct and went over to higher morality (94). Further, we know highly energetic people who suddenly give up in an effort and break down; the task would be easy if inhibitions had not been already present. If it is a matter of a shocking event, however, a deprivation or abstinence, the perception of grievous guilt or similar experiences, one cannot charge the illness entirely to the account of convenience, where simply the strength for normal reception and reaction to the impression is lacking. When a bullet perforates a person, shall we say: The body possessed too little capacity for adaptation to the bullet? The formulations of Freud, which anticipate the correct part of Jung's thoughts, deserve therefore the preference. Only, one must also include among the erotic needs, the denial of which makes the individual ill, the moral demands, which Freud does.

Finally, it may be pointed out here, that healthy and sick are exposed to exactly the same motives for repression. "We discover in the insane, not something new and unknown, but the substratum of our own being, the mother of the problems of life, on which we are all engaged." *

3. The Relation of the External and Internal Factors in Repression

The repression never proceeds from purely external or internal conditions but always from a disagreement of inner strivings, whether these have been excited by external or internal causes. In this disagreement, the internal forces must be recognized as the incomparably stronger ones. In mental equilibrium, in suitable utilization of the instincts and erotic demands, it should be noticed again that no external calamity, no stress of life conditions, can bring about a serious repression. Conversely, comparatively minor misfortune may result in the greatest disturbances when the mind is torn by grievous conflict. Thus, the external calamity is a provocative agent, the

---

* Same, p. 26.

light pressure on the electric button which shatters a mighty mass of rock.

A fourteen year old pupil jumps from the second story because he had a conflict with the teacher and received a bad report. The public gave itself up to spiteful condemnation of the teacher who "drove the poor victim to death." In reality, the youth has suffered unspeakably for years from severe repressions caused by the brutality of his father; the teacher merely did his duty.*

A teacher became ill with a severe anxiety neurosis because he could find no suitable dwelling and was disturbed by the noise in front of his house. He made written plans for departing from life. His wife discovered the writing and became so excited that she had to be confined in an insane asylum. Consideration for the children determined the father to save himself. He begged me to intercede spiritually for him. As an enthusiastic follower of Dubois, at the time, I sought by consoling and explaining to awaken new courage for life, and after some weeks, experienced a satisfactory result which strengthened my faith in the excellence of the method. Puzzled by later bad results, I investigated whether other influences had coincided with my ministrations, and sure enough, found that at that time an experienced physician had advised giving up coitus interruptus in favor of coitus condomatus and thereby established satisfactory sexual intercourse. I am convinced that the decisive factors in the cure belonged both to the physician and the pastor. After the treatment, the teacher found his dwelling very nice and declined to remove to a home offered him which he had long desired.

I defend the primacy of the inner life, not only because in ungoverned instinctive relations, an adaptation to the world is difficult of attainment, but also because the unsaved person unconsciously so fashions reality as to correspond to his mental complications and thereby often unfortunately brings about

---

* Compare the interesting 1st Diskussion der Wiener psychoan. Vereinigung über den Selbtsmord. Bergmann, Wiesbaden, 1910.

the necessity which renders the situations more severe. By disclosing this state of affairs, psychoanalysis has given us the key to the comprehension of countless acts otherwise incomprehensible.

From this standpoint, the psychology of unlucky persons becomes clearer to us. It can lead us to all kinds of unconscious motives and wishes which misfortune serves. When a boy is stricken with severe headache, always just at the time when he has to eat some distasteful food or work on a hated essay subject, that is certainly not intentional but still willed, even though willed unconsciously.* Thus, misfortune and secret tendencies often coincide.

A nervous boy of fifteen years had some misfortune every few days. Now he would fall from the planks, the wide opening between which, he wished to jump over, and be found lying with a broken leg, now he would receive a severe bodily injury while sliding down hill. He always kept his family in excitement. The analysis revealed loss of interest in life: the boy constantly carried a loaded revolver on his person and wanted to kill himself but was prevented by religious scruples. His misfortunes are disguised attempts at suicide and demands for affection.

Another youth of sixteen years, who for years seems to have striven for the record as an unlucky fellow, now falling from a wagon upon his head, now being struck by a mattock, etc., suffers from a painful hysterical point of pressure on the skull wall. The analysis revealed the phantasy, held for years, that he would crush his skull in at that point by a blow from a hammer. Since the analysis of these symptoms, neither boy has suffered from similar trouble.

Even with individuals who are in full health, the external misfortune often corresponds to an unconscious purpose. Much oftener than one would surmise, the person is situated as he has unconsciously prayed to be.

An otherwise exemplary young man disagrees with all his superiors and other important personalities, thereby endanger-

* Compare the examples on page 98.

ing his career which he had begun brilliantly. The analysis of his waking phantasies solved the riddle: Frequently, he runs up and down his room with clenched fists, contends with threatening voice against an imaginary enemy, as a rule, his superiors. From his dreams, however, it is seen with certainty that it is really his father who is meant, since the latter and the superior frequently appear as a composite figure. Thus, the pugnacious man wishes to vent on other objects the pleasure of his successful strife against his father, he wishes to realize now the hot, reckless, childish wishes, by which useless conduct he spoils his finest chances. The analysis saved him also.

The unconscious possesses a really refined virtuosity for molding people according to its tendencies. The husband, who has remained attached to his mother and lived in strife with her, knows how to bring a differently tempered wife unknowingly to the point where she will treat him as his mother did. So long as this fixation, which will be discussed later, remains in force, all good intentions are in vain.

4. THE RELATION BETWEEN REPRESSING AND REPRESSED FACTORS

Where two interests hostile to each other exist, a reciprocal action takes place, in which every active force will act as a repressing one. Often, one will be victorious for a long time, then the other. The oscillation can last for a whole lifetime.

A girl of twenty-two years now loved her fiancé passionately, now to her sorrow, found her affection gone. Especially striking to her was the circumstance that she loved him in his absence; as soon as she sees him alight from the car, she becomes cold, to become aglow again as soon as he has taken his train. From her dreams, it is evident that she thinks to find her father again in her lover and unconsciously confuses the two men. The father was the object of her longing so long as he stayed at a distance but repelled her by his cold behavior when he had returned. She hated and loved him simultaneously. Now love, now hate gained the upper hand, but the latter did not present itself openly in consciousness. The internal dissension was reflected in obsessional anxiety ideas. One day, she was stricken with anxiety which lasted two weeks until the analysis, that she would have a hemorrhage. Shortly before, she had visited a "beautiful," intelligent, lovable friend who was ill of pulmonary disease, who, because of the advanced stage of her disease, had broken her engagement. My patient suffered from the circumstance that her mother, when she was a child of six or seven years, had spoken of her in the presence of some ladies, as being of small intelligence, while she is justly proud of her mental endowment. She would like to be pretty and is so in fact, but she does not believe it because at home she was always depreciated. In all directions, she wishes to identify herself with the friend whom she recognizes as beautiful, particularly in the erotic situation as well. The obsession disappeared soon after her enlightenment. The anxiety over a hemorrhage showed that strong erotic longing was pent up. The changing of emotions ceased after the overcoming of other, easily elucidated (compensatory) obsessions (obsessional ideas), phobias (anxiety conditions) * and hallucinations, when the girl had become clearly conscious of her attitude toward her father and his substitute, the fiancé. The young bride-to-be perceived how much she had to gain, how much to lose, and ended the see-saw of repression forces by real and lasting love suitable to the hardship and happiness of married life.

Often, one sees how the repressed material takes possession of consciousness until the relation changes again. In this, repressing and repressed exchange rôles each time.

Both go back ultimately to elementary instincts. Still, in general, this connection with the demands of nature is more direct in the repressed, and further, it may be more easily demonstrated here.

* The psychoanalyst distinguishes between fear and anxiety. With the former, the reason and object are known, and there is a normal relation between occasion and reaction, with anxiety, on the other hand, either no reason at all or an insufficient one is given.

CHAPTER VI

THE INFANTILE ROOTS OF THE REPRESSION IN DETAIL

1. Historical

"The unconscious is the infantile and that particular part of a person which has been separated from the personality at that time and hence has been repressed."* In this formula, Freud once expressed his provisional judgment concerning the origin and nature of the subconscious which is important for us in this connection. Never has a psychologist ascribed to the first years of childhood, not merely to the hereditary endowment, so great an importance for the whole future conduct in life, as the father of psychoanalysis. Not only the dreams and ordinary performances of every-day life but also the highest achievements of art and poetry—we might add in his sense: also of morality and religion are dependent in high degree upon the impressions of childhood and outlined in these. Everywhere, he seeks to show infantile sources; even the thousandfold needs of the neuroses and psychoses, as well as the formation of character, take their origin in earliest child life and here receive their guiding impulses. As the tree has to suffer for a lifetime, for injuries done to it when just pushing its shoot above the ground, so also the human mind. And more: All neurotic troubles, so far as they proceed from mental causes, have an infantile previous history, without which they could not have come into existence.

From the medical side, a great objection was raised to this estimation of childhood and childhood impressions. They overwhelmed their Viennese colleague with angry accusation,

* Freud, Bemerkungen über einen Fall von Zwangsneurose. Jahrb. I, 373.

caricaturing irony, malicious jest, and did so much in that kind
of polemics that they thought argument and actual observations could be dispensed with as entirely superfluous. Other
physicians took a calm and expectant attitude toward Freud's
announcements.

To the pedagogue, Freud's accentuation of the first years of
life may seem less startling. At least, he will lend an attentive
ear with the greatest earnestness to the investigator, who, on
a basis of substantial works in his own field, discovers valuable
springs which take their origin in the domain of education. If
psychoanalysis is correct, then there beckon to the pedagogue,
perspectives such as scarcely one of its official representatives
would dare to dream of. The art of education appears as
savior in the constantly swelling flood of nervous maladies, it
gains a large influence in politics, morals and religion, it even
plays an important rôle in the genesis of artistic genius.
Guarding and directing, as giver of the law and of the saving
gospel, pedagogic activity rules over humanity, invested with
a power little dreamed of, if the psychoanalysis of Freud is
correct.

These promises, to the pronunciation of which, Freud, in
his modest, matter-of-fact manner, would never allow himself
to be transported, sound so exuberant that we critical pedagogues need to be admonished to prudent foresight. But if
the beautiful things which are inferred as consequences of the
analytic investigation were facts, what educator who is still
ready to learn something, would deny a priori the great new
resultant possibilities? Of course, he who dislikes something
new and great because it explains a bit of the things previously
done as incomplete and erroneous, will also be compelled to
declare war on Freud as an abominable disturber of the peace.

(A) THE IMPORTANCE OF INFANTILE IMPRESSIONS IN GENERAL

It is worthy of note that the psychoanalytic investigation
came upon the importance of the events of childhood entirely
by following its own paths. Every dream, which one had

occasion to analyze to its profoundest depths, every neurotic symptom which was followed back to its hidden source, disclosed a bit of the childlife of the first four years.* Freud came to the conjecture "that the impressions of earliest childhood (the prehistoric period, about to the end of the fourth year) in and for themselves, perhaps without depending upon their content, longed for reproduction, and that the repetition is a wishfulfillment." †

Only afterwards was attention called in analytical circles to the fact that sharp-sighted students of human nature had already given expression to these facts, of course, more with the help of an instinctive clairvoyance than on a basis of scientific investigation. I will give the words of one of the greatest students of the mind among the poets, Friedrich Hebbel: "When one sees himself compelled to speak concerning things which will be quite unintelligible to any one without inner experience, one cannot guard enough against misinterpretations. . . . Even men of insight themselves do not cease to quarrel with the poet over the choice of his material and thereby show that they always consider the work, the first stage of which, the conception, lies deep under consciousness and sometimes goes back to the dimmest distances of childhood, as a mere product of work, even though of noble kind, and that they attribute in the mental birth an arbitrariness which they would certainly not assign to the physical birth, attachment of which to nature is of course plainly visible. One may scold the small artisan when he brings something which does not please the lord and master; the poet, on the other hand, one must excuse, when all goes not well, he had no choice, not once does he have the choice whether he will produce a work or not, for once this has become alive, it may not be redigested, it may not be again changed into blood, but must appear in free independence and a suppressed or blocked mental delivery can cause destruction just as well as an abnormal physical delivery, whether in death

* Zur Ætiologie der Hysterie. Kl. Schriften I, p. 171.
† Traumdeutung, 3rd ed. p. 177.

or in insanity. One recalls Goethe's youthful companion, Lenz, also Hölderlin and Grabbe.'' *
I could not refrain from repeating in detail these words of farseeing wisdom which anticipate some of the chief thoughts of psychoanalysis. That in Hebbel's own creations, the traces of childhood may be discerned, has been shown already by Kuh † in his excellent biography.

That other mortals, too, remain under the sway of the influences of childhood for their whole lifetimes, the psychoanalysts have not discovered first. Hammer rightly says:

> "Touch not the dream of the children
> When a pleasure caresses them:
> Their grief hurts them not less
> Than thine hurts thee!
> Many an old man
> Whose heart no longer glows,
> Bears in his face a wrinkle
> Which out of his childhood came." ‡

Especially in the hours of stress, does the childhood reawaken, the mind harks back to its first Garden of Eden and calls longingly for the consoling figures of that age, inspires them with new life, becomes again just a child to be coddled and led about, in order to reappear with new energy in the stern reality. K. F. Meyer expresses this in his song "Heperos":

> "Over the dark and fur-clad hills
> Shone on me in my evening walk
> A love I feel go down
> In thy setting,—
> Unnoticed hast thou come
> From the pale air begun to glow.
> Thus with unheard steps

* Hebbel, Vorwort zur "Maria Magdalena" (1844). Sämtl. Werke, herausg. v. Bartels, Stuttgart und Leipzig, p. 822. O. Rank, Das Inzest-Motiv, p. 125.

† E. Kuh. Biographie Friedrich Hebbels, Vienna and Leipzig, 1907, Vol. II, p. 74 ff. (Maria Magdalena).

‡ Cited by Stekel, Zbl. III, p. 52,

Through the dusk agliding
Came the mother, who laid
On my shoulder, her firm hand
So that I could not conceal from her
What I suffer, what torments me.
And why without complaint
I am gnawed and consumed.
And I am silent, and in tears
Let her comfort me.
Has she a dwelling, now, the gracious one,
There in thy fields of light?
Of thy rays, I drink up each
Through the darkness I hear speaking,
—And it seems to me as if
I feel the cool hand on my shoulder,—
Speak, not of sweet beatitudes,
Only of the memories of old times!
Now she understands without more telling
Who I am in heart's reality.
This and that must she scold
Other things leaves she contented
And she means, so I conclude,
Be satisfied yourself.
Evening star, hasten quickly
Let her visit with her child!
Twinkling friendly, you go down . . .
Mother, Mother, come again!"

Even if we were not acquainted with Sadger's valuable, tactful and scientific monograph,* we would detect in these verses, the grief of the unhappy poet, whom the fixation upon the mother long held under the yoke of unproductive dreamer, whom the recognition withheld by the mother once thrust into mental darkness. Similar examples from the mouths of poets might be multiplied indefinitely. Why, precisely in inhibitions, the flight into the infantile becomes so striking, we shall see later.

In order to define the share of the infantile more exactly, we turn now to the psychoanalytic investigation. After Freud

---

* Sadger, Konrad Ferdinand Meyer, eine pathographisch-biographische Studie. Wiesbaden 1908. Adolf Frey mentions infantile impressions in the works of the poet, C. F. Meyer. Stuttgart, 1900, p. 36.

had shown the processes of the childlife to be the earliest determinants of disease, he found early infantile remnants in the dreams. He succeeded, indeed, in discovering in dreams, entirely forgotten impressions from the earliest years of life and in determining the correctness of these by external substantiation.* He found, to his astonishment, "in the dream, the child with its impulses coming to life." † For him, the dream is "the substitute for the infantile scenes changed by transference to recent material." ‡ What he says concerning the significance of sexuality as the nourishing soil of the higher mental activity (besides the ego instincts) must also be considered here, for he traces back the achievements named, to the early infantile sexuality. He finds the poetic endeavor outlined in childish play and phantasy play.‖ It reflects the deepest wish of the poet. "A phantasy floats as it were, among three periods of time, the three temporal possibilities of our imagination. The mental work joins an actual impression, an occasion in the present which was in a position to awaken one of the greatest wishes of the person, from there, it falls back upon the memory of an earlier, usually infantile experience, in which, that wish was fulfilled and creates now a situation related to the future, which situation is represented as the fulfillment of that wish, thus the daydream or phantasy." ¶ In the same manner, the poem comes into existence,§ poem and daydream are continuation and substitute for the onetime juvenile play. Myths are distorted wish-phantasies of whole nations, the secular dreams of young humanity.**

In the life of Leonardo da Vinci, Freud sought to show †† how the whole career and life-work of a great master was carried out under the influence of juvenile sexual affairs. Leon-

* Traumdeutung, 3rd ed. p. 137 ff.
† P. 139.
‡ P. 365 f.
‖ Freud, Der Dichter und das Phantasieren. Kl. Schriften II, pp. 197–206.
¶ P. 201.
§ P. 205.
** P. 205.
†† Freud, Eine Kindheitserinnerung des Leonardo da Vinci, 1910.

ardo's poverty in love,* his obsessional compulsion to investigation, which thwarted the artistic endeavors,† the origin and content of certain paintings, his ideal homosexuality,‡ are explained by the aid of individual and folk psychological parallels as products of a phantasy which absorbed the great artist in his cradle days: He wishes to remember that at that time, a vulture came to him, opened his mouth with its tail and struck his lips many times. According to Egyptian and Church mythology, the vulture was the bird which reproduced only in female forms, fructified by the wind. Leonardo, an illegitimate child, was taken from his mother when five years old. These relations are reflected in the phantasy, yes, in the whole life and activity of the artist. One can only properly judge this surmise of Freud's if one has become certain of the interpretations of dreams. What is especially important for us now is this: Where formerly, one spoke of inborn tendencies, and because of the precarious position of the hereditary theory, had to renounce individual explanation, Freud promises to carry the causal necessity a few important steps further and prove partially directable experiences to be the powers of fate. Still, he too, fully recognizes the ultimate power of the constitution.

The keen statements of Freud have been tested and substantiated by numerous analysts. Nevertheless, since I must assume that these witnesses are objected to, it should be remembered in this connection that almost every good description of life and analysis of artistic works, long ago pointed to the infantile remnants. I mention, for example, the biographies of Gottfried Keller and Leo Tolstoi.

That early dispositional attitudes were of great influence for the shaping of the life, has been shown us by psychoanalytic means in the lives of many artists: Sadger encountered much ill-will in 1908 when he traced back the delayed development and mental disease of Ferdinand Meyer to an early fixation upon the mother. His method of consideration was even

* P. 12.
† P. 13.
‡ P. 34.

at that time too new. Stekel too aroused much hostility when he brought Grillparzer's "Der Traum, ein Leben" (The Dream, a life) into connection with infantile family impressions.* It is easy to see that the poet's typical motive of the man standing between two women expresses his own erotic attitude toward his "eternal bride" and his sister. Further, the enormous influence of the mother is not difficult to discern: Just one trait shows enough: The poet, when twenty-eight years old, after the suicide of his mother, broke off the thread of his poetic production, in the midst of the composition of the "Golden Fleece," to take it up again only later when he played the G-Moll-Symphony of Mozart with a mother-substitute (Karoline Pichler) this being the last composition which he had played, four-handed, with his mother before her tragic end.† That early infantilism is exhibited here, is not proven.

New materials were provided by Sadger in his monographs on Kleist ‡ and Lenau.‖ I myself pointed out in the grotesquely colored piety of the Graf von Zinzendorf, plain aftereffects of the first years of childhood.¶ Max Graf furnished successful proof, in the eyes of anyone who does analytic work, of the infantile origin of the favorite theme of Richard Wagner: The woman standing between two men, who tears herself free from the first, the husband or fiancé, and throws herself into the arms of the second.§ In Chapter XII, section 10, we shall come to speak of this and likewise of the very scholarly and sharpsighted investigations of Otto Rank.

(B) THE CONTENT OF THE INFANTILE REPRESSIONS

When we ask concerning the content of the infantile roots buried in the unconscious, we find that they are exactly the

---

* Stekel, Dichtung und Neurose. Bausteine zur Psychologie des Künstlers u. des Kunstwerkes. Wiesbaden, 1909.

† K. Macke is in error when he explains the origin of the poet from the spirit of music. Biogr. Einleitung zu Grillparzers Werken, XI.

‡ J. Sadger, Heinrich von Kleist, Wiesbaden, 1909.

‖ J. Sadger, Aus d. Liebesleben Nicolaus Lenaus. 1909.

¶ O. Pfister, Die Frömmigkeit des Grafen L. v. Zinzendorf, 1910.

§ Max Graf, Richard Wagner im "fliegenden Holländer," Leipzig and Vienna, 1911.

same ones which we encountered as the proximate motives of repressions in adults, only undeveloped, corresponding to the age of childhood. It is our task to determine as well as possible from the analytic materials, the nature of the things which were once conscious and then repressed, before we present our own observations to the reader's consideration. Freud's assertion that sexual experiences and phantasies of the first years of life determine very strongly the later mental tendency, with its normal and abnormal expressions, met violent opposition. Even scholars who had studied the sexual life extensively and without prudery, like August Forel, flatly denied a sexual life in the first years of life. So experienced an analyst as Jung thinks that the libido, the desire, may be invested in the stage of childhood, at first exclusively in the form of the hunger instinct. "The ultimate, and in its functional significance, predominating field of application (of libido) is sexuality, which seems at first to be extraordinarily attached to the nutrition function." * Of incest, the child, on account of his undeveloped sexuality, is not yet capable.† The deepest foundation of the socalled incestuous desire runs not to cohabitation but to the wish for the protection enjoyed in the mother's womb and for rebirth.‡

We will first question the students of minds who are free from pretended infection with the mental epidemic of analysis. It has been shown that sensual childish wishes directed toward the parents, which are of undisputable erotic nature, were known and described by many poets. Stendhal confesses: "I was always in love with my mother. I wished always to kiss my mother and wished there were no clothes. I detested my father when he came to us and interrupted our kisses. I wished to give them to her always on the breast. One should deign to realize that I lost her when I was scarcely seven years old." Baudelaire testifies: "What does the child love so passionately in his mother, his nurse, his twin sister? Is it

---

* Jung, Wandlungen und Symbole der Libido, Jahrbuch IV, p. 180.
† P. 279.
‡ P. 267.

simply the being who nourishes, combs, washes and rocks him?
It is also the tenderness and sensual delight.'' Rosegger remarks: ''I admit indeed that in the love between mother and
son there exists a bit of the sexual—unconscious of course.
A mother loves her son quite differently from her daughter.'' *
Ganghofer reports a slight attack of anxiety which he underwent in his fourth year in an erotic experience: ''A girl of
eighteen years stepped over the little fellow as he lay in bed.'' †

Such confessions do not prove the universality of such emotions. The extensive material on which Freud based his well-
known thesis of the importance of the infantile sexuality, is
not published. The only two detailed analyses of children
which our literature affords, those of Freud and Jung, contain
extremely important material but they do not prove Freud's
thesis that all eroticism is derived from sexual pleasure or is
built on the pleasure of taking nourishment, as Jung has recently assumed. Maeder speaks of two types of women who
may be differentiated even in the third and fourth years of
life: the mother and the coquette.‡ But he does not publish
the analytic material.

One cannot be surprised that well-meaning but superficial
critics cannot make anything out of the important theory of
infantile sexuality.

2. PERSONAL OBSERVATIONS

(A) CLEAR SEXUAL ROOTS

A sixteen year old pupil suffers, among other things, from
anxiety that his nose (otherwise quite normal) excites unpleasant comment. Only by strong self-control, can he go
upon the street and he carefully conceals the anxiety-provoking
member with his hand. The anxiety had appeared very early:
At ten months, it broke out on various occasions, for example,
upon the sound of rattling wagons, then in the second year,

---

* From Rank, Inzest-Motiv, 32 f.
† Zbl. I, p. 165 f.
‡ Über zwei Frauentypen. Zbl. I, pp. 573–582.

it concentrated itself upon pigeons and children who could not yet walk and were just learning, as well as on snails. For years, a little dwarf persecuted the youngster in dreams. I had him first describe more exactly the anxiety over pigeons and heard with astonishment: "I was not afraid of being bitten by the doves but was anxious lest I be touched by the thin skin on the feet." The children excited anxiety because their little legs represented sexual symbolism. It required no special sharp-sightedness to assert with much certainty the cause of the phobia. The little dwarf who constantly persecuted him, was what is called in popular speech, "the little man," which is rendered still plainer by the cowl of the dwarf. The half stiff legs of little children, as well as the snails, must refer to the same object. The skin on the legs obviously refers to the prepuce; the anxiety over touching it, corresponds, like every anxiety, to a repressed wish. That the child, a little over a year old, had noticed the foreskin, must be explained on the ground of special irritation, and likewise the anxiety at ten months of age. I therefore explained to the astonished father that his son was suffering from the after-affects of a phimosis-operation undergone before the tenth month and probably also from later threats of castration. My conjecture was entirely confirmed. At seven years, and probably earlier, the boy's mother had threatened him with amputation of the penis because he was masturbating. More recent occasion for the anxiety regarding the nose came from the harmless remark of a comrade that he, our patient, had a potato nose. Urged to think clearly of the nose and give all his associations, he said: "The nose is thick, round, sticking out in front." That the feeling of shame applied to an organ with similar characteristics, which had played an ominous rôle in his earliest childhood, he saw at once.

A little lad of nine years become ill with twitchings of the arms. I refrained from analysis and sent him to an elderly neurologist with the report that the lad had spread the report among his fellow students that his mother practiced fellatio with him, while the woman accused, asserted that she had taken

into her mouth only the nipples of her child. I reported
further that the boy wished constantly and impatiently to go
to his mother in bed and exhibited erections in the bath. The
physician answered that we were dealing with "epileptoid attacks" which certainly have nothing to do with sexuality. To
my second inquiry if it might not be hysteria, I received an
angry tirade against Freud's psychoanalysis, while his own
psychoanalysis, which he had practiced for twenty years, was
extolled, and also the concession that only after a week's
observation could it be determined whether hysteria or epilepsy
were present. Naturally, I did not allow myself to be easily
diverted in this particular case from my pedagogic and pastoral rights because a little conflict with a physician sprang
from my analytic activity; I impressed on the mother, firmly
though with considerate restraint, the inordinate desire of her
little son. The boy recovered at once from his attacks while the
jealous neurologist, with his painful prudery and materialistic
method of consideration, in spite of electrical apparatus and
dietetic treatment, would probably have helped neither the
mental nor physical health of the child. The last report I
received concerning the boy was five years after the conversation; he had remained well during that time.

A merchant aged thirty-three, married for one year, suffered
from psychic impotence, which could not be cured by the physician consulted. The family life threatened to be disrupted
since the wife had an unbounded longing for children and
told her husband that she could no longer love him since she
felt herself deceived by him. It turned out that his sexuality
was entirely infantile: he loved to cling to his wife but otherwise behaved purely passively. Often, he wished to carry his
wife on his back. If, after great exertion, a premature ejaculation occurred, he felt pain in his penis. Although he had
never masturbated peripherally, he accused himself of onanism. Justly, for the phantasies to which he had given himself
were extraordinarily loaded with emotion.

The causes were at once revealed by simple questioning:
When three years old, my patient was taken into bed by the

maid and pressed ardently against her. When seven years old, he carried a little girl on his back. The maid called him a nasty fellow and threatened to tell his mother, whereupon, the youngster got the impression that he had done something terribly improper, which belief he powerfully repressed into his unconscious. The wish, to carry his wife on his back, is accordingly clear to us; naturally, in the presence of his wife, he did not recall the childhood experience. A sanctimonious young man, pupil of an extreme theological institute, practiced fellatio with him, during which the pain in his penis at the time of ejaculation first made its appearance. More important than all this was the fact that he once surprised his mother undressed. From his dreams, strong homosexual tendency was evident. In the waking state the patient showed only a strong desire to see bathing boys or the sturdy calves of young peasants. After this unsuitable utilization of instinct had been recognized and inhibited, normal potency appeared, his wife's love returned and soon a strapping child crowned the newly concluded union.

The example seems to me especially instructive for our investigation in one point. One can ask whether the cuddling of the three year old child was already of a sexual nature or whether pleasant experiences of an earlier period, memories of the taking of nourishment besides the body warmth now felt, created the pleasure, which then came to repression. But that the boy perceived clear sexual innervations when he carried the little girl, I consider excluded. Almost all boys have experienced similar things. But the prudish and brutal maid exaggerated the bagatelle into a grievous sexual trauma, she forced the harmless experience into the center of the sexual life, just as unskilled educators, by false threats concerning masturbation, help to overaccentuate it and strengthen its injuriousness.

I could easily give from my records a very long series of further examples to prove a sexual root for neurotic processes. When one sees a well educated, upright girl, of socalled good family, one at first considers it unthinkable that evil things could have taken place even under the protection of the parental roof and the parents are usually the last persons to believe it. But the stubborn facts cannot be eliminated from the world by well meaning wishes.

(b) EROTIC SOURCES

A lad of eighteen years suffers from melancholia, pains in his arm which often make writing impossible, further, from violent cramps in the thigh and especially from erotic obsessions. He falls in violent love with a number of girls, only to very soon lose his love instantly if he receives favor. To extremes, he does not allow it to come. Still he is forthwith irresistibly driven to another beauty, no matter how great reproaches he makes against himself because of his perfidious conduct. The arm trouble broke out when he had to confess to his father a crime against property and a foul love story tormented him. The pains in the leg formed a defensive measure against new love affairs. The beginning Don Juanism refers to the mother: she suffered from his third year until her death, for a period of seven years, from pulmonary tuberculosis and had to reside in various sanatoriums and many health resorts. Often, she returned to her family; then the child's nurse would be dismissed. As soon as the mother went away again, another was hired. The child, therefore, transferred his love to many female subjects, but at the same time, constantly sought his mother. The youth now repeats the same thing. He seeks his mother with fervent longing, often thinks he has found her, and then, disillusioned, sees his error.

The lad was free from masturbation and possessed good principles. The sexual root which lurked behind his eroticism soon came to light, however. One day, as he was ascending * the stairs, terrible asthma with palpitation of the heart seized him, together with a crick in the back. Commanded to fix his attention on this occurrence, he reported that his father had shortly before written to him of his intended visit. Further, it occurred to him that a year before, he had received a letter

* See above, page 94.

with same content but had averted the visit by telegraph, which, this time, did not go easily. The pain in the back reminded him that in the afternoon, a rendezvous in the forest had taken place. During the caressings, the youth bent over his girl, whereupon a tree-trunk hurt him painfully in that part of his back. Therefore the hysterical symptom transports him by way of wish into the situation, so pleasant at that time, to which he has now fled upon his father's announcement. Naturally, he could not guess this meaning of his crick in the back. Only when I had him fix his attention sharply on the symptom, did the reminiscence come. The asthma took us back to the first years of childhood. As a small child, our patient frequently had hallucinations ("sexual apparitions"),* upon the appearance of which, he fled anxiously to the bed of his elder brother. He saw two panting figures: One, a man armed with a knife or revolver and the other, a woman ordinarily carrying a broom. The boy had (like the one mentioned on page 68) observed his parents in the conjugal bed and thereby suffered one of the most frequent causes of the neurosis. Without analysis, it would have been impossible to discover these facts.

All symptoms, with the exception of the cramp in the thigh, disappeared quickly, unfortunately too quickly. The remaining pain also subsided to a minimum and therewith also the interest in the analysis. The attitude toward his father and along with this, his attitude toward humanity in general, was still not normal. After an insignificant conflict with the well meaning and estimable man, he joined his brother who had wandered to a distant part of the world. Perhaps this step redounded to his advantage, still he can scarcely avoid a hard school. The hysterical pains disappeared immediately after his departure.

The erotic conflict seems also to predominate in the following case which I will sketch because of its valuable pedagogic material, in spite of its fragmentary character: A woman of twenty-seven years has been for three years entirely incapable

---

* Compare Häberlin, see foot-note on page 13.

of working and has wandered from one sanitarium to another. Besides many hysterical symptoms (blinking of the eyes, stomach disorders, etc.), she suffers from an enormous feeling of insufficiency, constant mild twilight states, often extending over months, and from the feeling of not being really alive but being only an onlooker at life.

When five years of age, she lost her mother, when seven years old, her father. Immediately after the death of her mother, she was taken by her mother's sister. The intelligent patient described excellently the factors which chiefly determined her attitude toward life: "As a little human being, I brought with me into the world strong instincts in every regard, which were, however, immediately and forcibly suppressed, by a strict, nervously ill mother.* I still well recall from this period a rebellion against this coercive compulsion, at the same time, however, also an overstrong love, or better, sympathy, for my mother. This compulsion was continued from my fifth year on, after the death of my mother, by my foster-mother, also a nervous, religious, entirely masochistic character, striving toward the noblest things but violently suppressing in herself and others all life instincts. In spite of the fact that I hated this compulsion with my whole soul, my whole power to love is still inseparably bound up in her. Now, however, all my instincts, my childish egoism, are suppressed and repressed. I have from earliest childhood led a sham life, my longing for love never found gratification and met with only severity and hardship. Thus, 'I cannot,' became the fundamental tone of my life. I was always tired and miserable, loved sickness because of the loving duties connected with it. Envy and jealousy tormented me, all the repressed instincts developed into hatefulness.

"Then, after many years, came the breakdown. And now, when I clearly recognize the facts, I perceive that a gigantic power for love and life lives in me, but, and that is the shame, I cannot now utilize it for my fellowmen. My egoism

* Combating sexual acts is not meant here.

which has been repressed and denied all my life long, breaks forth in all its power. I have had nothing from life, absolutely have not lived, naturally only a part of my ego speaks thus and now should I work for my fellowmen who have had things far better than I, whom I envy, of whom I am jealous? I, the one who am so very tired and miserable, for them, who are so much stronger and fresher than I?

"I become almost insane in this state of indecision: my one ego loves people with an almost consuming power, which would devote its entire self,—my other ego wishes all for self. And now I ought to fight; but one fights only for some sort of an idea and this I have not—any longer. Once, I believed in a guiding, loving, helping omnipotence by whose favor it was easy to fight. Now, all that is destroyed in me.

"My first childish recollection is of the episode, when as a child of three or four years, I thought I offended my own mother. Wherever I should be in the world, I would have the feeling in everything which I might do, it had no value since I must make good this great injury against her. And yet I can, when I am with my foster-mother, I really do nothing at all for her but am so inhibited in my efforts as never before. As a child when I did something good and clever, I very often had the thought: 'If my mother could see this, then she would no longer find you bad!' And at the same time, the hypervalent thought to consider the bad, perverse and improper as belonging to me. Thus I had, and often have, resistance against the good, some such a feeling as: 'That is indeed not your place, what are you doing there?' That is simply ridiculous!"

After the first breakdown, she visited a sanitarium for four or five months. Immediately thereafter, she had a happy state which lasted a half year. The writings of Trine and Johannes Müller awakened in her a phantastic piety which is reflected in the following views: "I am God, a part of the great whole, thus certainly of some value. Therewith, the heavy load which had thus far forced me to be worse and of less value than others for my whole life, was lifted. This true nature is good, for it is of God. You must live every moment conformable to your true divine nature, then all the miserable, petty, unhealthy part of you, which really has no reality, will disappear."

During this time, she was, nevertheless, outwardly very ill and enjoyed, besides the care of the foster-mother, the admiration of a neurotic youth. Because of the latter, she got into strife with her mother and now came the catastrophe. One day, her friend stroked her hand affectionately, she became excited and resumed the masturbation which she had practiced when five or six years old and then repressed under the influence of her sister until a half year ago. Immediately, her faith in the beneficence and purity of nature disappeared. "Why is my view of the world, in which, I sought, from a child up, the beautiful and good, only embittered? Because I discovered sensuousness in the world? Perhaps! I cannot place it in the whole, I shudder before so much filth. Never has anyone (until the last year) spoken to me of it. In the home of my foster-parents, that is something never mentioned. Nothing but religion—a religion which makes me tired and sad."

"The man who loves me, loses my esteem entirely. Although my subconsciousness seeks to force this love (I received three marriage proposals in this manner), this love kills my own! It seems to me as if that must be otherwise if I could obey." This much from written communications before the beginning of the treatment.

The analysis was rendered difficult by the fact that the girl could undertake the tiresome journey to me only every two weeks and had to fill an unpleasant position secluded from external interests. Everyone would get the impression at first that we were dealing with an erotic conflict. The over-strict mother and foster-mother killed in the child the joy of living and the courage for her own enjoyment and endeavor, the belief in loving and being loved. The analytic conversation strengthened this surmise but also plainly revealed a sexual undercurrent. I can show this best in the origin of the twilight state: The first attack occurred immediately after the departure from the sanitarium. The girl related: "One day, I was pondering on the text, 'There is no fear in love but perfect love driveth out fear' (1st John 4:18). I said to myself: "Let everything go, yield yourself only to the father!" Half unconsciously, I did the evil deed. I was not ashamed, I went right to sleep. I found myself in the twilight state." For a half year, there was no repetition of this condition. Then the fanatical friend stroked and kissed her hand. The patient became excited and relapsed, on the average every fourteen days. "I was afraid of this end and of that which according to my fixed idea, would set in. But now the twilight states came often." At the same time, the phantastic piety broke down, the motivation for which was clearly disclosed.

At the begining of the analysis, the twilight states belonged to the worst symptoms, they appeared daily for hours at a time. During this condition, she had the feeling of being bad. Especially, when she came into a strange neighborhood or when something was changed in the house, the twilight state immediately appeared. She thought: "Yield yourself entirely to the twilight state and submit to everything." Often she had the distinct impression: "During this mental state, it is again like the time when I did the forbidden thing; at that time, I was as if in another world. When I performed the evil act, the world and nature seemed different to me. I often said to myself, I would like to be in another world and know nothing of instincts." I impressed upon her to hold these words fast.

Fourteen days later, in the next consultation, the symptom had almost disappeared. The patient saw that it merely realized the wish for this masturbation by yielding herself to the instincts without knowing of them. Still, the occasion for the outbreak of this symptom showed that the erotic need, in the broader sense, lurked behind it. The patient remembered plainly when ten years old to have experienced a deep, inexplicable sadness because some benches stood differently than ordinarily. Later, every change in the surroundings brought sadness. The benches signify that the corpse of the mother lay on the bier, the sadness with the feeling of strangeness, refers to the pain over removal to the new mother and the homesickness felt at that time, which expressed itself among other things also in ordinary dreams of the earlier home.

Thus, we find also in the twilight state, the erotic need as the driving force, as may be plainly seen from peculiarities in the general attitude toward reality. The sexuality, in addition to the eroticism, afforded the way for the flight from reality: the half sleep which each time excused the masturbation. Also, the whole exquisite masochistic attitude toward life showed a sexual undercurrent. When seven or eight years old, the child phantasied that she was tormented by a witch (= foster-mother) during which, she had to hang on a trapeze and felt sexual pleasure and afterwards anxiety. In the description of the tortures suffered, she ran riot in forms. After the acquaintance with the youth, masochistic ideas again appeared, plainly sexually toned, with subsequent anxiety. Thus, again in this case, I could not demonstrate an asexual eroticism as the cause of illness.

The analysis was not pursued to the end. Her external conditions were unfavorable, the case belonged to the very difficult, probably there was catatonia; her brother suffered from a severe form of this disease and was cared for in an insane asylum. Further, I still knew too little (as at that time, most analysts) of the treatment of the relations between educator and pupil. Nevertheless, considerable improvement was attained. The chief symptoms (twilight states and feelings of inferiority) disappeared almost entirely.

In the following case, sexuality in the narrower sense, was not spoken of at all:

A native of Holland, aged eighteen, complained to me that he suffered from severe pains, twitchings and often from pseudo-paralysis of the right arm and shoulder so that writing and piano playing were rendered well nigh impossible. The trouble was ''nervous.''

Upon being questioned, he said that he suffered from severe emotional ill humor. The problem of suicide occupied his thoughts a great deal, especially since he has read Goethe's "Werther," Ibsen's "Gespenster" and some similar gloomy literary works. Still, he would yield to no suicidal impulses, which turned out later to be an untrue assertion.

A year later, the youth succeeded in mastering his resistance to analysis and analyst. The exploration of the symptom proceeded with such ease, because of this circumstance, that the more involved analysis of resistance, which is usually unavoidable in severe cases and always much more penetrating and in which, the analyst leaves to the patient almost entire direction of the conversation, could be omitted.

The patient said that two years before, he read Goethe's "Werther" without knowing the reason for his reading it, as he at once added spontaneously. A short time later, there broke out on one hand, severe pains, which, beginning in the upper arm, shot through the whole arm, and on the other hand, suicidal impulses, which, but for the love of his parents, would probably have led to an act of desperation.

Obviously, that dimly perceived reason for identification with the suffering Werther, was in an unhappy love affair. For about five years, the youth has had Platonic relations with a girl of same age, who attracted him and pleased him immensely but also angered him by moods and pretended exaggerated reserve. He constantly wavered between being joyous and sorrowful. The quarrels, in which the little dame showed her love in the best form, were followed by sweet reconciliations. The Werther mood proceeded from a final separation, which, according to the assertion of the patient, had come from the circumstance that the young lady upon occasion of a walk with her lover, had withdrawn in rude and cowardly manner. Thus the suicidal impulse corresponded to the damming back of erotic emotions.

Longing for death and refusal of suicide formed a compromise in numerous dreams in which the youth, tired of life, escaped from life without guilt to himself, for instance, by falling from the window. The erotic background is plainly discernible to the experienced observer from the typical symbol of falling.

While the patient put the blame for the rupture upon the jilted friend, he was silent concerning the real motive and the burning self-reproach. Only the analysis elicited from him the confession that some comrades had represented to him that the girl possessed too little charm and too few talents and that he should have far higher aspirations, etc. The anxious attitude toward the one formerly so hotly desired justified the brusque jilting so little that he had to accuse himself of ungentlemanliness. Too proud to pick up again the severed threads, he inwardly renounced love for girls in general and surrendered to worldweariness. Hysteria at once intervened as the avenger of the injured amor.

The analysis of the pains in the arms proceeded rapidly. Keeping the symptom in view, the young man recalled that his father had asked him during one of his attacks of pain, "in especially gentle tone" what ailed him. In this, the patient betrayed his father-complex which frequently caused the production of the symptom in order to extort sympathy.

In the second place, the patient remembered while associating to unpleasant innervations in the arm, a scene which he had experienced with his esteemed music teacher. The latter said to him, several years ago, on account of bad arm position in piano playing: "I wouldn't have thought you could be so clumsy," by which, the incipient artist thought himself wounded in his honor.

Finally, the decisive trauma came to view. Seven years before the analysis, the patient had one day driven away several girls who sat on a wall, by throwing stones at them and then sitting on the wall himself. After awhile, he wished to bring still more stones but in so doing, fell so hard that he broke his collar bone. The reduction of the fracture was successfully accomplished only on the third day, accompanied by severe pain.

This confession made intelligible to us, why the break with

his girl friend caused hysterical phenomena in the arm. That familiar identification process, which may be included in the formula, "it is again as at that time," came into action. As the eleven year old boy had considered his pains in the arm a just punishment for his ungentlemanliness against the fair sex—the accident clearly had the meaning of an unintentional, even though subconsciously desired, self-punishment—so the sixteen year old youth saw himself branded as ungentlemanly and brutal before the bar of his conscience. The memory of the earlier ordeal did not come to clear consciousness. But the need for expiation, which gave the faithless more to do than the loss of the once beloved maiden, obtained satisfaction by creating the painful symptom which may therefore be recognized here as a wishfulfillment. To self-accusation, the memory of the piano-teacher also points; this would say: "You, too, were no virtuoso; how then could the lack of talents in your girl friend give you the right to cast her off? You are just as much in the wrong as that time on the wall when judgment overtook you." Consequently, the hysteria represented the expiation-complex, just as the anxiety symptom did the blocking up of the eroticism.

A short time after the beginning of the suicidal impulse and the physical phenomena accompanying the same, which increased as we know, even to paralysis, there came the downfall of his faith in God. Formerly, he had thanked God fervently for his love for his girl friend. Since the gift proved to be delusive, the giver must also fall—a psychological process which may be often observed where the erotic disturbance leads to renunciation of every love which has marriage in view.

Again, after a short space of time, the youth fell out with his father, who for the most part had been little concerned with his love affair. When the son, in his distress, occasionally showed his distaste for life, the father became terribly excited, called suicide pathological and unreasonable, a sign of deficient faith in God and moral fickleness. As the only means of help, he recommended work and prayer.

After about a year had passed, there came into the hands
of the young atheist, who was completely dominated by his
skepticism, some beautiful Madonna pictures. The impression
was so overwhelming that he immediately began to pray to
Mary. His good Reformed conscience, which had been developed by the spiritual influence of his religious teacher who
excelled in critical acumen as well as in sympathy, he soothed
by a false conclusion: since there was for him no longer a
Christ and he believed in no God, then he need make no reproach if he now lifted his heart to the Heavenly Virgin.
Shortly before this sublimation, the sister of his former sweet-
heart had greeted him most graciously, at which time, the
similarity between the sisters struck him and the noble bearing
of the girl inspired him with a secret longing, the desire for an
ideal sister of the lost fiancée.

In this adoration of the Madonna, the father-, mother- and
bride-complexes are all manifested. The longing for the ideal
Virgin takes the place of the earlier inclination toward the
loved one. To love Mary, the beautiful, pure, spotless one, did
not subject him to the danger of later disillusionment and
harsh interference from the side of father and friends. Further, the God-Mother, with her boundless love for her misunderstood, suffering son, provided a substitute for his own
mother who allowed him to miss the tone of loving consolation.
Finally, however, the Queen of Heaven represented divine
supremacy without bearing the fatal name of father or otherwise recalling the austere, uncomprehending father. In the
background, there naturally lurked the pleasure in avenging
himself on the Creator by pious adoration of the Madonna
and on the strict Protestant father, by the Catholic cult.

Thus, Mary represents the beloved one, yet, being without
physical and mental defects, she stood for the mother and
further, being without human shortsightedness, she takes the
place of the earthly and heavenly father and that without
tormenting austerity.

What a rich substitute, the divine Virgin afforded the
shattered hysteric, is shown by the following event. When the

pains became unbearable, the patient felt himself compelled to travel to Einsiedeln. He appears before the famous altar of Mary and will say his prayers, when, in an instant, the pain has gone. No wonder! The sufferer has found his beloved again and in the person of the graciously forgiving one. His self-accusations have therewith become groundless, he is no longer the unchivalrous person who cruelly left his beloved in the lurch.

That, in spite of this, the sublimation miscarried, is shown by the quick reappearance of physical and mental troubles. Painfully, the youth dragged himself through life, his achievements suffering great loss.

More than a half year, he remained under the sway of the Madonna. Then he fell in love with a young girl whom he informed at once, in characteristic fashion, of his suicidal thoughts. The sublimated libido, which the damming of the primary eroticism had raised to heavenly heights, flowed out to the new object, while for Mary, there remained only modest admiration without any especial ardor.

On the other hand, the relation to the father continued strained. The son, longing to be understood, felt ungratified. Hence, a sincere attitude toward God, the Heavenly Father, was also impossible. As usually happens in such cases, the sulking youth constructed all kinds of objections to God's purposes and fortified himself behind the unfathomableness of the idea of God, but was, nevertheless, himself not at all sure of the validity of his objections and suffered from internal desolation. Occasionally, also before the analysis, he prayed to a higher power whom he would under no consideration call God. My task consisted less in refuting the threadbare theoretical arguments than in soothing and conciliatory conversation concerning the relation toward the well-meaning father, whose error was not greater than that of thousands of educators who lack all neurological understanding.

Three weeks before our conversation, the hysteria had flared up again, though in diminished intensity. The analysis brought to light the circumstance that the lovesick youth, on one occasion, heard music poorly rendered, on another, saw poor handwriting. The reader probably surmises already that the new girl friend plays and writes badly, thus presenting the danger of a new estrangement. The discovery of this connection was not necessary to convince the patient of the correctness of our interpretation but it brought a surprising and significant confirmation of telling force.

As there was still some time remaining, I informed myself concerning some other traces of "nervousness." It turned out that the youth became terribly frightened and trembled violently when he was called suddenly. The most important trauma proved to be a peevish call of the father who could not allow the boy to show himself on the street with his first girl friend. To-day, the youth is afraid that his father may interfere to destroy his new affair. Since with him, as with so many neurotics, his superiors and teachers represent a substitute of the father, his fright is easily explained.

The effect of the conversation, which, because of its superficial nature, scarcely deserves the name, analysis, was pronounced. The talented young man was strongly affected by the glance into the causal connection of mental processes which had caused him such frightful suffering. With his father, whom he had caused so much concern, he became reconciled by a free confession. The cultural deficiency of his girl friend, with whom an ideal relation existed, he made light of. After a week, he reported triumphantly to his former pastor, to whom he again brought unbounded confidence, that he had now found peace with God and felt himself again a completely healthy, happy and fearless man. This fortunate condition has continued to the present (three years), an indication that even a somewhat ordinary symptom analysis, which is not to be altogether recommended for imitation, may work efficiently in the absence of much resistance.*

Similarly, sexual motives were lacking in the anamnesis of

---

* From my article: "Zur Psychologie des hyster. Madonnenkultus." Zbl. Psa. I, Part 1, reprinted in Z. f. Religionspsychologie V (1911), pp. 263–271.

the following case: A woman, at the beginning of the menopause, reported that she felt twitchings in her hand and feared that St. Vitus' dance, which she had had when fifteen to seventeen years old and which had been treated at that time with electricity and hydrotherapy, would break out again. The cause of that illness lay in a frightful experience: She had boasted (in self-tormenting provocation) that she could not be scared. A boy, to test her, threw himself from a tree into the snow right in front of her. The infantile root of the trouble was easy to find: the drunken father had pushed his three year old daughter through a glass door, of which episode, a scar under the eye remained as proof. Before the recent outbreak of twitching, a new fright had occurred: The son of our patient had been taken home by the police because of a theft. The mother fell in a faint from fear that the detective's dog would jump in her face. Whether sexual factors also aided, I do not know. A real analysis, I would not undertake because of the critical age of the woman. When I met her three and a half years later, she was well. Probably she would have visited me long before if the symptoms had not disappeared soon.

(c) NON-EROTIC SOURCES

No matter how strong objections I raise against deriving the whole mental life from sexuality and eroticism, I cannot disguise the embarrassment which now seizes me when I must name the roots of repression outside of the love-life. For the child, the attributes derived from the ego-instincts are most intimately intermingled with relations to parents, brothers, sisters and friends. But we emphasize the fact that by no means merely sensual affection binds the child to father and mother. Even the one year old child shows an outspoken instinct for self-assertion. Proudly, he shows how big he is. My experience shows that Alfred Adler generalizes too strongly the significance of organic inferiority for the origin of the feeling of inferiority, the overcoming of which causes the neurosis, and underestimates the effect of erotic obstacles.

But no one denies that many neuroses rest on the vain attempt to create self-esteem or on the effort to avoid a one-time suffering of childhood (compare 143f). There, too, a gratifying love seems to be able to compensate for the deficiency. Further, according to my experience, the feeling of intellectual or moral inferiority presses just as grievously on the spirit and determines just as strongly the outbreak of neurotic suffering. Let us not forget that the distinction between sexual and ego instincts (Freud *) is an abstraction. In reality, there exists in ambition, which, on account of want of appreciation, loss of means, etc., may come into severest repression, a considerable amount of eroticism, perhaps the wish to impress the father or the ladies. Therefore, one can often help such perplexed ones, analytically. But also, in the eroticism, there is often, probably always, a certain amount, even though small, of instinctive desire for self-esteem or self-accomplishment. Sexual traumata often occasion feelings of inferiority.

Adler's denial of the etiological significance of the sexual life in general (Adler & Fortmüller, "Heilen und Bilden," Munich, 1914, page 102), I consider a fundamentally false view. (See my article: "Die Pädagogik der Adlerschen Schule" in *Berner Seminarblätter* VIII, pages 159–173.)

That the ego instincts may be repressed, is admitted; this is a possibility but I have never seen it. But we are already beyond the bounds of our discussion.

* See above, page 72.

CHAPTER VII

THE REPRESSION PROCESS

THE observations given above enable us to understand more exactly the nature of the repression process and its general conditions. So far as possible, therefore, I shall omit new foundations for induction.

1. THE TRAUMATIC REPRESSION

In the beginning of the psychoanalytic investigation, it was thought that there must be assumed, as the cause of every neurosis, a shocking occurrence, a so-called trauma. Breuer and Freud said in their first publication: "Our experiences have shown us that the various symptoms, which pass for spontaneous, one might say idiopathic (primary) manifestations of hysteria, exist in just as strict relation to the causative trauma as those of the above-named (so-called traumatic hysteria)." * The painful memory of the shock remained in the unconscious and produced its effect from there "in the manner of a foreign body." It was only necessary to allow the reminiscence to be "abreacted" by full oral expression with accompanying affects, to put everything in order.† This was the view of the followers of the "Cathartic Method."

Though the widest field was thus granted to the trauma, still, Breuer at least, limited the psychological method of consideration by asserting that a great number of characteristic phenomena went back, not to ideas, but to physical irritations.‡

This method of consideration was historically necessary so long as we were not in a position to penetrate the deeper

* Studien über Hysterie (preliminary report), p. 2.
† P. 255.
‡ P. 166.

mental strata. The connection between shock and symptom was right at hand, the hereditary defect of the nervous system was also recognized. Hence, it is not surprising that the demand for causality was satisfied for awhile with the discovery of the trauma.

It is only to be regretted that even to-day, many who speak in detraction of psychoanalysis consider that view, which was certainly a valuable transition stage in its way, as the complete and final position of psychoanalysis.

Our consideration of the infantile roots of the repression has shown us that also behind the traumatic hysteria there exists infantile material. Since that material was somewhat scanty, another example may be given:

Before I knew Freud, I treated an hysterical girl, twenty-one years of age, who had suffered for some years from increasing melancholia, irritability, diminished capacity for work and chronic pains in the stomach. The latter trouble had been treated in vain for five years with powders, pumps and dietetic regulations. Further, the consolations, exhortations and prayers of constant pastoral attention availed nothing except to gain me the confidence of the patient. One day, she confessed voluntarily that five years before, her drunken mother pulled her daughter by the hair to the floor, held her head over an ash receptacle and threatened to kill her with the axe. After this confession had been made, accompanied by much affect, the stomachache disappeared, not to reappear up till now (five years). A half year after this cure, which astonished me greatly at the time, I learned to recognize unconscious motives for the first time, being taught by Freud in the meantime. The girl had often said: "The scene with the mother lies hard on my stomach." Still later, her considerably older sister reported to me that many years before she had been through an entirely similar affair with the alcoholic mother. It is fairly certain that something of that kind had befallen my patient with the stomach trouble in the early years, at all events, something similar.

Anyway, an analogous event always precedes the shock.

Hence the neurotic symptom has several determining factors, at least two. Therefore, it is called over-determined. Freud speaks of the experience ''that no hysterical symptom can proceed entirely from a real experience but that every time, the memory of earlier experiences awakened by associations, collaborates in the causation of the symptom.''* The same phenomenon occurred later in the trauma and other normal performances. We have often had opportunity and shall have it many times again, to show these over-determinations.† If I do not point out all of them, it is usually because the demands of brevity prevent, often also, because the analysis did not penetrate so deep. I can only assert that in general, where one has opportunity for searching exploration, the messenger of the earlier determinants may be detected.

As the trauma has gained a part of its importance from the overdeterminants and must yield to these, so there came a further backward pressure from the observation that the trauma is often brought about by unconscious intention.‡ We introduced some examples when we spoke of the psychology of unlucky persons and related phenomena.||

Finally, one often notes that the event causing the shock-is, in itself, really of insignificant nature, but has gained an immense importance from its previous history. One sees, even in daily life, how an indifferent remark, a trifling event, can call forth a disproportionate discharge of affect. The folk-saying regarding such events is: a ticklish point has been touched. The analysis gives us the motive for the ticklishness: To the present irritation, are added contributions of affect which have been prepared from previous analogous experiences. We shall be able to picture this after we have examined trans-

* Freud, Zur Ætiologie der Hysterie. Kl. Schriften I, p. 155.
† Also more recent impressions may determine, where the infantile prerequisite is given.
‡ K. Abraham, Über die Bedeutung sexueller Jugendtraumen für die Symptomatologie der Dementia præcox. Zbl. f. d. Nervenheilkunde u. Psychiatrie, 1907, No. 238.   C. G. Jung, Neue Bahnen der Psychologie. Raschers Jahrbuch, Vol. III, 1911.
|| See above, p. 110.

position of emotion, symbolic representation and other processes.

In the end, the precipitating circumstance becomes so irrelevant that we can no longer speak of a trauma.

An example in this connection: A youth of twenty years sees, four days before he must devote himself to military service, a funeral procession which disturbs him. Marched to the school for recruits, he is seized with terrible anxiety that he will never leave the place alive. With difficulty he crowds back a suicidal impulse. Only toward the end of his service, does the trouble find an end. A few days after his discharge, I undertook the analysis. [The funeral procession.] "I see only the hearse with the coachman. Now, there occurs to me something of which I had not thought: The coachman formerly lived on the same street as we. When I was six years old, I witnessed an accident to him. The horses ran away and a passenger fell from the wagon. They laid a black cloth over the man and took him to the hospital. I ran weeping to my mother."

[The coachman.] "My father. I carried his photograph in my pocket before my military service and also when received there; the photograph showed him in uniform."

[The coffin.] "Now I think of that of my former local preacher G. This man was my Sunday School teacher. He died at about fifty when I was about six." [Your father now?] "He is also fifty years old."

In the night before his furlough, he dreamed: "I came into our room in X Street (where the coachman lived). My parents and other black clothed persons were present. By the cupboard, stood a coffin. They were discussing serious things. I heard the words: One must go. I showed my train ticket. The glances of all fell on me. My father looked at me earnestly and said: You have such a ticket; with that, you cannot go back. The others wept. I replied that I had asked the conductor several times whether the ticket was right and he had said: "Yes, with that you go farther."

[The room.] "Here, the funeral of an old member of the

household took place. I saw the coffin carried by the cupboard which figured in the dream." (We leave aside the symbolic significance.) [The content of the coffin.] "It was covered." [Whom do you think was in the coffin?] "My grandfather died a year ago. Mother wept as now in the dream." [One must go.] "I can only think of myself." [The pale faces.] "I saw my father thus after an earthquake. In service, I had great joy when a letter or message came from him. Of my obsession, I said nothing to him."

Before the obsession which broke out during his service, another had prevailed for some days: Namely, the doubt whether the free interpretation of the Bible, to which he had been devoted might not in the end be sinful.

In explanation, it is to be added that the father of the patient is a strict, orthodox man of austere piety. His son feared him and in his presence suffered all kinds of constraint of gait, concerning which I will report in another place.

Some days before the outbreak of the anxiety, the youth had to lament the departure of his beloved. The separation pained him deeply for he feared to lose the girl entirely.

The interpretation of the incomplete associations seems to run something as follows: The coachman means the father; that he lost a passenger is repressed. In the coffin, a substitute for the father was phantasied, a man who, from his position as teacher, his age and his piety, now refused by the day-dreamer, could serve very well as representative of the repressed father. Behind this phantasy, lurks, as we shall show later, the wish for the death of the father. This wish cannot surprise us because of the resentment present. (A similar example, I have published previously *: Upon reading the description of a funeral procession, a youth became violently excited. He, too, phantasied the hated father and his substitute in the coffin.) In the photograph carried in the pocket, the father like the coachman wears a uniform; the son will also wear one in a few days. Thus, the primary wish is the unpermitted death-wish

* Ein Fall von psychanalytischer Seelsorge und Seelenheilung. Evang. Freiheit, 1909.

which is repressed. The obsession represents, as so often, a sin. The sacrifice by his own death is illuminated by the common possession of the uniform and the position of the son. The dream shows how the expectation of death is changed. The conductor promising salvation represents the colonel who consoled the excited recruit in friendly manner. The strikingly strong joy over news from the father is comprehensible to us in view of the repressed death wish. The obséssion receded when a young girl had sent him a friendly postcard.

Of a trauma, there can be no mention but only of a recent (just appeared) irritation or actual impression (Freud).*

2. THE PHANTASTIC REPRESSION

Our results, we find expressed by Freud in the "Traumdeutung" in the formula: "Not on the memories themselves, but on phantasies formed on the basis of memories, depend the hysterical symptoms." We can say the same of all other repressions. Often, phantasies which give veiled expression to a strong desire, precede the outbreak of a pathological symptom † in which the latter points by its aspect to the phantasies. It would not be correct to say: it is the phantasy which calls forth the neurotic malady; rather, the phantasy is only a symptom of a blocking of an instinct, which, under certain circumstances, must lead to illness. The phantasies are often produced on a basis of a definite disposition by the accumulation of little events which bring about conviction. In some analyses, we saw slights by the parents which caused painful, hence to be repressed, conviction (83, 112); at other times, sexual incitements occurred (88, 94); hate led to inadmissible death phantasies (83, 145, 296), the unallowed longing worked stealthily, etc. (178).

This insight, that a phantasy lies between reality and the repression, is of great importance for the comprehension of the repression. The deeply planted instinct, according to this

---

* See above, p. 152.

† Freud, Hysterische Phantasien und ihre Beziehung zur Bisexualität. Kl. Schriften II, p. 138 ff.

fundamentally important knowledge, goes back not directly to reality but to reality expressed in the phantasy, which reality is real only in imagination. Thus, when a person suffering from obsessional neurosis, has anxiety concerning a father who is long since dead,* or prays for him (see page 70), this is not the real father, but without the person's knowing the fact, it is the father-image still living in the imagination which has attracted the eroticism to itself. The father-picture (according to Jung's expression accepted by Freud, the father-image, Vater-Imago †) is the object of the repressed desire. Or, when an hysterical individual is attached to his mother, and drives his little ship of life in unbelievably rocky courses in order to find her, he does not usually proceed to her as she is, but to her, as she lives in his unconscious as the guardian of his childhood days, to the mother-image.‡ Hence, the influence of the parents is in no way interrupted by their death. On the contrary, we see a person ruled by a dead person and that indeed for his whole life-time.

Thus, the neurotic struggles with ghosts and even the normal individual stands continually under the sway of unreal forces which guide him now to injury, now to gain. Getting free from Maya, the illusion, is in fact an essential part of the problem of salvation, though not as Buddhism teaches it. The emancipation from the unreal, so far as it inhibits life, forms the requisite for all highest development of the noblest mental powers. Most normal individuals also suffer from inhibitions which rob them of a considerable part of their efficiency.

The content of the phantasy can also be a theory invested with affect. A girl of sixteen years suffered regularly at the menstrual epoch from vomiting. It turned out that when she was small, she had believed that children were born by the

* Freud, Bemerkungen ü. e. Fall v. Zwangsneurose. Jahrb. I, p. 362.
† Jung coined this expression in connection with Spitteler's psychological novel "Imago," as well as the ancient "Imagines et lares." Jahrb. III, p. 164.
‡ When a young man seeks a considerably older woman for a wife, it is not quite the mother of his first years of life who floats dimly through his mind.

mouth. After she had gained insight in this connection, the symptom ceased immediately. Especially do creation- and birth-theories seem to be of great importance for the later development of the individual.* In an elderly woman, I found the cause of her frigidity, etc., to be a shocking experience of childhood: She saw, under the bed of a parturient woman, a string and came to the conclusion that children were pulled out of the mother's body by the aid of this string.

3. The Degree of Repression (the Unconscious and Foreconscious)

The strength of the repression depends on many factors: The intensity and contradictoriness of the factors of repression with their affects, the suddenness of the conflict, its preparation by practice or some kind of experience even as far back as infancy, the effect of related processes, the further directability of the sum of excitation, the more or less clear conception of a painful idea, the resistance against the mastery of reality imposed by conscience and many other conditions may be mentioned.

One expects at the beginning that the repression would run through a whole scale of degrees. In the common course of ideas, we see one content of consciousness appear in the place of another. The narrowness of consciousness presupposes that kind of "repressions," I use the name in this sense reluctantly. Behind, there remains a disposition, the strength of which can be measured by means of various methods. I mention those of the retained members, those of chance, the saving method, the method of aids and whatever they may all be called.† Further, the memories which were lost without saving discomfort cannot all be reproduced, even where they undoubtedly have a powerful effect. Freud points out that just our most important memories, those which influence character so inten-

* Freud, Über infantile Sexualtheorien. Kl. Schriften II, pp. 159–174.
† M. Offner, Das Gedächtnis, pp. 38–43.

sively, which go back to the educational impressions of earliest youth, almost never become conscious to us.*

The stimulation and operation of the dispositions, the so-called reproduction, takes place in ordinary forgetting quite differently than in that where a repression in the narrow sense, a violent putting away of a painful idea, has occurred. If we will speak of the expressions of the repression, we come to speak of the cases in which a known idea resists reproduction in a striking manner (Chapter XII). Especially strong apperception of the idea sought for often helps over the difficulty.

Not so by strong repressions. Ever so intensive attempts to find the subconscious motive result at first fruitlessly. It avails not at all that the patient racks his brain, the idea sought for is not ready for consciousness, no matter how certainly it may give notice of its presence in pathological phenomena. The psychoanalytic method, too, though it penetrates under the surface smoothly and easily in favorable cases, possesses no magic formula which opens all doors at a touch, nor cleaves all overlying strata. Thus far, I have given particularly simple examples. But even there, I could not always disclose the byways which led to the goal. Months and even years of work would be, and often are, demanded to bring back the banned idea, the elimination of which many times requires the most tremendous efforts of the moral consciousness and all the affirmative forces of personality, and then the task would be performed only in part. Mountains of obstacles must often be removed, before a repressed group of thoughts, a so-called complex, an expression introduced by Jung and Bleuler and approved by Freud, is made accessible to clear consciousness. We shall hear that this exploration must not always be pursued to the deepest roots.

May definite degrees of repression be distinguished from one another? So long as we cannot measure the energies of the instincts, of the individual functions of these, and of the relation of individual instinctive activities, an exact statement

* Traumdeutung 2d ed. p. 333. 3rd ed. p. 361.

of the degree of repression is not to be thought of. Further, we have no psychological characteristic for the marking off of different stages. An apparently harmless symptom may have proceeded from strong repression or from a great sum of lesser repressions, a seemingly doubtful sign often rests on a weighty but still less deeply founded denial.

Freud emphasizes only one distinction: that between the foreconscious and unconscious. Because of their psychological character, we may discuss these at this point, although according to the relations of origin, this discussion would regularly come under the effects of the repression. The foreconscious is, as a non-conscious, also an unconscious. Still, Freud recommends keeping the two expressions sharply differentiated (see page 46). The excitation processes present in the foreconscious may, according to him, "appear in consciousness without further delay, provided certain conditions are fulfilled, for instance, the attainment of a certain intensity, a certain distribution of that function which one has to call attention and the like. It is, at the same time, the system which holds the key to voluntary motor activity. The system behind this, we call the unconscious because it has no entrance to consciousness except through the foreconscious, in which transition, its excitation process must have been subjected to changes." *
In the child, the separation of the two functions does not exist.† In adults, on the other hand, there is a sharp boundary between them, over which boundary, a sharp censorial control is exercised.‡

Concerning the products of the foreconscious, we are taught: It alone can afford the means for the transfer of the unconscious, instinctive impulse to consciousness and to the control of motor function.‖ It inhibits the impulses present in the unconscious.¶ It longs to sleep and when irritations occur which would affect the sleeper, it diverts a part of its attention

---

* Traumdeutung 2d ed. p. 334, 3rd ed. p. 362.
† P. 370.   ‖ P. 377.
‡ P. 377.   ¶ P. 386.

to these.* In neurotic maladies, the unconscious impulses are subjected to the foreconscious and thereby gain their way to the motor function. Every neurotic characteristic shows a conflict between the foreconscious and the unconscious.† "Proceeding from the foreconscious, the unconscious impulses control our speech and action or compel hallucinatory regression, and direct the apparatus not appointed for them by means of the attraction which the perceptions exercise on the distribution of our mental energy. This condition, we call the psychosis." ‡ In the hysterical symptom, a foreconscious motive must always be added to the unconscious motive in order that both wishes may be realized simultaneously in the pathological phenomenon. The foreconscious causes cessations of memories and affects.‖ In wit, a foreconscious thought is subjected to unconscious elaboration.¶

Thus, according to Freud, the unconscious falls into two divisions: That of unconscious, incapable of attaining consciousness in the narrower sense, and that of the foreconscious, which under cumulation of intensity can enter consciousness. "The foreconscious exists like a screen between the system of the unconscious and that of consciousness. It bars not only the entrance (of the unconscious) to consciousness, it controls also the approach to voluntary motor activity and rules the sending out of a mobile distributable energy, from which a share is entrusted to us as attention." §

4. CONCEPT OF THE COMPLEX

Under the term, "emotionally toned complex," Jung originally understood "a group of ideas held together by a definite affect." ** If, however, already at that time, we spoke of a "pregnancy-complex," †† a "money-complex" ‡‡ and

---

* P. 382. ‖ P. 375.
† P. 386. ¶ Der Witz, p. 141.
‡ P. 377 f. § Traumdeutung, p. 410.
** Jung, U. d. Verhalten d. Reaktionszeit im Assoziationsexperiment.
(4. Beitr. d. diagnost. Ass.-Studien), p. 14.
†† P. 18. ‡‡ P. 23.

others, it was assumed that the inclusive bond existed not in the affective field but in the intellectual. This speech usage has persisted. Freud describes the complex in agreement with Bleuler and Jung as a "group of ideational elements, belonging together, invested with affects" * and distinguishes in this conception, conscious and unconscious parts.† Of these parts, the unconscious factor is the more important. If one speaks of the "father-complex" of a person, one means not only that he loves or hates the father, but one thinks of its unconscious connection. It is indeed a surprising fact that in analytic research, at the point where complete indifference toward the father and mother seems to exist, an intense dependence may appear, against which dependence no intention can prevail.

I use the term complex, therefore, for a coherent group of ideas, emotionally toned, which has fallen, wholly or in greater part, to the unconscious.

5. Retention and Repulsion

With many persons who have previously developed normally, the repression is occasioned by extraordinarily severe and painful events. They are hurled back by paths which are discussed under the subject of so-called regression (Chapter X, B. 5), to infantile forms of activity. With others, and indeed with persons who in other affairs, display abundant energy, the denial of the actual performance demanded and the repression appear from insignificant external causes. Among relatives of the age of puberty, one frequently sees this sad change occur when the eroticism, so far occupied with parents and brothers and sisters, should turn to another love-object.

For example, a girl of sixteen years was taken ill with severe headache and was therefore removed from school by the physician. As no improvement occurred, she complained of her condition to me and added that she was tormented during sleepless nights by the fear that she would become insane.

* Freud, Über Psychoanalyse, p. 30.
† Freud, Zur Dynamik der Übertragung. Zbl. II, p. 169.

The confession was introduced by the following remark: "I suffer because there is no love among people." An exaggerated attachment to her brother was disclosed with ease. All other youths are dunces and fops. The dreams betray love-phantasies which were certainly only meant symbolically. Every thought of love and marriage aroused disgust. The brother, on the other hand, desires that his sister address him formally before strangers and is extremely jealous of her. He suffers from suicidal impulses. It was easy to break down the inhibition and to dissipate the headache as well as the obsessions.

Here, too, it would be unjustified to make indolence culpable for the arrested development. Of course, every transition to a new stage of development hides difficulties and demands sacrifice, but the free, healthy person takes care of his inner imperative without the injuries of repression and performs his task in reality. Grillparzer describes the transitional difficulties surpassingly well in his "Jüdin von Toledo":

> Still children grow and wax in years,
> And every critical age in development
> Gives notice of itself by a discomfort,
> Or often an illness which warns us
> We are the same and at the same time, also different,
> And the other is suited to the same.
> So it is with our inmost self,
> It extends and describes
> A wider circle about the same center.

Where an attachment from the past is present, a task easy in itself, becomes an enormous, impossible demand.

In reality there are many transitions between the retention and repulsion types (more detailed discussion of this subject will be found in the article: "Psychoanalyse und Jugendforschung," *Berner Seminarblätter* VIII, J. 1914, p. 194 ff. and in *American Journal of Psychology*, 1914.

CHAPTER VIII

THE GENERAL CONDITIONS

As we now prepare to determine the general conditions under which repression occurs, as well as the laws by which we have arranged the individual processes with an aim toward explaining them, we are met by a difficulty which compels a troublesome concession. In order to obtain by strict induction a theory of the special processes of the repression, we would have to introduce an immense number of observations. I recognize that in the two to three thousand hours of my analytic work thus far, enough results have not accumulated to enable me to give by examples, with sufficient thoroughness and completeness, the elements of the repression forces, the changes and inner connections of these. The temptation is great to take on faith a great master like Freud who has devoted to psychoanalysis his incomparable talents for observation eight to ten hours daily aside from vacations and Sundays for almost two decades. But this appeal to him would only be permissible if he could expose his immense material to testing, which is possible only in the smallest part. Thus, I must put down much as provisional hypothesis which I might assert as certain if my experience were larger; indeed, I fear, because of my restraint, to be looked at askance by more than one older analyst.

Nevertheless, attention must be given to the differences of opinion prevailing in competent circles. While ignorant persons may jest over the present uncertainty, earnest readers will feel themselves called upon by the deficiencies of our knowledge pointed out, to aid in overcoming the great difficulties.

1. THE INSTINCTS SHARING IN THE REPRESSION IN
GENERAL

(A) FREUD'S SYNTHETIC SEXUAL THEORY

We recall that Freud, although he recognizes beside the sexual instinct also the ego instincts, believes that all the higher emotions of sympathy, artistic enjoyment and religion develop from sexual desires (see above page 80). It is, therefore, our task to present his sexual theory and subject it to criticism.

According to Freud, the sexual instinct, which is also designated by the term "libido," * is composed of a number of partial instincts which are active even in the child. "The sexual instinct of the child reveals itself as highly composite; it permits a separation into many components which arise from various sources. The instinct is, above all, still independent of the function of reproduction, in the service of which it will later take its place. It serves for the attainment of various kinds of pleasurable sensations which we include together, according to analogies and connections, as sexual pleasure. The chief source of the infantile sexual pleasure is the suitable excitation of certain particularly irritable body zones which are in addition to the genitals, the mouth, anus, urethral orifice and in particular also the skin and other sensory surfaces. Since in this first phase of the child's sexual life, the gratification is found on his own body and is oblivious of a foreign object, we call this phase, according to a word coined by Havelock Ellis, "autoeroticism." Those places which are important for the gaining of sexual pleasure, we call erogenous zones. The pleasure-sucking of the smallest children is a good example of such an autoerotic gratification from an erogenous zone; the first scientific observer of this phenomenon, a pediatrist named Lindner of Budapest, has already rightly interpreted this as sexual gratification and written exhaustively of its transition into other and higher forms of sexual activity. Another sexual gratification of this period of life is the masturbationary

---

* Freud, Drei Abhandlungen zur Sexualtheorie, p. 1.

excitation of the genitals which has so great importance for the later life and in many individuals is never completely overcome. Besides these and other autoerotic activities, there come to expression very early in the child, those instinctive components of the sexual pleasure, or as we prefer to call it, the libido, which presuppose another person (than self) as object. These instincts appear in contrasting pairs, as active and passive; as the most important representatives of this group, I name the pleasure of inflicting pain (sadism) with its passive opposite (masochism), and the active and passive pleasure in looking (Schaulust) from the former of which (active Schaulust), later, the desire for knowledge branches off, as from the latter (passive Schaulust = pleasure from being looked at) the impulse to artistic and dramatic exhibition. Other sexual activities of the child come already under the viewpoint of the object-choice, in which another person becomes of chief importance; this person owes her importance originally to the consideration for the instinct of self-preservation. The distinction of sex plays in this infantile period no preëminent rôle; thus you can assign to every child without doing him an injustice, a bit of homosexual endowment.*

We will pause here to allow the critics a word.† Freud's sexual theory, since it builds the sexual instinct out of a group of partial instincts, may be designated as composite. A priori, one would wonder how it is possible that from such entirely separated sources, there should result a functional group which serves the one aim of reproduction so excellently. Is this polyphyletic conception not similar to an analogous one which would conceive of the hunger instinct as built up from pleasure of looking, grasping, chewing, swallowing, etc.? The theory of evolution shows us how organs are refined by progressive

* Freud, Über Psychoanalyse, p. 47 f.
† The following thoughts first came to expression in a seminary conducted by Dr. Jung. How much is his mental product, how much I added in dependence on Herbart's combat against the theory of the mental faculties, I cannot to-day state. The principal differences between his views and my own will come to expression later in several places.

differentiation, thereby, however, ever becoming more complicated. Never, however, so far as I know, does biology suppose the complicated structure of an organ to have been formed from a number of separate partial organs. Further, psychology has stripped off the old faculty-psychology which would derive the higher achievements from a number of separate faculties. Further, it recognizes the law of progressive differentiation.

Freud seems to represent the opposite view. This is only appearance, however. He adheres throughout to the phenomena and for good reasons, provisionally refuses the phylogenetic and metaphysical methods of consideration (in contrast to Jung). The partial instincts are not elementary forces for him, but are, according to his explicit explanation, susceptible of a further reduction, which leads on the one side, to a non-sexual "instinct" (compare Bergson's 'elan vital') and reactions to organic stimuli (Drei Abhandlungen, page 30). Nothing prevents retaining the evolutionary theory of the origin and selection of organs, the sensations of which appear within the sexual instinct, unhindered by Freud's psychology. Similarly, the phenomenological psychology of Freud can very well be broadened and enriched in the way of an evolutionary method of consideration. Freud has not spoken the final word.

But may all parts of the body, which Freud has called erogenous, be now considered as sexual sources or creators of sexual feelings? As an example, sucking may be named. It consists in sucking motions which do not serve the taking of nourishment. Its object is a part of the lips, the finger or the toe. "The pleasure-sucking is joined to complete occupation of the attention, leads either to falling asleep or even to a motor reaction in a kind of orgasm. Often, there is combined with the pleasure-sucking the rubbing of certain sensitive parts of the body as the breasts or external genitals. In this way, many children pass from sucking to masturbation. Of the sexual nature of this act, no observer (except Moll) has doubted. Still in the face of this bit of childish sexual activity, the best theories derived from adults leave us in the lurch."* "It is plain that the action of the sucking child is determined by his seeking for a pleasure which has already been experienced and is now remembered. It is also easy to surmise on what occasions, the child obtained the first experiences of this pleasure which it now endeavors to renew. The first activity of the child and that most important to life, the sucking at the mother's breast (or its substitute) must have made it acquainted with this pleasure. We might say, the child's lips have served as an erogenous zone and the stimulation by the warm milk stream was probably the cause of the sensation of pleasure. Originally, the gratification of the erogenous zone was united with the gratification of the need of nourishment. Whoever sees a child sink back from the breast satisfied and fall asleep with rosy cheeks and happy smile, will be compelled to say that this picture also remains a standard for the expression of sexual gratification in later life. Now the need for repetition of sexual gratification is separated from the need for taking nourishment." †

According to this exposition, the sucking serves at first for the gaining of pleasure in taking nourishment. Why is this motivation not sufficient to repeat the motion on objects which are similar to the source of drink? If one considers the sucking as automatism, why should he not put away the pleasure agency of the drinking as realized, as the piano player unconsciously drums out a melody? It is of course probable that the phenomenon of the pleasure-sucking is overdetermined. But may not the pleasure of the muscular movement also have a share? Every kicking could just as well be interpreted sexually. The similarity of the satisfied child to the sexually gratified man proves nothing for the sexual pleasure of the former. When a child energetically desires an object and obtains it, his gesture is similar, only the blood is not directed to the intestinal region and the need for sleep does not appear so quickly. If we assume with Freud that the child

---

* Freud, Drei Abhandlungen, 40 f.
† P. 41 f.

creates his reality in an hallucinatory manner, then the intensity of his motions will also not surprise us. That the mouth has an erogenous character from the very beginning, I cannot therefore consider as proven.

To be sure, under certain conditions, the mouth sometimes acquires the significance of a sexual organ.

A boy of fourteen and a half years hates his younger brother and torments him in spite of all punishment. Every morning, he awakens him by sticking his finger in his mouth. All educational means have been powerless against this habit. The analysis afforded aid: It found that the evildoer, who had been misused pederastically by his comrades, repeated those scenes in an obsessional manner by symbolical displacement, as he had once irritated the brother to fornication. The finger served again as penis-symbol. The hate proceeded from denial of the homosexual love. It was possible without trouble to free the seducer and endangered one and improve the attitude of the hostile brother. But here we are dealing with an effect of repression, the mechanism of which we will have to speak later. If the sucking is connected with other motor acts then the association might be called forth by the common motor pleasure, whereby the sexual sensations would be awakened only later.

Further, I cannot consider it proven that the irritation of the bowel-ending is originally sexual. Certainly the tickling occasioned by it can attract sexual libido, the same as the hunger instinct and indeed, mathematics, but the pleasurable anal sensations need not therefore be of sexual nature. I have, at all events, often observed how pent-up sexual desire may take possession of the anal zone. A patient of thirty-eight years who had not been able to get rid of his tormenting hemorrhoidal itching by all kinds of physical and chemical means, lost it immediately with the aid of the analysis, although the nodules remained. It turned out that the irritation always broke out when the normal sexual gratification or even when merely the eroticism was inhibited by refusal on the part of his wife, causing a flight to his mother who had extracted an intestinal worm from him when he was a boy of about five years.* But there the erogenesis is only acquired. When children strive to obtain heightened irritation of the anus by holding back the stool (in which, according to Freud's important discovery which I have often confirmed, lies the cause of the frequent infantile constipation, often persisting for a lifetime), the desire for tickling sensations suffices for explanation.

Further, I cannot admit the eye as an erogenous organ. In itself, it is not once, like the mouth, intestinal or genital apparatus, an object of perception. Only that which is seen can cause sexual irritation. Still, the eye can be invested with the rank of a sexual organ by later reflexion.† I know many hysterical girls for whom the eye plainly represents the peripheral female organ. Two of them suffered for years from reddened eyes which defied the efforts of oculists when defloration- or birth-wishes brought these and other hysterical symptoms to expression. One of these girls was analyzed by me and cured of the phenomenon. Another hysterical girl of sixteen years was seized with violent anxiety lest she should stick herself in the eye while stretching the forefinger of a glove. The day before, she had been sexually enlightened. What finger and eye stood for, was easily revealed and the anxiety disappeared. Further, these cases, which are conclusively substantiated by the Indian mythology, do not speak in favor of the theory of the physical erogenous root of the libido: Indra, because of a sexual misdemeanor, was condemned to wear spread over his whole body, the picture of Yoni (vulva); the gods took pity on him so far as to change the Yonis into eyes.‡

Also, the irritation of the sexual organs by the suckling child, which appears later, is not proven to be a general occurrence. Recently, objection has been raised against this observation in

* See my article: Kryptolalie, Kryptographie und unbewusstes Vexierbild bei Normalen. Jahrb. Vol. V. (1913).

† Compare Freud, Die psychogene Sehstörung in psychoanalytischer Auffassung. Ärztliche Fortbildung 1910, No. 9.

‡ Jung, Wandlungen u. Symbole d. Libido.

analytic circles. Reitler asserted that Freud's observations were gained on the sick and should therefore not be transferred to healthy individuals because the psychoneurosis rests on the disturbance of infantile sexual development.* I do not consider myself competent to decide the question. But this much for the pedagogues may follow as important result of psychoanalytic investigations, namely, that onanism in children is much wider spread and signifies infinitely more than was formerly supposed.

If we cannot prove the "partial instincts" as elements of sexuality from erogenous zones, so also they cannot be shown to come from contrasting paired relations to the object. Such ambivalent functions (Bleuler) are:

1. Hetero- and homosexuality, that is, the attitude of the sexual instinct toward those of the opposite or same sex.

2. Sadism and masochism, that is, gaining pleasure from inflicting or enduring (self-inflicted) suffering.

3. Activity of the instinct for looking and exhibiting (Schaulust and Zeigetrieb).

Concerning these contrasting pairs, Freud points out that both members are constantly present together and in such manner that one is developed stronger than the other. Every person is bisexually or bierotically endowed,† so far that he sends out erotic desires toward both sexes. The heterosexual libido leads normally to marriage, the homosexual to friendship, still, an ideal realization of instinct in art, religion and other achievements may take place. Ordinarily, the boy feels himself drawn more to the mother, the girl more to the father. On the basis of his analyses of neurotics, Freud considers the background of this erotic relation constantly as sexual and speaks accordingly in every case of a fixation on the parents, of incest repression. He recalls the saga of Œdipus who killed his father and married his mother and finds that this same

* Die Onanie. Vierzehn Beiträge zu einer Diskussion der Wiener psa. Vereinigung, Wiesbaden, 1912, p. 91.

† Freud, Hyster. Phant, u. i. Beziehungen zur Bisexualität. Kl. Schriften II, p. 144. Drei Abh. p. 6 ff.

incestuous desire lies at the bottom of every neurosis. This attitude, which occurs regularly with changed sex rôles also in women, Freud calls the nuclear complex of the neurosis. Now, it is quite beyond doubt that countless nervous maladies, upon careful investigation, go back to this nucleus—one may strive ever so long against this assumption, but it is simply irresistible. But that all neuroses rest on this attitude toward the family, is for me not quite conclusively established. Perhaps Freud is right, perhaps he has generalized too early.

That sadism and masochism constantly occur together cannot be denied. Whoever investigates these two expressions of instinct receives the impression that two functions which belong together, and which when mingled are not striking, have been torn apart. Freud confirms this view in a letter and illustrates it with the apt comparison, there may be heaped up in one corner of the cake all the sugar, in the other, all the salt.

I have given an example on page 77. Here is another: On page 132, we heard of a girl of seven or eight years, who, during her phantasy of being mistreated by a witch (foster-mother) while hanging on the trapeze, felt sexual pleasure and then anxiety. The same child then liked to play with boys and girls games in which severe punishment was applied. Whoever was naughty, was scorched with a burning-mirror, which afforded our patient great pleasure, or had to kneel submissively. When the turn came to our little sadist, she felt an unpleasant emotion and wished always to submit.

Marcinowsky, a skilled analyst, contends that sadism is always hate. He considers sadism as pleasure-toned cruelty because it is a symbolical love act.*

There may, however, be still other motives working along with these: the wish for momentarily displaying his power, to brutally accomplish his purpose, vengeance for pain endured and more complicated motives.

So far as my experience goes, the ambivalent instinctive impulses of sadism and masochism appear separately and rule

* Marcinowsky, Zbl. II, p. 542.

the whole sexual activity when the normal erotic development is impeded, either through denial of affection or through strong irritation of pleasure in cruelty as result of corporal punishment.

It is worthy of note that in the inhibition of one of the ambivalent instinctive tendencies, the other undergoes an increase. The girl who lost her lover experiences, so far as the libido did not withdraw to the father or Savior, a strengthening of her friendship for her girl companions, the punished and converted tormentor of animals seeks severe tortures for himself.

May this reversal not be easier understood by assuming that one and the same libido has come to mastery in different directions and according to inhibitions present, turned more to this or that activity in order to realize its gain of pleasure? If we are dealing with separate partial instincts, then I do not see how such a reciprocal relation would be possible. Rather, the one sexual instinct turns from one activity to another, as the life-force (Lebensdrang), in positions where other outlet is denied it, for example in children who are confined, devotes itself to sexuality.

Extraordinarily difficult to answer is the question of the significance of the Œdipus wish. Freud represents the view that the repression of the incestuous longing for the mother and the corresponding hatred of the father forms the nuclear complex of every neurosis in the male sex. According to this view, every neurotic girl and woman is a secret Electra. Against this hypothesis, which forms the greatest stumbling block to the critics, the criticism has hurled itself with more passionate excitement than calm judgment of the facts in the case, and one can only be amazed at the ease with which some arrive at conclusions on this difficult subject who have never seriously considered it, while others who have worked on the problems for years, gain a positive opinion only with the greatest difficulty.

Let us first establish the fact that uncommonly many neurotic individuals display an abnormal attachment, indeed erotic attachment, to their parents. We did not observe this state

of affairs in all our cases by a long ways. If the analysis had
been pushed deeper, without doubt there would have been
found far more motives of that kind. Still, it is to be remembered that we interpreted a great number of phenomena as
causal, understood their formation, without finding among
the determinants the Œdipus impulses or their feminine counterpart. The latter, we met plainly in the girl who was persecuted in her dream by her father (67); more or less plain
resemblances to the Œdipus situation we saw in the boy who
was afraid of horses, steam rollers, etc. (68), in another
person who wore himself out in strife with the number 13 (70),
in the girl who slandered her foster-father (75), in another
girl who fell in love with her pastor (82), in the engaged girl
who lost her love on the stairs (94), in the other girl who
could love her fiancé only when he was absent (111), in Grillparzer (120), in the impotent husband (124), in the youth
who suffered from pains in the arm and leg, asthma and
melancholia (126), in the melancholy pantheist and masochist
(128), in the pilgrim to Einsiedeln (137), and others. Still
other examples will follow. The attachment was not always
a sexual one. It was a question, nevertheless, whether the
repression of incestuous wishes lurked behind these phenomena.

While I was writing these lines, a man, aged twenty-seven,
came in, who, after long years of study and the most diverse attempts to obtain a professional position, had failed. He suffers from tremendous anxiety so that he no longer ventures
out among people and doubts himself. The anxiety broke out
after some symptoms which we will pass over here, when he
was about fifteen years old, when the intention of becoming
a dentist appeared. In connection with this intention, the
patient related that he remembered clearly a grievous experience of his youth. Before he went to school, he found that
his mother had an improper relation with a dentist. He remembered this so vividly that he considered a falsification of
memory as excluded. If we have perceived that anxiety goes
back to desires, aroused but not gratified, then the coincidence

of the choice of profession and the anxiety is no longer mysterious. The boy wished, without knowing it, to put himself in the place of the dentist. This explanation of course will suit only him who has personally investigated a number of similar patients.

We venture now on the criticism of the Freudian Œdipus hypothesis. (1) Not every person who has an Œdipus complex is neurotic. Sophocles, to whom no one will ascribe predilection for psychoanalysis, writes: "For many people have seen themselves in dreams joined to the mother." Freud also does not believe that the neurotics are different in this respect from normal individuals. (Traumdeutung, 4th ed., 196.)

(2) Not every neurotic has repressed a conscious Œdipus phantasy as a result of the incest barrier. A proof of this assertion are the foundlings who, like Luccheni, were given to an asylum immediately after birth.

(3) Not every erotic attachment to the parents is incestuous. One often finds, for example, the wish to return to the mother's womb (see pages 200, 300, and my article, "Die Entstehung der künstlerischen Inspiration" in "Imago" II, page 490 ff.). One finds it, however, only in people who would withdraw entirely from reality or would experience a rebirth. The repressed hate against the parents is very often neither jealousy nor unrequited love but the reaction to improper education.

(4) Where the picture of the neurosis shows plain evidence of an Œdipus repression, where, for example, in dreams and symptoms, sexual wishes are directed toward the mother, it is questionable whether they were already present in childhood or only later when a regressive movement of the phantasy to the infantile stage occurred, newly developed sexual desires were displaced backward upon the same object. The mother is ever the trusted friend on whom a great part of the disposable love is concentrated. The transition to a new object of love cannot, according to the law of reference, which is applicable to repressed and non-repressed phantasies (see below Chapter

XVII, proceed differently than that the new object of affection is projected upon the old object, that is the mother, whereby, present sexual desires are naturally attached to the early object. A gross Œdipus phantasy does not prove, therefore, the existence of an infantile repression of a wish of like content. While this conception applies for the type of individual thrown back into the regression (repulsion type), still, we recognize, on the other hand, the Freudian explanation for inhibited persons (retention type) who have always been hindered in the transference of love to other objects by a strong sexual attachment in the sense of Œdipus. That such individuals are often seen, is not to be disputed and the fundamental sexual tones are frequently repressed. The discovery of these sexual desires always gives the patient being analyzed a great surprise but one not to be controverted.

With these statements, our subject is only partially discussed. Much work is still to be performed before it is satisfactorily explained from all sides. In so doing, we will separate the phantasy which we have received from the mouth of Sophocles, from the wish for return to the mother's womb, as it is expressed for example by Nicodemus in John's Gospel 3 : 4. The latter phantasy is, as already acknowledged, often only a symbolical expression of a sublimated rebirth phantasy but certainly not always.

In a word, the concept of libido should be made more precise. Freud considers it, as mentioned, purely empirically as identical with sexual instinct (Drei Abhandlungen, page 1) or sexual pleasure (Über Psychoanalyse, page 48). Jung gives it a metaphysical or asexual meaning. In so doing, he includes also empirical quantities, namely, all volition, for example, hunger, in the term libido, as well as energy of growth which in the ontogenesis causes the individual to divide and germinate (Jahrbuch IV, 178 ff.). Jung specifies thus: "Libido should be the name for the energy which manifests itself in the life process and which is perceived subjectively as striving and desire" (Jahrbuch V, 342). This libido is "nothing concrete or familiar, but rather an absolute X, a pure hypothesis, a picture or marker, as little concretely conceivable as the energy of the physical world" (342).

Thus the long-used expression "libido" receives an entirely new meaning. The consequence was at first a regretable terminological confusion even among Jung's nearest adherents. Thus, Schmid, in his work on Psychology of Incendiarism, uses the expression now in one sense, now in another (Psychologische Abhandlungen, heràusg, von Jung, Leipsic and Vienna, 1914). The libido which is asexual in itself, is much like Freud's likewise asexual instinct ("Triebe"), which only attains sexual character under the influence of an erogenous organ (Drei Abhandlungen, 30), except that Freud does not, like Jung, invade the field of metaphysics. Into the further criticism of Jung's conception of the libido, we do not need to go here.

Thus, I consider Freud's libido-concept as the one which should be used exclusively in psychoanalytic terminology. On the other hand, I include all expression of instinct and volition under the name "life-force" (Lebensdrang) or will-to-life (Lebenswillen). This latter is differentiated according to the conditions of the perpetuation of the individual and the race in progressive development as air-hunger, instinct to movement, nutritional instinct, etc. up to the highest mental activities.* For the energies existing within the propagation processes and determining these, I prefer the expression, propagation-energies, for the metaphysical tendencies belonging to these energies, the name, propagation-will.

From this basis, we can also fix the terms "sexuality" and

---

* Later, I find that G. F. Lipps in his monograph, "Das Problem der Willensfreiheit" which has just appeared, has elaborated a theory which sounds much the same. For him, the life-instinct is the "immediate cause of the actions of the living being, which are executed under the influence of external, present and past, actually demonstrable or hidden forces, which, however, can never be absolutely derived from these forces" (Willensfr. 79). It is "an indivisable unity" (79), "a condition presupposed by us in our thinking, which never submits itself as such to investigation, but betrays itself to observation only in the connection between the forces and the resulting conditions." (85). To all of this, I subscribe.

"eroticism" more exactly. Freud extended, because of psychological assumptions which we recognized as not sure, the former term far beyond the customary speech usage after he had not done this at first. Thus, it happened that he was mostly misunderstood, to the detriment of his work. In opposition to him, I consider it suitable to use sexuality and psychosexuality in a more original sense, one better commended by the history of language and a consideration for comprehensibility. Under sexuality, we understand the sum total of those physical and psychical phenomena whch are related to reproduction or the activity of the reproductive instincts and organs. From this concept, we distinguish eroticism which we compare with "love" and can consider as characterized either as sexual or non-sexual.

2. "Censor" and "Resistance."

When Freud, by the aid of his psychoanalytic method, began to penetrate the unconscious of his patients, he received the impression that the patients set up a resistance against his efforts which he had to overcome by his work * and this resistance, indeed, stood in the way of the repressed ideas becoming conscious. "A new comprehension seemed to open to me now, as it occurred to me that this might well be the same mental force which had taken part in the originating of the hysterical symptom and had at that time hindered the conscious perception of the pathogenic idea." † As motives for repression, he found the affects of shame, reproach, mental pain, in short, painful contents, so that the repression seemed to him a defence.

Thus in the resistance, we are dealing with a hostile defence against unpleasant ideas and emotions and therewith also refusal to allow these to return or be brought back into consciousness. The result of this renitence consists mostly in the continuance of those symptoms of disease which depend on the repression. It is not the complex which struggles against its

* Studien über Hysterie, p. 234.
† P. 234.

disclosures but the foreconscious which would spare consciousness a grievous experience. Likewise, the resistance is directed not against the analyst and the treatment but against the rendering conscious of the repressed material. The effect is really a holding fast to the malady.* The cause of the resistance is, according to Freud's opinion, fear of the father, defiance and distrust toward him.† But of this, we need not speak here. It is sufficient proof of the existence of the resistance to point out that one may often succeed in finding the motive for resistance analytically, and in eliminating therewith, the obstacles to the return of the repressed material to consciousness, so that the flow of communications suddenly breaks forth with force. We know for a certainty that the power which hinders the free speaking out to the analyst is simultaneously the jailer of the complex, only against the analyst, special forms of resistance appear. If Kronfeld misses the proof of this assertion,‡ then he must make the acquaintance of the fact of the transference from his own contemplation and pass from the study of books to direct observation.

By the help of the resistance, a censoring activity is now exercised. Freud even speaks of "the censor" as if it were a force endowed with special powers. At the boundary between the conscious and unconscious activity, he assumes a censor which admits only what is pleasing to it and represses the rest. In sleep or under other conditions, the balance of power between the two conditions (consciousness and unconscious) changes, so that the repressed material can no longer be entirely held back. In this stage, the censor is not entirely removed but nevertheless changed.‖ The sleeping state lowers the power of the intrapsychic censor.¶

* Freud, über Psychotherapie. Kl. Schriften I, p. 209. Die Freudsche psa. Methode. I, p. 221. Tatbestandsdiagnostik u. Psa. Kl. Schriften II, p. 120. über "wilde Psa." Zbl. I, p. 94.
† Freud, Die zukünft. Chancen der Psa. Zbl. I, p. 4.
‡ Kronfeld, Ü. d. psycholog. Theorien Freuds u. verwandte Anschauungen (In book form), p. 104.
‖ Freud, über den Traum. (Grenzfragen) Wiesbaden, 1901, p. 339.
¶ Traumdeutung, p. 351.

Kovàcs uses the expression ''censor'' in about the Freudian sense, ''namely, as the name for a process of discrimination which seeks to adapt the ideas and affects to the conditions of a cultivated human being and to repress those unsuitable to society.'' * On the other hand, it is to be emphasized that conscience and the demands of society are not entirely the same. An ethically independent character will very often be in position to repress the socially suitable.

Jung originally denied the censor.† Later, he said: ''The censor is nothing else than the resistance which prevents us from carrying out a consideration uniformly, day by day, to the end. The censor allows an idea to pass only when it is so clothed that the dreamer cannot recognize it again.'' ‡ Thereby, the censor is eliminated as a function. Likewise, Bleuler would replace it by the more general term of inhibition by counter-striving affective necessities.||

According to Silberer's view, we are not dealing with a contradiction between Freud and Bleuler-Jung but only with the difference between the teleological and causal methods of consideration.¶ Without doubt, he is right, since Freud derives his ''censor'' from the balance of power of the factors of repression. The name is purely a figurative expression and includes those functions of repression which exist in the struggle for the protection of consciousness from unpleasant excitation. Since in sleep, the apperception relaxes, the resistance and therewith the censoring faculty can undergo a diminution.

3. The Constitution

It is unjust to reproach Freud with having overlooked the hereditary endowment. Of course, he limits the convenient asylum of ignorance of the hereditary predisposition, and where the analogy between parents and child makes easy the

---

* Kovacs, Introjektion, Projektion und Einfühlung. Zbl. II, p. 258.
† Jung, Psychologie der Dementia præcox, p. 76.
‡ Jung, L'analyse des Rêves. L'année psychologique, A. XV, p. 163.
|| Bleuler, Die Psychoanalyse Freuds. Jahrb II, p. 727.
¶ Herbert Silberer, Über die Symbolbildung. H. III, p. 693.

assumption of an hereditary relation, he points out with sharp criticism the exogenous connections. The pedagogues will be only grateful to him for this service. Even in his earliest works (1895), the father of psychoanalysis stated heredity as a condition of anxiety-neurosis.* Gradually, he estimated the constitutional factor still higher. In 1896, he found heredity an indispensable prerequisite in the majority of cases of severe neurosis but not as determining the form of the malady.† In 1905, he considered the hereditary predisposition as indispensable.‡ In 1912, he defended himself against the criticism of having denied the importance of inborn (constitutional) factors because he emphasized the infantile impressions. "Psychoanalysis has said much concerning the accidental factors of the etiology, little concerning the constitutional, but only because it could bring something new to the former, while concerning the latter, on the other hand, it knew no more than was already known." ‖ "The psychoanalytic investigation has enabled us to point out the neurotic disposition in the evolutionary history of the libido and to trace this disposition in its active factors back to inborn varieties of the psychosexual constitution and influences of the outer world experienced in early childhood." ¶ Among the inborn variations of the sexual constitution, he conceives "a preponderance of this or that one of the manifold sources of sexual excitement." § At all events, lues in the father strongly predisposes to neurosis.**

Jung lays the emphasis on the more or less developed ability to continue the course of development prescribed by the inner peculiarity and outer relations, in spite of the sacrifice demanded by it.

---

* Freud, Zur Kritik der "Angstneurose." Kl. Schriften I, p. 109 ff.
† Freud, L'hérédité et l'etiologie des névroses. Kl. Schr. I, p. 139. Compare p. 199.
‡ Freud, Bruchstück einer Hysterie-Analyse. Kl. Schr. II, p. 14.
‖ Freud, Zur Dynamik der Übertragung. Zbl. II, p. 167.
¶ Freud, Über neurot. Erkrankungstypen. Zbl. II, p. 297.
§ Freud, Drei Abh. p. 80.
** Same.

Adler considers the inferiority of an organ as constitutional cause of the neurosis: "The digestive apparatus, the respiratory organs, the heart, the skin, the sexual apparatus, the motor organs, the sense organs and the pain paths become thrown into excitement according to their fitness for the expression of the wish for power, and show the forms of hostile, aggressive attack or of quiescence and of flight, inhibition of aggression, both in harmony with the "vital line" of the patient, with his secret life plan. To give in brief some examples of organ dialect: Scorn can come to expression by the refusal of normal functions, envy and desire by pain, ambition by sleeplessness, thirst for power by oversensitiveness, by anxiety and by organic nervous maladies." * To put it differently, from the experience of an inferior organ, there follows a feeling of inferiority which must be removed by aggressive endeavor. From this attitude, follow forced strivings toward strengthening of the value of the personality and from these forced efforts, the neurosis proceeds. We have discussed this theory and its exaggeration by Adler on page 139.

* Adler, Organdialekt., Monatsh. f. Päd. u. Schulreform IV. Year, (1912), p. 325.

SECTION 2

THE RETROGRESSIONS OF THE REPRESSION, FIXATION AND REPULSION

(THE MANIFESTATIONS)

CHAPTER IX

THE PHYSICAL MANIFESTATIONS

1. SYMPTOMS

THE repression does not occasion the submergence below the threshold of consciousness of an idea actually thought but rather the restriction of an instinct in a certain place, so that as a result of this restriction, certain ideas become incapable of coming into consciousness and in addition, the further normal development of that instinct is inhibited within a certain domain. Thus far, we speak of a fixation of instinct.

There is, however, no absolute quiescence of the instincts. If normal activity is denied them, they grow in an abnormal direction. Thus, by the repression and fixation, the instincts are deflected into paths deviating from the original direction and driven to new creations. We call these new formations, manifestations.

Under manifestations, I understand all phenomena which psychoanalysis shows to be direct effects of the repressed and fixed unconscious.

The fact that repression shows itself in a physical symptom, Breuer and Freud expressed in the formula: "The excitation proceeding from the affective idea becomes converted into a physical phenomenon." * Breuer's supposition that the foun-

* Studien über Hysterie, p. 180.

173

dation and condition of hysteria may be the existence of hypnoidal (sleeplike) states,* was soon given up by Freud. In place of these states, there were other conditions which we have already brought to the reader's attention. On the other hand, the riddle, why psychic processes can occasion physical ones, remains unsolved. The name "conversion" presupposes a transformation of psychic energy into physical energy, in which we, the followers of psychophysical parallelism, cannot believe. The thing itself is not a whit more enigmatical than the relationship between processes of will and action. In addition, I call attention to the fact that all pathological physical reactions to mental impressions are denoted as hysterical.

Some physicians gave themselves endless trouble to collect and describe the symptoms of hysteria. Naturally, it is impossible to conceive of completeness in this symptomatology and further, nothing would be gained by it. The same signs of illness may owe their origin to the most diverse mental conflicts. We educators are primarily interested only in the most important of the external characteristics but on the other hand, because of our profession, we are very eager to recognize the mental backgound. It should be remembered that we trouble ourselves concerning the bodily injuries only because they form the tell-tale signal of a mental complication which is of highest importance for the utilization of the intellectual, esthetic, religious and ethical powers and for the development of the whole character and because we cannot possibly solve the educational problem without also eliminating at the same time the physical suffering.

I shall refer first to some of the physical marks of hysteria which we have recognized so far. We will group them as motor, vasomotor and sensory phenomena and distinguish functional increase and decrease.

A. Motor Phenomena:

(a) Increased: clucking (33), twitching in the cheeks (41), asthmatic dyspnea (68), tic of eyelid (74), convulsions in the arm (123).

* Studien über Hysterie, p. 9.

(b) Decreased: dumbness, astasia (31), stuttering (84), writer's cramp (88), paralysis (90).

B. Vasomotor Symptoms:

Swollen lips (32), skin eruption (34). These examples contain only a small part of my observations.

C. Sensory Symptoms:

(a) Hyperesthesias: Migraine with feeling of hair being pulled out (32), itching of scalp (34), temporal migraine (35), two crowns of thorns (36), visions (angel, devil, Schleiermacher) (37), buzzing in the ear (41), innervations in the arm (44), tactile hallucinations in the hands and feet (81), neuralgia (98), pains in the arm, leg and back (126), in the shoulder (132), in stomach (142).

(b) Hypesthesias: Dimness of vision (31), deafness (34).

Since the sensory deficiencies and vasomotor symptoms were shown somewhat scantily, I shall give some further illustrations:

A patient of twenty-two years, who will come before us often again—we have already made his acquaintance as an asthmatic (68)—has suffered for some years from severe near-sightedness, although the physicians could find no myopia. A slight clouding of the cornea bears no relation to the visual defect as will soon show. The youth greatly fears becoming totally blind. Asked concerning the outbreak of the trouble, the patient recalled that he had first noticed the disturbance when he mistook an approaching trolley car with two signal targets for two men. (We recall here that the steam roller represented the father panting from coitus.) When the latter had discovered from traces in the closet the masturbation of his son, he had whipped him in great wrath and shouted at him: "You will become blind, you already have closed eyes, you pig!" The threat was occasionally repeated. Soon thereafter, the visual power diminished and the compulsion to look at himself continually in the mirror began, along with many other symptoms. Immediately after the disclosure of this fact, the young man, who had previously

worn strong and still stronger eyeglasses, read small print at
a distance of one meter without lenses and some days later,
laid aside the glasses entirely.

A man of about forty complained to me that for some time
he had entirely lost the sensation in one big toe. His wife had
previously been under my pastoral care suffering with distaste
for life and irritability. I knew therefore that her last par-
turition had been accompanied by danger to her life and that
she resisted sexual intercourse. I had referred her in this
matter to the family doctor who assured her that there was
no certain means of preventing conception except refraining
from intercourse. Under such circumstances, it was not easy
to cure the wife by way of sublimation (see below) and at the
same time, her husband was importunate. What kind of a
meaning the anesthesia of the toe had is at once clear to us
if we remember its symbolical significance: Phidias engraved
the name of Phryne on the great toe of Zeus.* The anesthesia
of the toe symbolized masculine frigidity and served also for
the subliminal refusal of this. That atrophy of the spinal
cord was not present is shown by the fact that for more than
three years sensation in the toe has been present again; other,
milder nervous phenomena predominate. I advised the man
to consult a neurologist but he did not take my advice. An
analysis was not performed.

That the unconscious manifests itself in physical expressions
which are neither connected with familiar motor nor with
sensory nerve functions, we know from the history of religion
and hypnosis. One may recall the monks with stigmata
(Francis of Assisi) and nuns with bloody sweat. Analogous
phenomena have been brought about by hypnotism.† Hys-

---

* Compare in this connection, Jung, Wandlungen u. Symbole der
Libido. Jahrb. IV, p. 166. L. Binswanger, Analyse einer hyster.
Phobie. Jahrb. III, p. 302 ff. (Folk-psychological references in Aigre-
mont, Fuss- und Schuhsymbolik und -erotik, Leipzig, 1909; the phallic
significance of the foot is here demonstrated without analysis, likewise
by Kleinpaul, Das Leben der Sprache, Vol. II, p. 490, cited by Stekel,
Die Sprache des Traumes, Wiesbaden 1911, 7.

† Forel, Hypnotismus, p. 27.

teria, nevertheless, proceeds gradually beyond hypnotic vaso-motor symptoms.

The girl with swollen lips (32) did the following trick: informed concerning the nature of her comical symptom, she resolutely undertook the treatment of her mother one day. According to her report, her mother recalled that she had suffered since her eighteenth year from a painful swelling on the tongue which had resisted all medical treatment, as also had been the case for a long time with her seventeen-year-old son. Now came the question whether this trouble might not perhaps be of hysterical nature. The mother reported that in her time, one rather thought of an infection, still it could scarcely have been such. Shortly before the onset of the swelling, a friend of her brother, who was suffering from the same trouble, had been in her house, yet he had neither touched with his tongue an eating instrument nor any other object. Triumphantly, the daughter, who was accustomed to use a very unceremonious tone, called out: "Aha! You have identified yourself with the young man, you were in love with him!" Now, this method of treatment was not even analytically correct. Still, it sufficed to dislodge the old trouble and the son promptly followed the example of his mother by eating.*

Besides undoubted · "automatic" signs, there are some in which a part of the unconscious motive passes over into consciousness so that one might speak of semi-automatisms if the analysis had not displaced that term which cuts the causal connections in the wrong place.

A girl of thirteen and one half years was attacked with trembling. Sixteen months later, she entered one of my classes with increased symptoms. She was unable to give anyone her hand and touched only the outermost finger-tips to draw them back very quickly. She could walk only in dancing steps, with hands raised, as if she were in a minuet. Street urchins often imitated her in derision. In one of her first

---

* The young man who exerts himself against the analysis, is also a clever imitator. When his sister injured her foot, he awoke the following night with severe pain in his foot.

years of life, the girl had lost her father and acquired a step-father whom she hated from her earliest days because of his severity. An uncle struck her on the back when she was four years old. When seven years of age, she had anxiety-dreams without telling of what she was afraid. In school, she was laughed at as a foreigner because of her speech, to which she reacted with immeasurable hate. Further she detested her mother. Some months before the outbreak of the tremors, she dreamed that as she was standing in a room, a knife was thrown at her through the open door by a workman. The man who did this, strongly resembled the wicked uncle who had chastised her and thereby plainly awakened sexual emotions. As every analyst knows from a mass of proof, knife and door signify masculine and feminine symbols (see below Chapter XI). Thus the girl wished a sexual attack from the uncle who stood for the stepfather. Details of the dream, she refused to give. The nervous malady broke out when the hysterical girl had got into strife with her only friend and all the girls expressed their displeasure in strong form. Two weeks after the trembling which accompanied the wrath phantasy, the dancing appeared. At that time, the little one received a visit from a brother, ten years older, who formed a positive (beloved) father substitute. The brother reported that his child had St. Vitus' dance, per-haps his sister might have it also. The hysterical girl imagined the chorea as a real dance. She had wished for a long time to be able to dance. From the newspaper, she was familiar with the positions in the minuet dance which she had assumed. During the dancing, she was afraid of falling.

· Striking was the love of finery of the homely girl, as well as her longing for caresses which she boldly sought for.

The meaning and connection of the symptoms are fairly clear: The girl did not know how to bring her love intelli-gently into use, since she had fallen out with parents and play-mates, had to renounce the love of her married brother and in her love-making was too little successful. After the damming up of the homoerotic instinctive activity, a physical symptom appeared which was directed into a new path by further determinants. The girl identified herself with the brother's child which had St. Vitus' dance; the brother, she raised to father and realized in hysterical manner her wish to dance. The position of her hands expressed however, two other tendencies: the intention of protecting herself from falling (morally) and the resistance against shaking hands. The wishes to fall and to be loved were repressed.

The analysis was not carried to completion since the girl plainly concealed energetically a part of her secrets; she entered the class of a minister who was making arrangements to apply psychoanalysis in a pastoral way. So far as I was concerned, I succeeded in stopping the dancing. The hatred of men and its symbol, the refusal to shake hands, persisted. The analysis did not come to pass, unfortunately, although the girl was earnestly urged thereto. A half year later, I saw the girl strolling with a peasant at a late hour under suspicious circumstances. What has become of the young coquette, I do not know, as she went away. I fear she will be dragged down to the depths by her untrained sensuality.

As foundation for physical manifestations, we often recognize a certain bodily weakness as for example in the following case:

A girl of nineteen has suffered for three years with some remissions, for one and one half years constantly, from a very severe, barking cough, against which the physicians can accomplish nothing. Upon questioning, I learned the following: A year after the beginning of her illness, the girl left her birthplace and moved into a pension where she was hospitably received. Soon, the cough ceased, to recur with rather lessened force when two other girls entered and took the lead as favorites. After the rivals had gone, the cough also disappeared completely. After a short time came the death of her dearest relative, the only one by whom she felt herself understood. From that time till the analysis, the cough dominated; the analysis eliminated the cough in two sessions and in some further ones, the ethical inhibition as well. The girl had a number of painful experiences and phantasies which concerned the parents, had repressed these and was prejudiced by the mood so created. The strongest impression had been made by the idea that in her twelfth year, a harmless love had been rudely destroyed. Even at that time, she said: "Father and mother do not love me, they wish I were dead." Four years later, she suffered from an acute bronchitis with much cough. As no one sent her to the physician or to bed, she thought she possessed absolute proof that her death was wished for and revelled in the idea that it would be discovered too late how much she had been misunderstood. Whenever the parent-complex ruled, the coughing broke out, as if to say: "It is again as at that time when I was seriously ill and no one bothered about me." The masochistic death-wish came to expression. Now we understand also why the cough, which went parallel to the attitude toward the environment, ceased under friendly treatment and appeared when she was put in the background.

How the denial of the suicidal thoughts was very prettily unmasked by the association-experiment, I will show later.

The patient at first resisted the treatment with the hypocritical pretext that she was being punished by God, in reality, however, because she would not renounce her hysterical gain of pleasure and particularly the hatred of her parents. I showed her this condition of affairs and her foolishness and after a few consultations attained not only the stopping of the cough but also a favorable change in her ethical relation.

This observation teaches us that a real organic disease can be taken over by the unconscious and continued on its own account.* Much more often, nevertheless, the reverse takes place, an illness which is apparently of undoubted organic origin, is traced back to nothing but mental causes. On this point, the physicians may discuss more profitably. I mention only a very frequent occurrence which happens to us educators.

Often, we have to deal with pupils who suffer from fatigue.

* We also saw organic inferiority as a disposing cause of hysteria on page 96.

The physician is accustomed to allow them to leave school and sends them to the country, from which they return, sometimes improved and sometimes unimproved. In the process, much time is lost and the exhaustion soon returns. How many a career has been cruelly blasted as a result! Physicians trained in psychoanalysis have noted that a great part of the tired pupils suffer only from mental conflicts. I, too, have obtained such results.

A talented girl of sixteen years, from North Germany, suffered for a year and a half from great lassitude and for the same length of time from convulsive laughter and weeping. It was also impossible for her to have wool or silk touch her. Previously she had suffered from somnambulism: she sometimes twisted her underclothes into cords and laid them on the floor.

The first convulsion came when one of her brothers snatched away some little thing which she had wanted to eat. The affect surprised and provoked the girl so much the more since she was not at all selfish. Another time, she asked her neighbor during the study-hour to make a D in round script. The other wrote instead of that, "Du," whereupon the convulsion with laughter set in and then passed into weeping. The analysis revealed at first that the fear was present that she would be written blockhead ("Dummkopf") or something similar. The very next session elucidated the anxiety: When a small child, our patient was called "Dummerchen" (little stupid) because she allowed everything to be taken from her without resistance by her brother, two years older than herself. The nickname became indeed her constant name. The intelligent little person did not seem to know stronger affects at all, at least she yielded quietly, to being plundered. That in reality, powerful emotions were present in the depths, the future made plain. Most striking was the absence of emotional reaction when the little brother perished: he snatched an object from the hand of his three year old sister in the laundry and in so doing, stumbled into a tub of hot water. Eight days later, our patient stood beside her brother's corpse without showing inner excitement. The pantomime carried out in somnambulism repeated the fateful scene under motives which we can now give only hypothetically: The girl suffered still from the feeling of being slighted, which, according to information furnished by her mother, had actually taken place in the early years of childhood, and repressed the wish arising from the unconscious that again, an event like that earlier one might remove her rival. Thereby, during all the years, the memory of the catastrophe was blotted out. Her mother's narrative first refreshed her memory but not for the tragic affair, merely for the harmless play which had taken place between them shortly before.

The analysis of the touching-phobia, we will describe later. Its result was as follows: The patient saw unconsciously in every bit of woolen underwear, the underclothing of the scalded little brother, in every silken stuff, the garment worn by an old lady who was present at the funeral. The feeling of inferiority was repeatedly satisfied in sadistic wishes.

The life of the well endowed girl was plainly centered about the overcoming of the inferiority, in which the strong pressure by feelings of helplessness was inhibited. Her relations toward the members of her family were entirely correct. As consciousness of helplessness, however, allowed no protest to come forward when she was slighted, there constantly resulted the regression to the neurosis and her vindictive wrath. The convulsions expressed joy in injury and anger which alternated that each might break out so much the more violently. I call this phenomenon, which is often found in hysteria, the polarization of antagonistic instinctive tendencies.*

The lassitude decreased, like all the other symptoms, after a few hours of analysis. It was a result of the severe, dimly recognized mental struggle and probably might also console when the results did not fully correspond to the ambitious efforts.† After my pedagogic efforts, the strikingly monoto-

---

* Compare my article: Hysterie und Mystik bei Marg. Ebner (1291–1351). Zbl. I, p. 484.

† For another example of psychogenic fatigue, see below, page 197.

nous, poor-in-affect speech· changed remarkably. The young girl realized much better how to express herself and took an honorable place in her class. In brief, she defended her rights courageously. Her attitude toward life became excellent.

2. THE EXTERNAL AND INTERNAL ASSOCIATIONS IN THE MANIFESTATION PROCESS

The representation of the physical hysterical symptom proceeds along two paths, namely, by that of the inner or outer association or by both together. Often, the manifestation reproduces simply one scene, the renewing of which by a present experience, is rendered desirable. A recent occasion reproduces a similar previous occurrence which makes the present situation appear in consoling light or else contains a relation to the present. Now an earlier situation is revived, now it is expressed by this: "It is again as at that time, when the event, which comes to expression here, occurred," the present recreates from the past, courage, guidance and hope for the future. In this process, the only absolute essential is that the connection between manifestation and complex may not become conscious. If this should happen, then the secret which occasioned the disguise, would be disclosed. Naturally, only a small group of characteristics from an earlier event can be reproduced.

Such reproduction-symptoms are exceedingly frequent. We have already found them many times (for example on pages 32, 44, 86). I will add a few other cases:

The girl mentioned on page 179, who allowed the complex to come to expression through the secret speech of the cough, suffered, after the cure of her violent barking, as for years before, from migraine which she would not place at my disposal. Finally, she concluded to sacrifice the private cult which she practiced at the altar of hysteria. Questioned concerning the first appearance of the trouble, she said that at the time of the first migraine, she had menstruated for the first time, but because her father, mother and some brothers and sisters were confined to bed with influenza, she had nursed her family in spite of the violent headache, while other girls were granted rest and protection under these circumstances. At present, the girl suffers under the often heard reproach that she is lazy and does nothing for her family. This unjust accusation, however, always produces migraine. In this way, the patient plainly revives that period during which she distinguished herself by heroic self-sacrifice and extraordinary industry, while the cough illustrates the meanness of her parents during the illness of their daughter. Both symptoms are, therefore, as is constantly the case, internally united. From the hour of this none-too-deep exploration, the headache remained absent.

A pupil of seventeen years, brought to my pastoral treatment by melancholia, blushed every moment or so, on the left half of his face, especially his ear. This phenomenon reminded him of a box on the ear which he had received from his father, the last time, a half year previously. At that time, he wished to run away from the parental roof and would have done so if his father had not turned him back. In the analysis, he now substituted me in the rôle of father, for reasons of transference to be discussed below. My command to speak corresponded to the earlier efforts of the father to get a secret from his son. The blushing corresponded to the wish that I, too, would be rough like the father, then the patient might run away from me or humiliate me. The symptom (erythromania) disappeared at once.

An hysterical man of twenty-two years suffered among other things from prickling sensations in the right half of the face. One proceeded from the teeth perpendicularly upwards, the other from the temple horizontally toward the parietal region. Both sensations go back to brutal punishment by the father. A band about a hand's breadth wide presses on the patient's neck and back after the midday meal. The jugulars swell and threaten to burst. When the youth was still a child, the father compelled him to rest on a couch after meals, shoved a cushion under his neck and loin regions and bent the head violently backward. In the new formations, the patient continually seeks new material for sweet phantasies of revenge and yet wishes at the same time to experience the father's affection. These phenomena also disappeared at the moment of the analysis.

Frequently, however, the symptom forms, not a mere reproduction, but a new formation and indeed a symbolical representation of an idea. Here, an inner association between repressed material and symptom takes place. Examples of this, we have already met in great numbers. I refer to the dumbness, the hanging by a thread (31), the clucking (33), the imaginary piece of coal in the eye (75), the crown of thorns (36), the anesthetic toe (176), etc.

Being partial to pedagogic material, I shall describe a few more cases which will show external and internal psychological productions of hysteria.

The teacher who had sent me his pupil afflicted with paralyses and convulsions (86), consulted me for a far more severe case. The twelve year old girl, who was the patient, had suffered now for the third time, from phenomena which the physician pronounced St. Vitus' dance (chorea). When seven years old, the child had a disturbance of writing, her hand began to tremble, soon the foot became restless, and with her hands, she pulled and tugged at the persons who would hold her. In her tenth year, the trouble which had disappeared after some weeks, returned in greater violence. The tongue could no longer be moved. A course of baths brought improvement, still the speech and writing remained greatly inhibited. A full year, school had to be given up. Five weeks ago, came the third and by far most severe outbreak. The well developed, but strikingly pale child displayed a far-reaching hysteria. Without cessation, she swung the distorted arms, of which, the right had become weak, the upper body turned hither and thither, the knees often gave way, the face continually made grimaces: the mouth drew apart, saliva was automatically forced between the teeth, the eyes winked abnormally often, the nose and brow were wrinkled. If the child wished to grasp an object, she invariably struck beside it. Spoons, pens, playthings, etc., were flung away; writing was not to be thought of. Drinking from a cup was also impossible. The tongue was often so paralyzed that no word could be spoken. Convulsive laughter and weeping frequently appeared.

In addition, there were mental anomalies, of which, I must mention at least the severe anxiety which had for years compelled her to look under the bed.

It is not possible to give in brief form more than the most important determinants of such a wide-spread hysteria. I could not find them all, since the child, although I avoided suggestion. as much as possible in the interest of a thorough treatment, had lost all symptoms after eight sessions. Such an outcome is very pleasant for the patient; the analyst who would like to throw light on all peculiarities feels unsatisfied, however, since he can explain many traits only ex analogia.

The first attack, which was essentially in the form of writer's cramp, was little elucidated: the child wrote poorly. At home, she excused herself by saying that her neighbor constantly pulled at her arm. Before she entered school, she had long had anxiety, with which she had long been inoculated. Considerable sexual traumata had preceded. The disturbance of writing corresponded every time to a strong wish to be freed from school and to be excused for bad penmanship.

The second outbreak resulted again in a cessation of the school-life. The teacher was a coarse, punishing pedagogue who openly said that the children should not divulge what took place in the school-room, especially if a child was whipped. Our patient although intelligent, was often struck, but did not venture to complain to her parents. The anxiety became constantly stronger. The stern man could not sing well. The spaces between his teeth rendered his enunciation difficult. If the frightened children did not sing correctly, they were treated to the violin bow. Many of them suffered from inhibitions of speech. Once, the children had to name the doors. One could not, because of fright, get the words "Zwei Aborte" (two water-closets) beyond the lips. In that locality, forbidden things had taken place, in which our hysterical patient had had a share. The latter was, therefore, likewise inhibited from speaking the words and received her flogging. Again, the girl wished to seek protection from her parents but was afraid of the vengeance of the tormentor. That since that time, the habit of looking under the bed has prevailed, discloses that a sexual inhibition must also have existed.

The last and severest illness occurred after the girl had been punished for masturbation by the mother, an otherwise sensible and affectionate woman. Even before the first attack of illness, the child had once received some slaps because she had asked her mother whence the children came. Without doubt, this mistake had shared in the malady with strong effect. During this report, the patient excreted a striking amount of saliva. A strong homosexual compensation had occurred: The child wished constantly to be taken into bed with the mother. By sleeplessness, she really attained this object of being kept the whole night by the mother.

Merely the opportunity of being allowed to confide these tormenting thoughts to the mother and me exercised a quieting action. Once when she had not been able to go to sleep, she had dictated to her mother the following little song which she had learned from a companion at school:

> "Mother, mother, what is that
> Which crawls in my belly?"
> "Child, that I cannot tell you,
> You must first ask your father!"

Similarly run the following lines, only here the doctor and midwife are the subjects; the midwife answers:

> "Child, this I can tell you,
> To-morrow you will have young,
> One dead, the other blind,
> One with a hole in the head." *

Craftily the girl sought to retain her evil habit. Both before and during the illness, a violent twitching of the part

* It is remarkable how often those children who are not correctly enlightened, fall into bloody sadisticism.

in question would occur. Making clear the meaning of this attempt at extortion sufficed to eliminate it at once.

The gimaces signified, among other things, in teeth-showing, derision of the toothless teacher and suppression of the sexual secret. The winking of the eyes referred to the repression of the sexual pleasure in looking (Schaulust) which was ever very keen. The grasping near objects showed on harmless objects what would happen toward dangerous ones. The objects hurled away called forth by symbolic meaning anxiety for touching things. The swinging of the arms proved to be composite: One motion was forward and ended in a menacing movement outward. Asked to think of this, the girl recalled that her grandmother once said that if one cannot speak, someone is plaguing him.* This someone was to be warded off by the gesture. Other determinants were added: When one and one half or two years of age, the child was lifted out of bed by the hands and suffered a slight dislocation. This information was given by the mother who was present during the whole analysis. Another time the father lifted his daughter by the hands and likewise caused a dislocation. Further, the refractory child did not wish to extend her hand to the bad teacher. Finally, she wished to protect herself from falling (compare page 179).

The following case describes an analytic experiment which was only partially successful: Into my pastoral care, there came a high grade imbecile boy, fifteen years of age, hysterical, who has been subject to convulsions in the arms and legs for eighteen months. Many times, for an hour, his feet twisted inward, then outward, his arms were drawn back at the elbow at the same time, the hands remaining beside the chest. A four months' residence in a sanitarium for nervous diseases had brought no improvement.

The convulsive attitudes proved to be determined by external and internal associations. They referred to scenes which the boy wished subliminally, but consciously refused. He belonged to a gang of boys, thirteen to fifteen years of age, who

* Beautiful peasant psychology!

had banded together for the purpose of sexual orgies and who had not even refrained from pederasty. They were fond of amusing themselves with obscene marching practices. Once they imitated a cripple whose feet were twisted inward. In so doing, they held each other by the genitals. Our patient advised against this practice since it was not right to mock a cripple. Another time, the youths imitated hopping birds by turning the feet outwards and again using forbidden holds with the hands. A man saw this and pursued the boys who fled. Thus, we understand that the patient on the one hand wished for the sexual scenes again, among all of which, however, he chose those in convulsions in which he played the finest rôle and escaped successfully from the scrape.

Therewith, however, only the outermost stratum is revealed. The dreams lead much deeper. Since we are not yet familiar with dream-formation, I have thus far given very few dream analyses, although in so doing I must have awakened an incorrect impression of the course of analytic work and one soon to be corrected. At this point, however, I cannot avoid giving a short dream interpretation. For many years, our hysterical patient has dreamed, with slight variations, something like the following:

"Someone crawls from under my bed. I spring upon him, he seizes me, I fall back and go to sleep. He wishes to run away, I again spring on him, a chase ensues and I call out; father and mother rush after the enemy with sticks and brooms. I seize the revolver which he left lying under the bed and spring after the intruder. I pursue him, striking him on the back, to the police-station; we all go home and lie down to sleep. I awaken with anxiety that someone is crawling from under my bed."

This hysterical patient also looked under the bed every night. The man in the dream held his arms in crawling as the dreamer does during his convulsion. The intruder was described as thin, clumsy, dark, of medium stature. This is the way his god-father appears, as the association now says. This person lacked a finger joint. Once, my patient hallucinated this uncanny man as creeping forth from under his bed. The assailant in the dream seized the sleeper to tickle him under the arms and lower rib borders, as his father often did in play of an evening. Also, the father's hands in so doing assume the attitude which appears automatically in the convulsion. Clearly, the crawling figure is meant to portray the father. The severed finger joint of the god-father which figured in one place, betrays a castration thought. The attitude of crouching on the elbows is also that of a person during coitus. The son imitates in his automatism the father and pursues him from the house in the dream as a sexual criminal with the aid of the asexual father. The blows which the fugitive receives, reminds our hero of those which he himself received. To this, comes another plot: The dreamer had read, shortly before the hallucination, of a murderer who lurked under the bed. Hence he phantasied himself in this rôle. At that time, he threatened his brother that he would strike him dead, for which, he was whipped by his father. Further, the repressed wish to destroy his brother, also exists in the symptom. Later when the convulsion had already occurred, still other phantasies were added: He gave to the man lying on his elbows, the face of a coal carrier who had asked him the way to the cellar. The position of the arms of the sack bearer, in its sexual symbolic meaning, thus strengthened the symptom.

After the first sessions, the contractures lessened to a minimum. Then a resistance asserted itself which I could not overcome. The boy refused to give information, his defects in intelligence probably served the repression in good stead. Hence, the convulsions became greater, but at their greatest, did not attain the intensity and frequency which they had had for the eighteen months preceding the treatment. I hoped to be able to analyze the boy completely later and spared the extremely tiresome work only for the time being. Unfortunately, after some weeks, the boy left my place of residence.

In conclusion, it should be remembered that normal individuals also very frequently show a slight physical manifestation. A minor or major headache or stomachache, a mild intestinal catarrh, a mild insomnia and similar incidents of psychogenic nature (mental origin) are thousandfold and belong to the every-day phenomena which may be eliminated by a little occasional analysis (often by autoanalysis). Who is not a little bit nervous? The famous neurologist, Möbius, asserts in all seriousness that every person has hysterical symptoms and no one has contradicted him.

CHAPTER X

THE MOST IMPORTANT PSYCHIC PATHS

EVERY repression restricts an instinct in such a manner that its activity in reality is rendered permanently impossible to a lesser or greater extent. Often, the inhibition of the instinct is so insignificant that it is either not perceptible or so only by the most careful analytic investigation; in severe cases, this inhibition can drive men into the most tormenting confinement; indeed a severe psychoneurosis or psychosis belongs under some circumstances to the most dreadful things which can happen in life. In every repression, the life-force comes into some state of inhibited development, it may be in its activity as reproductive function or as nutritional instinct or in other interests.

Whatever is inhibited by repression is, according to our psychological understanding (54), the instinct, but only in certain concrete performances, thus, those united to intellectual and emotional affairs. In their places, the life-force seeks new paths, which, when they do not appear on the physical side, lead just as easily to changed emotional processes as to altered intellectual phenomena.

I shall sketch these processes in detail, without regard to whether we are observing them in sound or sick persons. Particular considerations recommend reproducing the most important pathological types in their fundamental characteristics. The same laws hold for healthy and sick. Yes, the conflicts, too, which oppress the sick in their sufferings, are the same which make the healthy work.*

* Jung, D. Inhalt d. Psychose, p. 25.

1. The Paths of the Libido in Detail

A. EMOTIONAL PROCESSES

1. *Losses of Emotion*

(a) The repression often expresses itself very strikingly in the decrease of such emotions as have been present and the non-appearance of expected new emotions. For the educator, these ellipses are of considerable importance for they may definitely determine the direction of the life. The pedagogue trained in analysis is greatly needed by those who are emotionless toward their fellowmen and hence despairing of life, or those who in pathological irritability, make enemies of everyone. Most portentous is the emotional loss, when, at time of marriage, the real sexual demand comes to an individual. Since the roots of the absence of love, which is often so tragic, go back to childhood, the educator must be familiar with these processes.

Frequently, lovers discover, to their deep pain, that their ardor grows cool without visible motive and indeed may cease. The judgment and estimation of the erotic object has remained the same or some tiny objection may have arisen which does not at all justify the refusal of love. In spite of all self-reproaches, of all autosuggestive arguments, love remains absent and in its place, inner disgust, anxiety, pity, perhaps despair have become active.

The traditional psychology which oriented itself almost exclusively according to the surface of consciousness, did not know what to make of this process, as it in general knew little how to deal with the wonderfully rich and varied, but also difficult to understand, field of the love-life. Does psychoanalysis solve the riddle?

Two very young girls, who were joined to excellent men in strong love and suddenly lost their affection apparently entirely, came under my pastoral observation. With one, vulgar sexual enlightenment by a girl comrade had caused distaste for marriage and therewith the disappearance of love. The other had shared the room of a somewhat frivolous companion for some time and become familiar with nasty things. In addition, she heard an older girl speak of "worldly love" as impure and impious and in contrast, praise the sweet adoration of Jesus in extreme pietistic form, as holy. The purity of heart, the quiet holiness of the pious exhorter, who, with the Apostle Paul, judged everything else as dross in order to win Christ, contrasted favorably with the foolish actions of the other companion. The very young little fiancée fled from the temptations of her despised sexuality into ascetic piety. To her lover, a worthy teacher, she wrote a farewell letter, sympathetic but energetic in tone, of being the happy bride of Christ and was deaf to all entreaties of her parents and of the troubled fiancé, as well as to all religious and moral teachings; hence they turned to me. I advised explaining to her the origin of her conduct. As a matter of fact, the fanaticism disappeared very soon and the earlier love returned enriched by purer ideas of the value of marriage.

A youth of twenty years complained to me that his feeling toward his fiancée, to whom he had been deeply attached for some years, had for a few months disappeared. He torments the girl by undeserved nagging, of which he is afterwards ashamed. Now he begs me to tell him whence comes his coldness and what he should do. In accordance with my wish, he reported his last dream. It ran as follows: "I dreamed that I stood in the Kasernenplatz and my lady friend went by." [Nothing else?] "Yes. The whole dream was: I am standing in the court of our former school-house. Someone commanded repeatedly: 'Stand at attention!' I obey each time and stand at attention. Thereupon, I find myself with my cousin in the waiting-room of a polyclinic." [The court.] "There, as a boy, I passed by with my present friend." [Someone.] "My friend." [Stand at attention.] "Thus we are commanded early in military service. That was especially painful to me. I cannot endure this physical obedience." [I obey each time.] "The motion, a sudden jerk, a drawing back of the shoulders and throwing out of the chest, then the sinking together, was rhythmical and reminded me of something which you can already imagine. I was much excited. I spoke with my friend of free love. Before I explained to her, she knew nothing of sexual things and became suddenly eager to assume all the consequences of love since we both suffer, love each other and are destined to marry. I told her of my scruples. Then she became sad. Her love seemed to have gone, also she will no longer yield everything for others, while previously she was noted for altruism." [The cousin.] "She is of same age as myself and resembles my mother in many ways."

For the comprehension of the dream, it should be added that the youth had questioned me concerning free love some months before, probably shortly before the loss of his love. He had at that time almost decided to accept the offer of his fiancée but was convinced of the ethical objections to prenuptial sexual intercourse. His present communication allows the unspoken reproof to be perceived: "There, now see what you have done! I am betrayed in my love and debased to a moody man, the loved one too from a noble-minded nature to an egotistic creature!"

The interpretation is: "I obey (ironically) the beloved, who stimulates me in annoying manner to sexual intercourse (commands),* I prefer, however, to pass the time which I must wait while love-sick, with the upright, mother-like cousin."

Now we understand why the love failed: The youth wishes his unpleasant irritations out of the way. His absence of love is not necessarily genuine but signifies merely a defence neurosis (Freud) or measure of assurance (Adler). We observe at the same time the flight to the mother (modeled on the infantile). Noteworthy further is the so frequent double-faced character of the manifestation: It can express renunciation quite as well as longing. The youth would like to discover a

---

* The command "Achtung, steht!" (attention, stand!) naturally refers ironically to erection.

moral demand for sexual intercourse, the dream betrays a higher ethical tendency.*

A peasant boy of eighteen desired my help because he felt unable to work and was constantly cold toward everybody. The drunken father, whom he hurled to the floor recently in protecting his mother, and had to tie with a rope, he hates and despises. Also, for the mother who had shown him too little affection when he was small, he has no hearty feeling, no matter how much he tries to have it. His comrades are as a whole unfit for friendship since he must mostly refuse them or where he could be friendly, is rejected by them. The youth shows strong introversion (shut off from the outer world, turning of the libido inward) and cannot be approached with grounds of reason. His inner need is great. Analysis of his dreams shows: The young man is fixed upon his mother who outweighs companions of his own age. In the conflict between mother and comrades, he appears in the dream upon the mother's side. The faults with which he reproaches his comrades are exactly those with which he convicts himself (projections). The dream following this disclosure is typically homosexual and anal-erotic, as in the case of a man soon to be discussed (200). My patient was greatly surprised when I remarked to him that from the dream, I should conclude that his bowel functions were not in order; in reality, he has suffered since childhood from constipation which trouble disappeared from the day of the analysis. The next dream pictured the reconciliation with his father but at the expense of his comrades who came off badly. The following conversation affords the motive: "I have always been defenceless against them." Because unconsciously he feels inferior to them, he belittles them consciously. Finally, after eleven conversations, the libido was forced to apply itself to the surroundings in normal manner. Since then, the young man feels happy, contented with life, able to work and entirely

---

* One sees also from this example that the unconscious in no ways always represents a kingdom of the animalistic, unmoral and hostile to culture, even though this is usually the case.

healthy. Hate and inhibitions for work have disappeared. Other examples, we saw on pages 80, 94, 111. The pastor often has to deal with marriages in which the hearth-fire is out because love has failed. Naturally, love cannot be extorted by admonitions and good advice. On the other hand, I know a number of cases in which when the repression was eliminated, the pent-up love returned and brought a beautiful happiness with it. One must guard carefully against considering the loss of the emotion of love as absence of love. Under the threshold of consciousness, the inclination very often exists in great force and waits longingly for occasion to master consciousness.

Love often diminishes where in the substitute for the parents, traits appear which do not correspond to those of the parents. Once on a journey, I became acquainted with a young merchant who had been married only a month and had used this period to acquire a nice neurosis. He slept twelve hours at night and every midday from two till six o'clock, thus demonstrating very plainly his wish for a flight from reality. Hours at a time, he sat weeping and brooding over his misfortune before the funeral wreath of his mother. Love for his attractive wife had entirely disappeared. The anamnesis disclosed: The young wife was a niece of the dead mother of the subject. He had known her from a child but felt no deep affection for her. Only when the mother lay on her death-bed, did the cousin who was some years older than himself and resembled the mother in face, suddenly appear to him as uncommonly lovable. He became engaged to her very quickly and married her. Even on the next day, he felt that he had been deceived. It was easy for me to overcome the sleepiness but because of lack of time, I referred the patient to a neurologist for a thorough analysis. The latter cured the neurosis but also demonstrated a dementia præcox in the woman which gave a bad outlook for the marriage.

Similar perils to marriage from fixations upon the parents occur so frequently that one would earnestly wish that all those about to be married might know whether they are fooled by an injurious father- or mother-substitute. Only the analysis can afford conclusion on this point.

Other cases also occur: love can be repressed by the fact that infantile repressed hate comes to life again. This condition, the analyst in particular often has to trace (compare below, Chapter XVII, The Transference).

Where a love which was not simply a neurotic flood-wave (see following section) disappears, we are often dealing with a regression to an infantile condition. If there is no place for the ardent longing, then it seeks the parent-substitutes which occasioned the infantile condition.

(b) A second group of emotional deficiencies has to do with emotions hindered by repression. These inhibitions also are to blame for much unhappiness. Numbers of people come to every analyst who suffer shipwreck because the deepest longing either comes not at all or too late into consciousness. The motives are the same as in the rejection of emotion. Where it was formerly believed that the inability to love was to be explained as a primary disposition, we know to-day that every person who is not an idiot bears within himself sexual and erotic capabilities and that incapacity for sexual love depends without exception on repression processes. In proof, I can offer for consideration here only a limited number of observations from an abundant material.

An unmarried woman physician of fifty became ill from a severe obsessional neurosis. She had to add the street-lamps, square the sum and make that the starting-point for other, in part more complicated, computations. Still worse, however, did three obsessing ideas torment her and give her no rest: She constantly heard the melodies: "You are embraced, millions, this kiss of the whole world!" and "I know that my Redeemer liveth." In addition, she saw herself sitting in the snow in a pool of blood. The lady who told me of this case discovered the meaning of both obsessions herself: the patient had as a girl received a marriage proposal to which in spite of all high esteem for the lover and all friendship for him, she could not react with love. In the menopause, the love, long withheld, breaks violently forth and turns toward the man whom she really loved without knowing it. An analysis was not done. The visual phantasy, I am inclined to consider, because of analogous cases, as realizing the wish for birth in a condition of innocence.

From my own work I know of the following examples: A woman teacher of thirty-five years had earlier, on account of superior intellectual, esthetic and ethical talents, been courted uncommonly much but was not able to produce the eroticism necessary for marriage or a love affair. She is the ideal friend who charms everyone by her sympathetic nature. But the sentimentality of her expression was united, as so often, to the incapacity to realize her eroticism. While she dedicated herself to children with touching devotion, her innermost nature cried out for salvation and love. Still, for years, she felt happy since she successfully repressed the voices from the depths. Finally came the breaking through of the unconscious. Melancholia with strong suicidal impulses which led to an unsuccessful attempt to take her own life rendered analysis necessary. The analytic investigation revealed the evidence that the love of the patient was entirely attached to her father and her whole life filled with the wish to impress this important man, for whom, in consciousness, there was little inclination. Her whole activity formed an imitation of the father, without the person in question being aware of it; on this uncomprehended plan, her life happiness threatened to be wrecked. When the fixation was removed, the patient, now eager for life, returned to her friendships. Every morning she awakened in tears: The onetime lovers appeared one after another in her dreams and waking phantasies and she thought she could detect that she had secretly loved one or the other, only the former condition of being chained by her complexes, had prevented the deep-rooted emotion from coming into consciousness.*

The analysis, from which I present only a small fragment,

---

* It would also be conceivable that the eroticism, only now set free, projects a newly developed love upon the images out of the past.

gave her the ability to adapt her inclinations to reality. She regretted most deeply the blindness of her previous life which seemed to her in spite of admirable results rather a dallying with the realities of life. We are dealing here with a person who in the sense of the traditional pathology must have been called perfectly normal and yet she was restrained from her own destiny by subliminal restrictions. How many individuals are forced in similar manner with demoniacal violence to paths which prevent a free development of their highest, especially their moral, powers. How much poverty in love is not inborn but merely the expression of an infantile fixation which might be dissipated by analytic pedagogy!

Often, the eroticism is displayed in perverse formations. I will show in two examples how the barring of normal love-impulses precedes that kind of sexual abnormalities.

A wealthy merchant of twenty-six years, of superior talents, is incapable of loving a girl and founding his own household. The apparently completely normal man loves poetry and himself writes lyric poems of excellent content and admirable execution. Strangely enough, however, the expression of love is absolutely lacking in them. His sexual needs he satisfies without scruple by means of prostitutes. Thus, it cannot surprise us that he does not know how to gain much from life although he might be a real artist with his excellent talents. Without psychoanalysis, it would have been impossible to explain his condition. The dreams disclosed not only the extraordinarily frequent wish to return to the mother's womb, but also a strong interest for the lower back parts of his mother. The wish, to lie there, pushes forward strongly. To this wish there is joined a group of characteristics which Freud * first discovered and which have since been very often substantiated. Freud recognized in a considerable number of persons a striking love of orderliness, frugality and stubbornness, besides chronic constipation. This type is met frequently in shop people, teachers and scholars, who, in spite

* Freud, Character und Analerotik. Kl. Schriften II, pp. 132–137.

of a scrupulous overpunctuality, do not attain to a noble achievement corresponding to their talents. Freud furnished the proof that all these persons are neurotics who were robbed by a certain repression of a considerable part of their chances in life, and he disclosed the inner psychological connections of the symptoms. Thanks to analysis, that devastation of life can be eliminated.

The young man of whom I am speaking was analerotic * to a high degree without feeling anything of the homosexual or pedarastic wishes. In his toilet, he is laughably exact. It is terrible to him to be compelled to make a visit in a hurry because it is two days since he was shaved. Every minutia, the multimillionaire writes carefully down. A certain preference for peculiarities is unmistakable. With his parents, he is on bad terms, especially with his father who is still deeper in analeroticism than he. Twice, the youth attempted to fall in love, but he chose two cousins with whom he knew in advance, according to his testimony, that an alliance was absolutely impossible. Naturally, the love was insincere. It was a clever attempt to free himself from the mother by the aid of a mother-double.

The neurotic individual being on a journey, I could hold only two conversations with him. They sufficed to make clear his situation to him and awaken in him the decision to free himself from his inhibitions by thorough analysis in order to attain an efficient life.

As last example, I mention a woman principal of an institute, twenty-eight years of age, of high moral standing, whom a neurologist of my pastorate introduced. The lady suffers from severe melancholia since she thinks she cannot longer endure her homosexual needs. If she met a young girl on the street, she would be seized with an ardent desire to kiss her. Weeks at a time, she saw the unknown girl, who was perhaps not particularly charming, constantly before her, and could no longer sleep from grief over the fact that she cannot

* Anus signifies the end of the bowel.

satisfy her kissing passion as on some earlier friends. Especial pain was caused her by the fear that she had seduced to homosexual love a fourteen-year old girl entrusted to her care, by her sensual tenderness, although improper acts had never occurred. The little girl trembled with excitement when she was embraced and wept of lovesickness when she did not see the beloved one often enough.

Our homosexual patient had a father, physically handsome, but one who was insignificant and anxious, who left entirely to his energetic and intelligent wife the direction of the business and the education of the children. The little daughter admired her mother and, even early, judged her father as insignificant. As a small girl she was normal. She played equally gladly with boys and girls. With both, she encountered improper things: girls allowed themselves in the dangerous play of doctor, to be guilty of improper touching, and further, a little sickly boy with whom the child had to associate when seven to nine years old, allowed similar transgressions. When about eight years old, she fell in love with an adult cousin who often tossed her in the air, during which procedure she felt a "peculiar sensation." When ten or eleven years old, she was repeatedly misused by a woman housekeeper of forty years. Pronounced homosexuality broke out when the girl was thirteen years old. At that time, she went much with a teacher who resembled her mother in many ways but who surpassed her in culture. This passionate individual, who had outspoken homosexual tendencies, for two years overwhelmed the girl with excessive affection. At that period, there developed in the little one a genuine passion for kissing while the sexual desires awakened by the housekeeper receded. Some little love affairs with boys also led to kissing but passion was lacking in these affairs. Those affairs were undertaken more from imitation and vanity.

In the pension, the one-sided erotic direction was further developed in warm friendships. When nineteen years of age, she undertook two heterosexual erotic attempts which, however, failed. The first concerned a very young artist of feminine appearance. The love was very intimate, the young girl revelled in ideal conversation and liked to exchange kisses with the youth. After his departure, there came a correspondence filled with homesickness; promises were not given.

Five or six weeks after the separation from her beloved friend, she became engaged out of despair to a fine peasant boy since she got along badly at home with a relative and had to give up the plan of a higher education. She thought to develop love for her fiancé but immediately after the published announcement of her engagement, anxiety overwhelmed her that she had undertaken something impossible. The dull, retiring man plainly resembled her father. Seven months, she dissembled love; every morning brought gall and longing for death. Finally, she broke off the relation and concentrated her emotions entirely on relatives of her own sex. In this, she retained a refined, feminine attitude and gave the impression of having a genuine maidenly nature.

So long as she was homosexually gratified, she troubled herself little about vocation, nature, art and religion; as soon as her tendency underwent inhibitions, the ideal interests appeared in force. She herself compared these fluctuations to a balance.

When she was ardently in love, she was free from sexual excitements. Once with the unloved fiancé, on the other hand, she was sexually excited when he caressed her in an entirely proper manner.

The analysis could not be carried to the end, unfortunately, since the improvement appeared too quickly. Feminine inverted individuals have not so far been analyzed. I dare not venture to illuminate the darkness. Still, I can point out some spots of light.

The reaction attempt pointed to only the most superficial layers of the repressions present. The first dream led deeper: ''A cat bit me on the front of the left index finger and for a long time would not release me. Then the finger swelled up and burst open to the bone. The tendon was lacerated, much water flowed out. Then someone said I would have a stiff finger. I thought: 'What a shame, now I cannot play the piano any more!' I awoke and found my finger so fast asleep that I could not move it.''

Sleep was preceded by a despairing prayer which brought temporary rest. Before the analysis, the girl was extremely restless and longed for her loved ones but said that she only brought new misfortune on them.

To the cat was associated the house in which the housekeeper lived, after this, the child who was apparently seduced to homosexuality and a friend of her youth who loved the dreamer when she was eight or ten years old. The kitten had at first wanted to bite her in the foot. The swelling finger acquired on the underside a four-cornered appendix like a magazine rifle. Its sexual symbolic meaning becomes thereby still plainer: The patient dreamed herself in the man's position, her sleeping finger awoke the idea of an erect penis. The bursting open to the bone and the losing of water disclose that a feminine phantasy was also active in the unconscious. - The upper slit is like that of a gun.

Now the dreamer recalled that the water flowed down steps and that she ran with her wound to a woman physician friend. The latter met her suddenly in the neighborhood of a merry-go-round. Then said the sister of the injured one: "She can fix your finger in a minute." But the physician interposed: "I am sorry but I do not operate." She sent the patient to a male physician.

The associations were few: The intimate woman physician friend had really said to her shortly before that unfortunately she did not operate but would take an operative course. She had danced with her at a masked ball (hence the merry-go-round). The sexuality excited by the young seduced girl was to be gratified by the friend of like age. This wish is repressed in favor of a heterosexual one. The physician is the analyst on whom a weak transference (see below) came into existence. That the physician helped is therefore not dreamed. The sexuality conceived as masculine remains therefore as tension (the finger remained stiff). The earlier graceful love activity (piano playing) ceases. A solution of the conflict is not found, hence comes the flight to the waking state; still the longing for health prevails.

The peripheral sexuality of this homosexual individual has been repressed, as it seems, as a result of disgusting experiences. As substitute, the passion for kissing sprang up. The constitutional claims of the eroticism became fixed on the mother who was also apparently inclined to harmless, asexual kissing. The higher needs forced an intensive identification with the mother. The repressed sexuality, nevertheless, plainly entered into a comparison with the handsome but mentally unimportant father. Even in strongly heterosexual girls, we often find hysterical symptoms which show that a masculine sexual rôle has been assumed. But in the cases known to me, only the incestuous love, not the whole sexuality, was split off. Our present patient, on the other hand, fell into homosexual passion for kissing because a radical genital repression occurred and the infantile incestuous love for the imposing father was later thrown into eclipse by the recognition of his inferiority. The father lingers, so far as I can assume from analogous observations on other inverted individuals, for her in every man so far as he does not, like the young artist, have a feminine figure. Hence the passion for kissing must apply itself to the female sex.

The analysis of the dream quoted gave the inverted one * first of all the certainty that behind the apparently harmless and therefore tenaciously retained longing for affection from persons of the female sex, gross sexual wishes lurked. At first this unpleasant discovery caused fright but it also occasioned the passage to valuable sublimations.

The lady now voluntarily renounced the sensual tenderness, the loss of which no longer made her unhappy. Since we were dealing with a mild inversion, an entirely normal eroticism might perhaps have been attained if the patient had not been so highly pleased that she withdrew from analysis. It was

---

* Freud's expression for persons whose sexuality is directed exclusively to members of the same sex (Drei Abh., p. 2).

striking how the physical appearance changed: the face which had become prematurely aged from worry, again assumed a youthful appearance.

I could now show by a still further list of examples how the heterosexual emotions could not appear in normal manner toward persons outside the family because they were fixed on brothers or sisters. It might be shown that without exception this subconscious repression goes back to a deeper-lying fixation upon the parents. But in this book, we can offer only a few examples.

We have seen that not only insincere but also real repression-free emotions may be lost under the influence of the repression. That the libido knows how to create constantly a substitute in all this change, we shall have occasion to demonstrate later.

2.   *The Emotional Flood*

Just as little as physical energies which limit one another, change into nothing, even so little can psychic energies pass under the repression without leaving a trace. We shall see a great number of smooth paths into which the banished libido knows how to smuggle itself, often in wonderful disguise. First, let us discuss one of the most frequent: The contributions made to the conscious emotional life from the unconscious enable trifling emotions to attain a powerful emphasis.

We must console ourselves in the present illumination of the dynamic relations to general considerations. Later, we shall consider the particular processes and laws whereby the emotional flood appears.

The emotional investment can affect any functions or values. There is no emotionally toned performance, no valuation which may not suffer from conditions of the complex, either a loss or an overemphasis, that is, an exaggerated emotional emphasis not appropriate in itself.

I shall begin with some clear examples which deal with the distribution of emotion in the intellectual processes.

An Austrian lady of about thirty years suddenly began to take a passionate interest in astronomy and to despise the previously preferred poetry. She suffered from migraine in the forehead (identification with a Roman heroine who, because of an unhappy marriage, shot herself), from anxiety in tunnels and from vaginal pains which, according to the report of a woman gynecologist, were hysterically maintained under the pretext of a scar. The lady married without love. Towards her physically and mentally superior husband, whom she revered and admired, she acted erotically cold but was secretly passionate toward a strikingly ugly man. As a young girl, she had loved a handsome youth whom she could not marry; since then, she has fallen in love with several amazingly homely men. Before the appearance of her passion for astronomy, she had dismissed the last of her friends. The star science was preferred because it had nothing to do with eroticism.

Another lady living in ungratifying wedlock fled into postage-stamp collecting to which she applied herself until late at night if she would assure herself of rest. This same neurotic individual had a dread of long snails and earth-worms while she handled without discomfort small snails and other creeping things. She could not eat meat, especially unsmoked meat, but had a predilection for white orange peel and other indigestible food. I leave it for the reader to interpret these phenomena. To him who has worked analytically with symbols, this presents no mystery.

Frequently, the repressed eroticism escapes into eroticism in highly refined form but directed toward another object than the real one. A young lady of twenty-three years fell in love with her nurse so intensely during a short illness that she became cold toward her fiancé and all other male friends and relatives. She wept when the deaconess was long engaged with other patients. After her recovery, she thought day and night only of the admired nurse. The latter was neither particularly pretty nor charming in manner. Rather she was distinguished by an almost austere nature and also by a strong will. At the first meeting she seemed surly so that our patient felt almost hurt. To offset this, however, she proved trustworthy and well-meaning. The passion blazed up when the apparently disagreeable sister softly approached the patient's bed at night and looked after her. The young girl had felt since her childhood that she was slighted by her mother. In her mother, she missed the constancy, reliability in keeping secrets entrusted to her and real tenderness expressed in deeds. The sweet endearments of the mother have become repulsive to her. The deaconess makes a contrasting mother-substitute: behind the austerity of the person playing the mother, lurks trustworthiness and good intention. In the nurse, the longed-for mother is loved, the libido set free from the mother comes to her. In addition, the sister exemplified the virtues which the girl wished for herself.

The will, too, can be chosen as carrier of feelings from the unconscious. He who is charged in this way, feels himself seized by a demand for activity which is enigmatical to him who despises the subliminal region.

I analyzed a man aged thirty-nine who showed interesting religious phenomena. From a boy up, possessed of strong sexual needs, he hoped to find peace in marriage. His wife, however, refused in the first years of wedded life to bear children and caused her husband to practice coitus interruptus. After a short time, his inclination toward nature-cure methods, to which he had previously been moderately attached, became passionate, indeed even fanatical. He bought about one hundred books on the subject and had for other things only slight interest. To my question put after this report, ''Of what were you thinking?'' I received the answer: ''In all things, one must carry on things normally.'' This answer awakened, in the connection named, a surmise which I kept to myself for the time being. I heard further that after some years the wife became reconciled to normal intercourse. Immediately, the cult of nature-healing ceased, to recur again after the birth of the first child when the former bad habit, the immediate cause of countless anxiety neuroses and hysterias, because the sexuality was again inhibited, was resumed.

An example of increased emphasis on the religious life, we noted above (92). Further cases will come to notice.

When a young girl appears very sentimental and is characterized by excessive use of adjectives and by exaggerated sweetness, she is as a rule hysterical and incapable of a great and true love. Such natures can stimulate like personalities who suffer similarly from a kind of "psychic diabetes," to ardent love and themselves rave in love until the real demands of life begin, when all has vanished.

Whenever the educator sees such emotional outbursts appear without external cause, he may conclude with infallible certainty that there is a previous repressive process.

The emotional flood shows us a reinforcement of certain emotions by other emotions foreign to them. If the repression ceases or if the falsification of the emotions is explained, the delusion dissolves. The person on whom we transposed emotions really belonging to another then becomes of no account to us. Following the flood, comes the ebb, following the erotic ecstasy, comes erotic desolation. The person who was hotly loved yesterday, may have become of no importance to-day if the delusion has vanished. Further, the emotional flood causes much unhappiness especially when, under its influence, important decisions are made, for instance, a marriage contract (see page 197). Many times, the repression lasts for a lifetime and the emotion which happened like a cuckoo's egg remains unchanged. It may happen that a man devotes to his wife all the time the affects which really belong to his mother. Certain it is that all persons carry within themselves many such erroneously harbored emotions while all education and the entire higher civilized life rests in part on such invaders which came from the land of the unconscious and were falsely assigned to this or that post in our consciousness.

3. The Transposition of Emotion

The investigation of certain striking emotional amplifications which are not explainable by conscious processes, (only those of this kind are under discussion) revealed to us the fact that that kind of phenomena may be interpreted as the influx of another repressed process.

This transposition of affects is violently assailed by opponents of psychoanalysis. Kronfeld assumes that Freud deduced this conception from a definite theory concerning "the nature of the associative explanation of psychic events" and other hypothetical constructions.* With the aim of contradicting, he engages in logical discussions concerning psychological principles. Over the psychological facts brought forward by Freud, which must be and are known to him,† he does not trouble himself. Still less does he interrogate reality as to whether the transposition asserted by Freud and the imposing company of his adherents, occurs. With him who refuses to exercise his own observation, knowledge gained from experience is not to be discussed. The opponents of Galileo refused to look through his telescope; a certain Mr. Bouilland, on March 11, 1878, sprang at the throat of the physicist, Du Moucel, who introduced the phonograph and called him a lying ventriloquist. On Sept. 30, 1878, the same Mr. Bouilland "after a thorough trial of the Edison apparatus," explained the pretended invention to be a swindle, for one could not assume that such a measly bit of metal could reproduce the noble tone of the human voice.‡

He who is inclined to overcome the aversion which clings to all of us toward things which are at first mysterious—and I include Kronfeld also with these seekers after truth—may reconcile himself with the results described below. We will permit ourselves to be warned once more by the critics to avoid hasty hypotheses. Proceeding from the facts, we shall accord to theoretic construction only so much place and right as is unconditionally necessary for the gaining of a causal connection. The assumptions stated provisionally we shall abandon every time that new experiences contradict them.

We have already pointed out transpositions of emotion in a considerable number of cases. In the last section, we spoke of overemphasized pleasure in astronomy, postage-stamps, in a nurse, in nature cure, that is, pleasure which cannot be ex-

* Kronfeld, p. 61.   † Same, p. 44.
‡ Kemmerich, Kultur-Kuriosa.

explained from the value of the object itself. Earlier, we recognized Scheffel's "Ekkehard" as a remedy for clucking (34), washing became a great ceremony (68), machines, horses, the nose, legs of doves and children, cockroaches assumed the character of fearful objects (68, 122, 103), a rubber tire and a clamp which held a bicycle pump attained irresistible attraction (76), a kitten and gas mantle stimulated the pleasure in aggression with obsessional force (77), the figure of Jesus became, as result of unfortunate love, invested with enormous emotion which disappeared after the disappearance of that deficiency in love (92), sympathy assumed a pathological degree (102), a moderate scarcity of available dwellings became the destroyer of life's happiness (109), the Madonna gained the character of a beneficent goddess of love (136). The sight of a funeral procession led to an obsessional idea (144), the mouth of a brother attained irresistible attractive force (159), the eye became the female sexual symbol (160), harmless wool and silk developed into untouchable, horrible objects (182).

Whoever has done analytic work for any length of time is not confused by dozens, perhaps hundreds of observations. But I am almost afraid of tiring the reader by further cases. Still, the fear of facts displayed by certain critics, on whose fairness I place great hopes, may serve as my excuse for presenting for consideration a few more observations.

The sixteen year old girl mentioned on page 160, who, while knitting, feared to stick herself in the eyes, had a similar phobia two years earlier. She feared for a period of several weeks when she lay in bed to strike against the bedside table. If she turned toward the wall, her anxiety did not become less. [Put your mind on the table.] "Nothing." [Put more attention on it.] "I was anxious then because I knew from comrades that something would soon happen to me. I was fearfully ashamed of this and thought if only no one would notice it. I wished to give no offence. Yet I put the matter out of my head." We understand now why the bedside table was feared: it is the article which gives offence.

Another girl aged fourteen and one half years, had for a number of years had a pathological fear of beetles. When she saw one, she betrayed the most violent agitation. All possible suggestions had been tried to free the girl from her phobia by educational influences but without result. Even a soothsayer had tried her skill and brutally compelled the little one to touch a painted beetle; naturally, the anxiety only increased. The analysis attempted at first to define the symptom more clearly. It turned out that the skin of the beetle inspired her with greatest horror (see page 122, the masculine counterpart). Then appeared the anxiety that the animal might crawl up her back or be injured on its thin wing membranes. Finally, the chief determinants appeared: the little girl had been shamefully seduced by a servant maid and her lover. Both instructed the child in improper acts and assured her that she would have a tickling sensation as if beetles were crawling on her body, which the child found interesting. Further, they explained the significance of the hymen to her. In the beginning, they made the child drunk when they indulged their appetites, later, they let her look on unceremoniously. After repression of the masturbation, the anxiety appeared which we have already met so often as expression of dammed-up sexual desire and attached itself to the idea of beetles. The girl often imagined that she lay decaying in the grave while beetles crawled about on her. The phobia diminished at once but returned as result of later severe sexual irritation, whereupon an infantile stage of the phobia was discovered (227).

Freud long ago pointed out that anxiety which has become free, the sexual origin of which is not remembered, changes to the general fear of animals, thunderstorms, darkness, etc.* Thus is often explained the vertigo on stairs and near precipices. I once climbed a mountain in company with a patient aged twenty-two years; the mountain was crowned by a terrace with a splendid outlook. My patient kept himself eight or ten steps from the balustrade and explained that he was subject to extreme vertigo. I bade him (experimentally) to

* Freud, Die Abwehr-Neuropsychosen. Kl. Schriften I, p. 53.

practice self-control but in spite of evident effort, he was held back. Then I commanded him to reflect upon what we had found in probing his anxiety in the presence of machines and horses (68) and left him to himself. Some seconds later, he stood beside me and quietly looked into the abyss. How are we to interpret such experiences if we deny that a sexually conditioned affect of anxiety which has arisen elsewhere, reinforced the insignificant asexual excitement?

Of pedagogic interest is the transposition of the feeling of guilt. The pupil described on pages 31 and 102 had stolen from his mother since he was six years old without having any remorse from so doing. At this point, he allowed himself to be seduced to onanism which he practised a single time in the morning before school. From that time, the sexual complex expressed itself in automatisms: For three weeks, he experienced every morning an automatic sexual act. To the onanistic activity, he ascribed no significance, on the other hand, since the slip into masturbation, his conscience has tormented him violently over the theft. Here we see the sexual anxiety transposed to another reaction of conscience.

There is not only crossing of affects but also such an one of emotions. One sees this best in a series of transpositions. I will be content with a clear example: A sixteen-year-old girl was brought for my pastoral treatment because of pathological grief, refractoriness to most housework, unmannerly behavior toward parents and melancholia. The sadness broke out continually in the society of children when any love-song was sung or danced. It was plainly evident that behind this, an affair of childhood lurked: When twelve years old, the little girl was in love and had been compelled in brusque manner under harmful reproaches to send her friend away. (During the grief which compelled violent weeping, she did not think of that event.) From the time of the departure of the friend, she hated the God of love whom she had named as protector of her tender covenant. This did not, however, prevent her from praying passionately to the creative power, but of God she would know nothing at all since the Bible said that God is love and love was loathsome to her.

The distaste for housework led to a great surprise. I asked: "Do you hate all housework?" and received the reply: "Yes, all." [Do you hate any particular work more than the rest?] "Yes. The most distasteful to me is dusting, setting in order, cutting the flowers and caring for canary birds." [What do you do less unwillingly?] "I am glad to set the table, make the beds, water the flowers and run errands." [Thus, it is cleaning work which excites you mostly to misbehavior?] "Certainly. But no, the flowers!" [What do you do with them?] "I must cut off the ends of the stems because the sap-canals are stopped up."

Here, the girl became greatly embarrassed. I knew that she had suffered since earliest childhood from severe constipation which had been combated with enemata and countless laxatives. Immediately, the girl grasped the connection between the difficulty of bodily purification and household cleaning work. How the causal connection is to be considered, we cannot now say. Enough, the stubborn little one yielded her anal-erotic gain of pleasure from enemata and hardened masses of feces and therewith also the symbolic expression of this repressed desire, the aversion to cleaning work and was changed with little trouble and to the astonishment of her family, into a proper, industrious little house-mother and reverent, obedient little daughter.

Further, the resentment transposed from love (and from the father) upon God disappeared very soon, together with the pathological sadness and the girl confessed great joy in the Christian God of love.

The girl felt entirely well for three months. Then her mother wished that the child might be freed from another bad habit which dated back many years. She was fond of tearing the skin from her thumb. I knew, naturally, what this habit betrayed, especially as the mother reported that her trying child had masturbated when eight years old. From extra caution and because the religious ethical relations left nothing more to be desired, I refused to treat this symptom although I must have known at that time that I was going out of the way of my pedagogic duty. A far more skilled neurologist than myself, to whom, however, my patient brought no frankness, succeeded in overcoming the obsessional movement by exceedingly arduous work. Yet scarcely had it ceased than the girl began to eat raw carrots with ravenous appetite. With enthusiastic gestures and exaggerated emotional expressions, she described the sweetness of carrots. Encouraged by the physician's example, I allowed the little one to find the sexual meaning of carrots, their symbolical identification with the finger, whereupon, the ravenous desire disappeared.

Somewhat later, during a violin concert, there awoke an ardent desire to learn to play this instrument. Asked for the motive, she openly confessed that she connected a curious feeling with the wish. She wished a violin, for as she remarked with enraptured, plainly erotic, facial expression, "One can put so much into it." Whoever is familiar with Swiss children knows what fiddle (Geige) means in their jargon. When the eager little daughter accompanied by her father, bought the violin, she began suddenly after a long remission to pull off the skin on her finger again so that even the most skeptical person must see how this automatism, the desire for carrots and playing a violin, betrayed the same unconscious, and that the same affect passed over to the different ideas. The pulling at the skin ceased at once again, for one manifestation relieved the other. When I showed the girl, who played very prettily on the piano, the meaning of her extravagant passion for the violin, this symptom disappeared also.*

Are we now warranted in speaking of transposition of emotion? Let us state the two criteria and postulates of causal connection established by us. As criteria, we found that of relationship by content and that of constant result. The synthetic postulate ran: The establishment of a causal connection

* Further examples by Freud, Kl. Schriften I, p. 54.

may contradict no other experiences concerning causal connection. The analytic postulate was that the dictum must be as simple as possible.

In our cases, we often saw an affect, for example, anxiety or consciousness of guilt, which belonged to one idea, split-off from it and appear attached to another idea. Here, the causal criteria and postulates of causal connection plainly coincide. At other times, we saw an emotion which would be enigmatical to the consciousness-psychology, disappear and another similarly inexplicable one appear. We have already recognized that the emotion does not reappear attached to any special favorite idea, but that the carrier of emotion must have some relationship (positive or negative) or even a relation of external association to the earlier idea. Of this we shall have more to say later. Enough! We find all the conditions at hand for the assumption of emotional transpositions.

The question may be asked whether instincts can also be transposed. The fact is that the hunger instinct, for instance, can act vicariously for the sexual instinct. One example, we have already seen. Inversely, the revulsion against sexuality may manifest itself in refusal to eat in general or against certain foods. Only the instinct itself is not transposed, but the particular instinct is joined to certain functions by the aid of particular organs. Rather, we will say in accordance with our explanation of the concepts, life-force (Lebensdrang) and instinct: The life-force invested in an activity of instinct devotes itself, as a result of a repression, to another activity. Therefore, instead of speaking of a transposition of instinct, we speak more correctly of a reversal or transposition of life-force.

Likewise, we consider the transference of emotion and affect as "new canalization" of the life-force. Only in this way, does it become comprehensible to us how mathematics or religion may attain an increase in emphasis as a result of sexual repression.

The transposition of emotions and affects is also an everyday phenomenon among healthy individuals so that Kronfeld's denial of its existence surprised me. Bleuler recalls the familiar phenomenon that the angry person is inclined to destroy things which are quite innocent of his affect; "the woman unhappy in marriage takes out her anger on the servant maid; she herself knows not at all the real cause of her dissatisfaction with her husband and seeks it in the conduct of the maid." * To what teacher are similar smuggling of affects unknown? One strikes the sack and means the donkey, one admires the beautiful toilette and transfers the admiration to the wearer, the old rheumatic patient transfers his rage over the pain upon the innocent cat. Is that really so absolutely new that Freud should be called theorist and juggler of terms?

Even the preanalytic psychology,† which certainly no one will accuse of any too keen perception, has noticed something related to transposition of emotion. Höffding observes that the same things and circumstances seem quite different to us according to our various moods. He formulated the statement: "The emotion does not change immediately with the ideas but spreads over the new ideas, even if these bear no relation to that which caused the emotion." ‡ This "expansion of emotion" is something different from the transposition by which the previous carrier of emotion is unburdened. Nevertheless, it approaches the phenomenon described by us. In Wundt's three-volume standard work, I could not discover even this much consideration of the poor emotional processes. On the other hand, Witasek recognizes an emotional transference of which he gives good examples: "An object which reminds me of a person dear to me, becomes likewise dear and precious, no matter how worthless it may be in itself. A place in which I may once have undergone a really disagreeable scene, inspires me at once when I come upon it again, with a mild discomfort, even if I do not recall that scene at all

---

* Bleuler, Die Psychoanalyse Freuds, Jahrb. II, p. 695.

† I would ask that the word analytic be understood as psychoanalytic. I am far from asserting that the prefreudian psychology did not analyze at all, it has really produced a series of such works, from which psychoanalysis itself has made grateful use.

‡ H. Höffding, Psychologie, Leipzig, 1893, p. 417.

clearly."* Ebbinghaus also calls the attachment between emotions and sensations and ideas, a free one; he recalls that to a person on a bitter winter day, everything feels gray, while on a pleasant spring day everything seems rosy.† But instead of going into the conditions of these variations in emotion in detail, he makes use of the vague statement that the particular nature of the emotions which attach themselves to sensations and ideas is outside the content of those influencing the relation of the objective emotional causes in the weal and woe of the mind.‡ Störring, in his investigations concerning the approval and disapproval in volition, develops the view that emotional states which have appeared in the experience of more remote effects of the will, may be transferred to the idea of a nearer effect of the same; ‖ his whole teaching of the summation-centers of emotions, so important for pedagogy, rests on transposition of emotion. Under summation-centers, he understands "intellectual processes (ideas and judgments), to which in the course of life, a great number of emotional states have attached themselves, so that with the reproduction of such ideas and the reappearance of such judgments, emotional experiences from the most diverse temporal divisions of the life come to re-echo." Thus for the individual with good intellectual and emotional endowment, the idea of the parents, then perhaps the idea of a friend, the idea of a life companion and in a religious individual, the idea of God would become summation-centers of emotion. I say: for the individual with good intellectual and emotional endowment, for the emotional states which have attached themselves in the course of life to those ideas and judgments, are, as one may easily see, set free only in smallest part or not at all by the ideas or judgments themselves, but are rather only transferred upon these

* Witasek, Grundlinien d. Psych. p. 340.
† H. Ebbinghaus, Abriss der Psychologie, 3rd ed. (Dürr) Leipzig, 1910, p. 78 f.
‡ Same, p. 79. Compare Ebbinghaus-Dürr, Grundzüge d. Psych. I, p. 562.
‖ G. Störring, Moralphilos. Streitfragen, Leipzig, 1903, I, p. 57.

ideas.* In this statement, a transposition of emotion is correctly described. Psychoanalysis added only the important invasion of repressed, thus unconscious, emotional energies and showed that the transplantation takes place also upon very much more remote ideas. Psychology which preceded psychoanalysis has recognized irradiation but not the transposition of emotion in its significance.

B. INTELLECTUAL MANIFESTATIONS

1. *Reductions (Anesthesia, Inattention, Amnesia).*

Like emotions, intellectual processes may also, under certain conditions, be inhibited, weakened or completely frustrated.

(a) **Anesthesia.** How an organ of special sense can be deprived of its functional capacity, was shown in a sufficient number of examples. I described complex-occasioned limitations or entire loss of sensation of sight (31, 175), hearing (96), tactile sensation in the toe (176). By far the most frequent phenomenon of this kind is the sexual anesthesia in women, which has such a fateful effect and devastates so many marriages. That it depends almost always upon repression and fixation, no one can deny, who investigates the unconscious of persons afflicted by it and eliminates the absence of sensation, which is often a very difficult task; the treatment of this condition need not be described in this pedagogic book. It is sufficient that the educator should know that this very serious evil depends on injurious influences which a correct education can avoid. In isolated observations, I found what Sadger asserts: "From my psychoanalytic results among sexually anesthetic women, I can assert that without exception the basis of lack of sexual feeling is formed by incestuous thoughts of the father which awakened at the time of puberty and then immediately underwent the sharpest suppression, that is, were completely forgotten." † In other cases, the sexuality has

* Same, p. 123.

† J. Sadger, Aus d. Liebesleben Nicolaus Lenaus, Leipzig and Vienna, 1909, p. 9.

been rendered loathsome as a whole or the husband was not really loved.

(b) **Inattention.** It is a known fact that one overlooks unloved persons much easier than loved ones. A striking example of inattention or overlooking is the following. A man of middle age discovered some years ago that he could no longer see the waning moon, while he often enjoyed watching the growing stars. He often undertook to look at the vanishing sickle but in spite of all resolutions, the attempt failed, since he regularly forgot his intention although every week in winter, he had to make a long journey at night just before sunrise. The analysis revealed the reason : The fugitive from the moon has a secret dread of every symbol of age and death. The waning moon reminds him of his own decline. The deeper motives remained hidden to him since he refused analysis. Thus he caught a glimpse of the waning moon only twice in the course of four years.

(c) **Amnesia.** In the example just quoted, we have observed besides the inadvertency, an amnesia, in that the resolution to look for the waning moon was always forgotten. Naturally, most forgetting depends on complexes. A repression in our sense does not take place, even though the narrowness of consciousness and the limitation of capacity for reproduction constantly make a separation. On a basis of analytic experiences, we conclude that there is a barring by resistance only where the forgetting is particularly striking.

A normal acquaintance in the home of a distant relative was asked for the address of his mother when to his astonishment, he could not recall the name of the street, although he used it every few days and frequently wrote it on letters. The analysis showed the forgetter that the first syllable of the lost word was the same as the name of his brother's fiancée. The mother furthered the engagement and often invited the young lady to her dwelling. Now, to the annoyance of the forgetful one, the engagement has been broken. The latter, at the solicitation of his mother, went to the seldom-visited relatives in whose presence the forgetting occurred. The relationship-complex was constellated by the vocation. The memory of the familiar street name remained absent because of the painful emotion which would have cropped out in this situation.

Above (181, 211), we mentioned a girl whose little brother burned himself in the laundry and who completely forgot the tragic event but remembered exactly how, shortly before, she sat on the steps and played with the child.

A young lady visited a book-store to buy ''Niels Lyhne'' by Jakobsen. To her astonishment, she could not think of the author's name. In its place, Petersen popped up, but she recognized this word as false. In the analysis, the name of the father of an editor friend came into her mind, which directed her to Jakobsen. That person was an intelligent but pedantic man who prevented his son from developing his poetic talent. Jakobsen likewise had to struggle to utilize his endowment. The young lady was herself a poetess and suffered from a pedantic father who hindered her mental development. She had seen that her infantile fixation on the once deified man must be given up. As a school girl, she passionately loved a cousin considerably older than herself, who read to her an article on Jakobsen. She freed herself from him because he was intimate with a married woman and turned out to be a woman-chaser. Finally, she came upon the thoughts, Petersen might be the given-name of the author of ''Neils Lyhne.'' Peter is correct.

As motive for repression, we recognize at once the intention to free the poet from his father as the girl would like to free herself and the editor friend from their fathers. She makes him, as it were, his own father by affixing to his forename, the ending, —sen. In addition, the one-time father substitute, who wrote the article on Jakobsen, is refused. Further determinants were not to be found since other matters seemed more important.

In very many psychoneuroses, an important event is split off and the analysis must remove a mass of obstacles from the way before the memory may become conscious. Often as we know, we are dealing only with phantasies in which repressed wishes hide. It is always amnesias, however, which lie at the bottom of the formation of neurotic symptoms.* Often, so-called cover-memories crowd forward which the skilled analyst may interpret as proof of a definite trauma. Often, it may be said with absolute certainty that this or that must have happened, perhaps in one of the first years of life, but the person being analyzed may not remember it, even though the parents confirm the surmise most decisively.

Very beautiful examples of forgetting occasioned by repression are afforded by Freud in his book, "Zur Psychopathologie des Alltagslebens." † To appreciate them properly, one must examine them in all their detail. Every abbreviation is a loss. I will give therefore, a not less instructive investigation by Jung: "A gentleman wishes to recite the familiar poem: 'Ein Fichtenbaum steht einsam, etc.' (A figtree stands alone.) In the line, 'Ihn schläfert' (He is sleepy), he was completely stuck, he had entirely forgotten 'mit weisser Decke' (with white covering). This forgetting in a verse so familiar seemed striking to me and I had him reproduce what he associated to 'mit weisser Decke.' The following series resulted: In a white covering, one thinks of a shroud—a linen cloth with which a corpse is covered—(pause)—Now, a close friend comes into mind—his brother has just died suddenly—he may have died of a heart attack—he was too corpulent—my friend is also corpulent and I have already thought it might also happen to him—he plainly takes too little exercise—when I heard of the sudden death, I suddenly became anxious lest it might also happen to me since we in our family likewise have a tendency to corpulence and further, my grandfather died of a heart attack; I am also too corpulent and have therefore in the last few days started in with a reduction treatment.‡ Thus the gentleman had unconsciously identified himself with the figtree which was covered with the white mantle."

* Freud, Psychopathologie d. Alltagslebens, p. 27.
† Freud, Same, pp. 1–23.
‡ Jung, Ü. d. Psychologie d. Dementia præcox, p. 64.

Of course Jung intentionally gives only the most important determinants. If the person being analyzed were sufficiently willing, one would certainly have come upon an infantile root in this case too.

In life and also in school-life, this simultaneous unintentional and intentional forgetfulness play a considerable rôle. A complicated example, but one which affords much insight, we gave on page 98 (missed rendezvous). When an analytic patient forgets the appointed hour, one never goes wrong in concluding that there is resistance against the analysis. In an evening party, the host went into another room to get some cigarettes for a guest. Nevertheless, he forgot his intention, visited the sleeping children and returned without the desired articles. A little analysis revealed the subconscious motive for this oversight. The guest owed his host a small sum of money and the creditor strove against asking for it. The repressed wish was able to obtain masked expression.

Just as much which analytic experience has brought to light had been recognized by keen observers by purely empirical and unscientific means in isolated cases, so the forgetting occasioned by discomfort had not escaped the attention of a brilliant discoverer. Darwin reports: "When I found a published fact, a new observation or a thought, which contradicted one of my general results, I noted it down word for word as soon as possible. For experience has taught me that such facts and results escape the memory easier than those which are pleasant to us."*

Still more clearly does Bulwer understand amnesia by repression. He says: "I repeat, therefore, it is an example of the all-destroying tyranny of everyday life that whenever a striking event disturbs the regular course of thought and endeavor, it hastens to bury in its sand the object which has become unpleasant to it; the mind cannot then push aside quick enough a riddle which may influence the reason pathologically; reason seeks to solve it, . . . and we are surprised how quickly

* Zentralblatt, f. Psychoanalyse I, p. 614.

such incidents, although they are not really forgotten, but can be voluntarily recalled again, . . . are, as you might say, repressed from the eye of the mind.'' *

Darwin and Bulwer thus have a presentiment of the mechanism of repression, though the former perhaps did not realize the extent of its field of application and the latter, its force which leads to complete forgetting.

Other examples may be found in the Zentralblatt für Psychoanalyse I, 407 (Freud), I-497 (Dr. Alfred Meisl), II-84ff. (Dr. Ernest Jones), II-632 (Dr. Karl Weiss), II-650 (Dr. Marie Stegmann), III-54f. (Dr. Jones).

2. Cover-Memories

An extraordinarily fine substantiation of the psychoanalytic exploration rule is to be found in the following circumstance: when a person is trying to recall a forgotten word or event, in the presence of too strong resistance against direct reproduction of the same and a stripping-off of the deviations upon constituent parts of the surroundings, an idea comes into his mind which is recognized as incorrect but which proves, upon closer inspection, to be related to the missing idea. Many times when memory is strained, an idea at once pops up which is considered the right one but really is not. In the second case, we speak of a cover-memory, since consciousness of a real memory is produced, while in the first instance, only a memory of a cover association.

Since none of my examples can compare with those of Freud, I shall this time borrow an illustration from him: Two men, one older than the other, who had traveled together six months previously in Sicily, were exchanging reminiscences of those beautiful and instructive days ''What was the name of the place'' asked the younger, ''where we passed the night in order to join the party to Selinus? Calatafimi, wasn't it?'' The elder refused this: ''Certainly not, but I too have forgotten

* Reported by Herbert Silberer, Zbl. I, p. 443.

the name although I remember very well all the details of our stay there. It suffices for me that I notice that when another has forgotten a name, immediately the forgetting is induced in me. Shall we not seek the name? No other occurs to me except Caltanisetta which is still certainly not correct." "No," says the younger, "the name begins with W or a W precedes it." "There is no W in Italian," replied the elder. "I meant V and said W because I am so accustomed to it in my mother-tongue." The elder struggled against the V. He said: "I think I have already forgotten many Sicilian names in general; it would be timely to investigate. What is the name of the place of high elevation which in ancient times was called 'Enna'? Oh, I know now, Castrogiovanni." The next moment, the younger had also found the lost name. He called out: "Castelvetrano," and rejoiced that the asserted V could be proven. The elder still missed for awhile the feeling of recognition; after he had accepted the name, however, he attempted to explain how it had escaped him. He said: "Plainly, because the second half, vetrano, sounded like veteran. I know already that I do not like to think of age and react in strange fashion when I am reminded of it. Thus, for example, not long ago I reproached a highly esteemed friend in most emphatic words with being long past the years of youth, because he had once said concerning me in most flattering words that 'I was no longer a young man.' My resistance to the second half of the name, Castelvetrano, proceeded also from the fact that the first sound of the same was inverted in the substitute word, Caltanisetta." And the name, Caltanisetta, itself? asks the younger. "That has always seemed to me like a pet name for a young woman," asserted the elder.

A little later, he added: "The name for 'Enna' was also only a substitute name. And now it occurs to me that this name, Castrogiovanni, sounds the same to giovane-young, as the lost name, Castelvetrano, to veteran, old."

The elder thought he had thus given the reasons for his forgetting of the names. From what motive the younger had come to the same exceptional phenomenon, was not investigated.*

In this beautiful example, various things are worthy of note. At first, it was not certain a priori that the forgetting was conditioned on a complex for it is nothing unusual when, a half year after an extensive journey, the name of a station is forgotten. But the one who forgot seems to have suspected the repression and this is important. It is interesting, how, that after the incorrect memory, the theme was left and transferred to another. And yet it approached the goal. Thus one proceeds in every analysis. Further, the circumstance that instead of the repressed word sought for (vetrano), its opposite cropped out, is often found. Even without being expressly mentioned, the cover word, "Caltanisetta" would be judged to have a repressed relation to a young woman and indeed a creature as sweet as ardent, since "Anisette" denotes a well known liqueur and "calt" contains the stem from "caldo" which denotes hot, hotblooded.

Whether with the younger man, we may detect from "Calatafimi" an emotional relation to some kind of "Galathe" we shall not investigate.

How important, a cover-memory can be pedagogically, a case from my practice will show. I treated a girl of fourteen and a half years for melancholia, severe stuttering and anxiety conditions. Even the first reaction-investigation pointed to the fact that the drunken foster-father maltreated the wife and children and had devastated the youth of the child. An enormous number of ugly scenes which had excited the hysterical child came to expression. The symptoms receded very beautifully. After four months of work (one to two hours a week), we stumbled on a phantasy which included the motive of the severest symptom, the stuttering.

The speech disturbance broke out on her first school-day. The child was terribly afraid of school, struggled to the street and had to be carried. Instead of the stern teacher she had

* Freud, Ein Beitrag zum Vergessen von Eigennamen. Zbl. I, p. 407 f.

been threatened with, the child found an extremely friendly woman teacher; nevertheless, she was so overcome with anxiety that she could not speak a word. The girl asserted now in the analysis that she had imagined at that time that beside every bench there was sitting on left and right a lion and a tiger and if a child arose or grasped at the pen-box, the beasts of prey hurled themselves on the transgressor to devour her.

Naturally, an intelligent girl of six and three quarter years can have had such an idea of school as little as Leonardo da Vinci, as a suckling in the cradle, had a phantasy of a vulture. Thus the phantasy must have been projected into that period.

. Even he who is not acquanted with the symbolism of lion and tiger may guess the approximate conditions of affairs when I make some further additions. The child had suffered at that time for some two and three quarter years from severe anxiety, uttered anxiety cries in sleep and crept under the bed while asleep. The father often came home drunk, late at night, the mother snatched her little daughter from the bed and fled from the monster to a neighbor's house. Often, she called to the raging man: "Don't roar like a lion or tiger!" The father repeatedly threatened the child: "Just wait until you come to a stern teacher in school, he will treat you quite differently from me!" In addition, other children utilized the child's anxiety for school and in jest related horrible things which were, however, taken in earnest. Thus the school became the embodiment of all that was terrible. The rough treatment on the first school-day brought the long-present hysteria to an open outbreak. How much suffering the rough measure brought on the girl, from whom, in her fifteenth year, no teacher could entice a word!

Before I interpreted the phantasy to the girl, she afforded a good substantiation of my assumption. In the night following her story, she dreamed she was pursued by a roaring lion and an elephant with uplifted trunk. From both animals appeared the figure of the father.

Unfortunately, the completion of the analysis did not occur. The recovery of the girl made splendid progress for a time, the stuttering, the headache, anxiety and melancholia disappeared almost entirely. Then a sudden deplorable change took place for the affairs at home became wretched.

The father, from whom the mother had lived apart for some years, again entered in his earlier rôle of tormentor of the family. The girl was constantly a witness of the intimacies of the parents who slept in the same room with her. The authorities intervened, the girl was cared for elsewhere and the analysis had to be interrupted.

We will later make the acquaintance of the lion and tiger symbols and therewith our causality requirement may be at least indirectly satisfied.

3. *"Déjà Vu"* (*Seen Before*)

Under a "déjà vu," one understands a falsification of memory in which the person thinks he has already experienced the present experience. The phenomenon is uncommonly widespread. In a mixed class of twenty-four pupils of seventeen years of age, I found sixteen who had had it; in a class of sixteen boys fifteen years of age, seven remembered having had it. Plato founds his theory of the preëxistence of the soul on this mysterious experience besides other grounds.

The analysis explains the phenomenon. Here, only one example which unfortunately I cannot show in its connection with other neurotic phenomena: It concerns a girl of thirteen and three quarter years who, upon her entrance into the women's clinic, was struck with the idea that she had certainly been there before and held fast to this belief although she saw the impossibility of this assumption. The feeling of acquaintanceship proceeds from a transposition: The pregnant girl had two years previously, in another clinic, met a man, swollen presumably with small-pox, by whom she was afraid of being infected. This patient she compared with her father who had once been similarly sick and swollen. Now she was herself as pregnant, an infected, swollen person, of course not by that patient or the father who was joined to him as a unity but probably by her elder brother who held in the family the position of the father who was now dead. Thus far, the feeling of recognition has its good ground; only, it is falsely transferred from the painful condition of the pregnant one to the idea of place instead of being applied to the proper condition. I can also give a further determinant of the déjà vu. Asked to describe the locality and give her associations to it, the patient reported: "The feeling of recognition appeared beside a long bench which stood in the hall. We had a similar one in the kitchen. Otherwise nothing." [More.] "I remember that at home I was often teased on account of a little episode. When I was five years old, I sat one day on that bench, laid my hands in my lap and sighed. The maid asked me the reason. I answered: 'I am thinking over whom I shall later marry.'" The marriage question must have occupied the girl much during her pregnancy. It is therefore very probable that right by the bench, the déjà vu came to pass. The scheme familiar to us: "It is now as at that time" came into application.*

4. Hypermnesia

It often happens that an apparently insignificant event is held by the memory with astounding tenacity. One finds as cause that that reproduced experience bears an important analogy at the moment of remembering and further that additions of libido have come to it by repression. The girl mentioned on page 221, who recalled how when three years old she played on the steps with her little brother, pushed this reminiscence forward because she wished to hide the consciousness of guilt for spiteful hatred. The picture of innocent playing children would deck the repressed death-wish with a mantle of love. Now and then, a real experience of slight importance gains, by symbolic interpretation, an important value.

Ludwig Binswanger has presented us with beautiful examples in his instructive "Analyse einer hysterischen

* Freud gives other examples in his Psychopathologie d. Alltagsleb.

Phobie''* (Analysis of an hysterical phobia). A girl of twenty years recalled that when five and three quarters years old, she saw how her boot-heel had become loose. This, in itself, certainly insignificant occurrence gained deep importance from the fact that a series of most important thoughts reposed in that idea. The most powerful longing, the most intense remorse, birth phantasies, death wishes, maximum love and hate, an unbelievably widespread material was concentrated in the separating boot-heel.

Other examples are found among the cover-memories and above on page 41 ("Pentakosiomedimnen"), under Chapter XII, 6b: dream of the Duchess of Angoulême, as well as in my article: "Kryptolalie und Kryptographie bei Normalen." †

It often happens also that an idea has disappeared from memory, which cannot be wondered at much, but has reappeared as manifestation, for example, as obsessional idea or dream.

5. The Regression

If internal or external obstacles block the path of an active instinct, the libido flows backwards. The backward-flowing movement is called regression. It appears in various forms. It is always a return to the infantile (status) and indeed either the material bringing to life of juvenile ideas, emotions and strivings or the formal renewing of forms of activity which were suitable for the juvenile stage.

a. The regression to infantile contents (mental). This is often conscious. Persons who see no hope before them and are inhibited in their endeavors, busy themselves much with their childhood, for example, persons who are aged and seriously ill. Much more frequent still is the subconscious return to the first years of life.

When we dug out the infantile roots of the neurosis, we saw old events in the significance of the determinants of the pres-

* L. Binswanger, Analyse einer hyster. Phobie, Jahrb. III, pp. 228–308.

† Jahrbuch V, p. 142 ff.

ent condition. I described particularly plain examples in my investigations of religious glossolalia and automatic secret writing.* I give below the analysis of the first speech of a religious fanatic aged twenty-four. It runs:

"Esin gut efflorien meinosgat schinohaz daheit wenesgut när wossalaitsch enogaz to lorden hat wuschenehat menofeite lor; si wophantes menelör gut menofeit hi so met dä lör."

Most of the words call forth associations without difficulty which I repeat in the following paragraphs:

1. [Esin.] Nothing.

2. [Gut.] My grandfather always said I was a good boy. When a child, I always had the word good (gut) in my mouth, for example, good mother, good apple. (I left this word too quickly.)

3. [Efflorien.] My father's employer once said he would take me with him to Florence. That made me glad. When I was prevented, I was disappointed. [Efflorien.] Perhaps I have a dim recollection: That gentleman said, in Florence we shall visit the zoo, there we will see an elephant. "Eff" refers to elephant. The elephant in Basel is still fresh in my mind: When we were standing in front of him, he took the hat off a girl and stamped on it.

4. [Meinosgat.] Something quite clear comes to mind: When eleven years old, I lost a very dear friend by name of Oskar, whose death overwhelmed me, so that I went around for awhile like a shadow. [Meinosgat.] I said "Osgar" not Oskar. [At.] I often accompanied him to a studio (Atelier) in which I admired the beautiful things.

5. [Schinohaz.] Refers to my school time. We had a teacher who beat us terribly and made us learn fearfully. Once I said to a friend: "Der Lehrer tue einem fast das Herz 'abschinegeln.'" That is a common expression in that region. My friend complained of me to the teacher who gave me four blows. "Haz" refers to heart. I was also fearfully

* Jahrbuch III, also separate imprint by Deuticke, Leipzig and Vienna, 1912.

tormented by the boys because I went to the meetings. They persecuted me, fleeced me of my goods.

6. [Daheit.] Perhaps also on account of school time. We had a new pupil who was always saying: "Da heit me gseh" (Swiss colloquialism meaning "Da hat man gesehen" = There was seen), "da heit me gha" ("gehabt" = had), etc. We found this funny; we rushed after him calling "Da heit, da heit." He turned and struck me on the ears.

7. [Wenesgut.] My mother was always saying, for instance, to a good report: "If it goes well, the father will give you thus and so." Once I received from a teacher an honor-reward of two francs for the best composition, another time I won a first prize in climbing. More often, however, it did not go well; in a swimming race, I would have been drowned in the middle of a pond if someone had not helped me. [När] I think that belongs to the following.

8. [Närwossalaitsch.] That is a little difficult. I think of everything so childish. We once had a visit from a negro who spoke his mother tongue. Each of us pupils would repeat something after him. I was nine or ten years old. Perhaps the word given (närwossalaitsch) was among those words. All the others could repeat a little piece, I could not. I was afraid of the negro on account of his teeth and lips. He had a beautiful watch of which I was very covetous. In general, I longed for everything which I saw. That was a great vice. I was often tempted to steal. Now, no longer.

9. [Enogaz.] Might one associate this word with a cat? When I was eleven years old, we four comrades went over the country and came across a cat. Two put it in a bag and explained that they would strike and kill the animal. My comrade and I protested but they did the deed nevertheless. We turned around at once and informed the teacher about it. [Eno.] Might one not write that, eine (= one)?

10. [To lorden (English expression from lord).] The "lord" reminds me of an experience from my thirteenth year. Because of nervous weakness and pains in all the nerves, I had

been taken out of school. A distinguished English preacher came along and delivered a sermon in which the ever-recurring word "lord" struck me. He spoke also of the Lord Mayor of London and his splendor. The latter, he compared with the glory of heaven. This impressed me powerfully. I read also in a newspaper of a lord. My mother taught me, however, that God is greater than all the lords of England. I dreamed from that, that I also possessed that splendor.

11. [Hat.] I think that word stands for itself. My grandfather took me once into a church tower. While he was ringing the bell, the clapper struck me on the head and I was almost killed. Hereupon, I was dismissed with a stick. That, I have always before my eyes. [Hat.] I think of "hat" as "hat gethan" (have as have done). (Postscript five months later: Evil mouths persecuted me at the time of the speaking with tongues, but their effort reached me not.)

12. [Wuschenehat.] Wusch means wash. We had a servant maid whose name reminds me of the second and third syllables of the word. Once she played with me during the washing and the linen scorched. That caused a great fuss because of which, she left us. I was innocent.

13. [Menofeite.] Is not that an English word? It seems to me that I have heard it in the previously mentioned English sermon, still it is quite hazy to me. "Men" is English, for instance, good man = guter Mann. [Menofeite.] Now it comes to mind. The Englishman spoke of different sects, also of that of Mrs. White, then of the religious war between Spain and England and of the destruction of the Spanish fleet. By this, he wished to show that we also have to fight with invisible forces. [Mrs. White.] The Adventist. I find she cannot defend her position. Many Adventists wished in vain to convert us. The Englishman called them dependent because they were led by women. My mother was angry at this because she felt herself attacked.

14. [Lor.] If it is "Lora," I can interpret it. The employer of my father had a horse named Lora with which I was

very friendly when a child. One day it kicked when the groom tormented it and hit me on the leg. [Si.] I can't make anything out of that.

15. [Si wo.] Perhaps that refers again to a child's game. One day we played hide and seek. "Si wo" means: "See, where are you!" I lost myself in the forest and wandered around for three hours.

16. [Phantes.] Phantasy. The teacher scolded us when we spoke falsely: "You phantasy." Once he wrote under a composition: "Nice phantasy." That bothered me.

17. [Menelör.] Mene, is it? One might translate that, meine (= mine). In the factory, I helped my father on a Saturday afternoon. There I had to pass with needles through lowries, that is, trucks. A needle point penetrated deep into my finger and broke off. The physician could get it out only with difficulty.

18. [Gut.] As before. If it was good. [Gut.] At a wedding feast, I retained the cover after each course. Suddenly I had a whole stack of eating utensils lying about me and was laughed at so much that I was fearfully embarrassed.

19. [Menofeit.] That, we have already had. "Man of the White." The mother said afterwards that she did not think it proper for the Englishman to be so personal, one might also expose much among his adherents. [Hi.] Nothing.

20. [Hiso.] A half-witted workman in the factory always said: "Hi, hi" and "So, so." The others mimicked him, I, however, protected him.

21. [Met.] One might translate it: mit (with). Once I went out with my father and the baby carriage. When we were far from home, a heavy hail storm came up. We could still quickly find shelter in a barn. Tiles and windows were broken. We were greatly afraid.

22. [Da lör.] Again the scene in the factory. The chief severely reprimanded my father because he gave me such a difficult task. Since then I can no longer do it.

Later additions:

1. [Esin.] I could almost trace that back to recent time.

When I expressed doubt concerning the speaking with tongues, one accused me of being an intellectual fancy-monger. ''Esin'' means ''ein Sinn'' and refers to the fact that I will brood over everything with my mind.

2. [Gut.] I worked on a written article, the conclusion of which I did not find for a long while. Now, however, all is well.

3. [Efflorien.] The journey to Florence came to naught like the elephant's hat.

4. [Meinosgat.] Memory of my friend Oskar.

Since the subsequent words brought nothing new to light, I broke off, certainly much too early to gain the complex which was already peeping through and to which the various associations point back as to the common point of convergence, as the rays which break forth behind a wall, in spite of their diverging directions, point to a central place. I asked therefore: [Has a common characteristic of all your associations become clear to you?] All concern the period of my youth. [Pleasant experiences?] No, rather unpleasant. [Certainly, only all finally turn out well. What do you say now? Do you wish to console yourself with that, because at present you have trouble on your heart?] It is so! I am in trouble because of my future, my existence. I have an inclination to study, to have a theological education and do not know how to begin. Thus I suffer from a constant internal strife.

From results which we will later submit to the reader, we assume the right to formulate the meaning of the regressions to childhood in the following manner:

Word in secret speech	Idea conditioned by complex	Relief for complex
1. Esin	I foster doubts of my secret speech.	Never mind. Only your brooding mind doubts.
2. gut	They doubt my kindness of heart (necessary in ministerial profession) (later expressly confirmed).	You were always a good son and man.

3. efflorien — The disappointment regarding Florence; an unlucky man cannot study. — Nothing to it; it was only as if an elephant destroyed a hat.

4. meinosgat — You poor thing, you lost your truest friend. — You possess the true heart necessary for a minister. (Over-compensation for internal accusations of unworthiness for the profession.)

5. schinohaz — Persecution by teacher and fellow pupils. — I was innocent, suffered for my uprightness and pious conviction.

6. daheit — Persecution by fellow pupils. — There was no guilt, only harmless jest.

7. wenesgut — Misfortune in a swimming race. — Fortunate salvation from death; virtuous deeds.

8. närwossalaitsch — Deficient talent in speaking, covetousness. — Genius for secret speech. Freedom from covetousness.

9. enogaz — Persecution by fellow pupils, deficient authority among comrades. — You suffer on account of your fondness for animals.

10. to lorden — Ambition, love of splendor. — Now I long only for the Lord of Heaven.

11. hat — You were careless in a church and came into mortal danger. — That childish carelessness has long been atoned for. (The verb denotes in Swiss German the preterite, for which in this dialect, there is no simple form; perhaps there is also a contraction of "hart" since there may be a play on the harshness of the bell striking on the head.)

12. wuschenehat   The dallying with a   The guilt was entirely
                  girl brought unpleasant   on the girl's part.
                  things.

13. menofeite   I allow myself to be di-   I have refused the Ad-
                  rected by women and am   ventists directed by a
                  accordingly   dependent.   woman, thus am inde-
                  (This reproach appears   pendent; for the rest,
                  plainly later.)   that reproach against
                  those   influenced   by
                  women is exaggerated.

14. lor   You suffered a misfor-   The groom alone was
                  tune from a trusted   guilty, the misfortune
                  horse.   had a good ending.

15. si wo   I am in the wrong.   I corrected myself.

16. phantes   My phantasy was des-   (Phantasy is also a val-
                  pised.   uable talent.)

17. menelör   My clumsiness in the   That work which was
                  factory injured me.   too hard for your age
                  should not have been
                  assigned to you.

18. gut   You have already made   That was only a social
                  a fool of yourself.   bagatelle.

19. monofeit   You   are   ruled   by   Others have perhaps
                  women.   still greater faults.

20. hiso   You were mocked as a   You have gallantly taken
                  fool.   the part of the feeble-
                  minded, hence the mock-
                  ery against you.

21. met   A storm threatened.   You were protected.

22. dä lör   Again the accident with   It was not mine, but my
                  the lowries.   father's mistake.

The memory of one-time adversities and the harmless character of these is plainly called forth as in dream, hallucination,

hysterical symptom, obsessional neurotic phenomenon and other automatisms by present needs which possess similarity to those infantile experiences. It is not difficult to derive these present tormenting impressions which have taken flight in the secret speech and there manifest themselves in suggestive manner from the secret speech.

The thinking of our subject is forced back into childhood by the circumstance that the young man sees himself inhibited in his career. He must satisfy himself with his infantile repressions. His wish is plainly to become a regular minister. Against this wish, there arise grave doubts which, under the threshold of consciousness, awaken memories of youthful experiences, which memories, by the relationship of these experiences to the present situation, seemingly strengthen those doubts; but by the favorable outcome of the experiences and upon closer consideration, the memories support the opposite view, indeed, at times, change into fortunate results supporting the present wish.

In brief, the secret speech says: You possess the necessary religious, moral and intellectual qualifications to be able, with God's help, to become a minister in spite of persecution and misfortune. That in delusion, all earlier ideas of a person are reflected, has already been recognized by the poet Hebbel.*

When we have opportunity to analyze thoroughly the dreams and manifestations of normal individuals, we find constantly, such infantile traces, to which they have gone back because the present was opposed to a passionate wish.

Poetry is full of such regressions. In Johann Schlaf's "Frühling," we read these lines: "Here I lay, now, under my hawthorn, playing and wandering to my heart's content." "And now I am a child again." "Putting the head deeper in the grass. Now making my longing, perceiving mind smaller and ever smaller and now I am quite wee small again." † Does this not remind us of Jung's patient in the

---

* F. Hebbel, Tagebücher Vol. I, 3 (March 29, 1835).

† Cited by Richard Hamann, Der Impressionismus in Leben u. Kunst. Köln, 1907, p. 92.

climacteric, who felt as if her arms and legs were all the time growing smaller and who wished to be carried and felt how she let herself go?* Hebbel says very truly in his "Genoveva": "It is life's worst malady to still know what we were, when we are that no longer. There, would we creep back into our roots, but in vain." †

This longing often expresses itself as longing for the mother with those who strive against the delusion, for example, Hölderlin and Lenau.‡

Further, infantile acts are resumed in the regression. A gentleman, aged thirty-six, who was undergoing analysis on account of impotence, reports that he brought candy home to his wife, something he had never done during a married life of ten years and afterwards regarded as childish. The forces of libido freed in the analysis, he cannot at once utilize properly. As a child, he often brought his mother similar delicacies.

An important variety of the process under discussion is the symbolizing regression. Freud gives the following example of this phenomenon: "In the parent-complex, we recognize the root of the religious need; the almighty, just God and kindly Nature seem to us to be perfect sublimations of the father and mother, still more as renewals and restorations of the early infantile conceptions of these two persons. Biologically, the religious life goes back to the long persisting helplessness and need for assistance of the little human child, who, when he has later recognized his real destitution and weakness in comparison with the great force of life, feels his position just as in childhood and seeks to deny his wretchedness by the regressive renewal of infantile protective measures." ||

Thus, this would be a regression which sets up, instead of the infantile parent-image, a symbolical representative of the same. From this circumstance, follows the very important fact that

---

* Riklin, Wunscherfüllung u. Symbolik im Märchen, page 13.
† Hebbel, Genoveva, Act III, Scene 4.
‡ Lenau, Sonette (Der Seelenkranke.)
|| Freud, Leonardo, 57. I scarcely need to add that I cannot consider the problem of religious truth as solved therewith.

the contents of the regression do not necessarily disclose former ideas and wishes but later elaborations and investments of these ideas and wishes. Nothing prevents, therefore, considering incestuous regression ideas as such and interpreting them the same as other symbols so long as the infantile incestuous wish is not shown to be an universal human factor. On this point, more exact investigations are to be awaited.

b. Regression to Infantile Forms of Activity

The child is not capable of a scientific mode of thinking. He thinks in pictures, likenesses. The adult, too, who goes in pursuit of scientific prey is, under circumstances when he does not attain his goal, thrown back upon this infantile thinking in pictures; such circumstances are fatigue, weakness from disease or toxins, for example, alcohol) and other injuries to consciousness. For a beautiful example, we are indebted to Alfred Robitsek who subjected one of the most important of the more recent discoveries in the field of chemistry, that of the benzol ring by Kekulé to an analytic investigation. Kekulé described at the twenty-fifth anniversary of that discovery, how he sank into a dreamy state on the roof of an omnibus: The atoms flitted about before me, many times two smaller ones joined to form a pair, larger ones embraced two smaller, still larger, three and even four. He spent part of the night in putting this dream structure on paper and thus sprang into existence the celebrated structural theory. It happened similarly with the benzol theory: Again the atoms danced before his dreaming eyes. A snakelike movement began. "And see, what was that? One of the snakes seized his own tail and mockingly whirled the structure before my eyes. I awoke as by a stroke of lightning; this time too, I needed the remainder of the night to work out the consequences of this hypothesis." * The great chemist added wittily: "Let us learn to dream, gentlemen, then perhaps we shall find the truth;

* A. Robitsek, Symbol. Denken in der chem. Forschg. Imago I, 83–90.

"And he who thinks not,
To him it is sent,
He has it without trouble."

but let us guard against publishing our dreams until they have been tested by the waking reason."*

Silberer, who first investigated this kind of hypnoid hallucinations, describes the mechanism in these words: "The psychic content produced by the meditation, or in broader sense, by the disturbance, is perceived, because of the sleepy confusion, not in the form corresponding to its normal apperception, but in a distinct picture converted into a symbol and hallucinated as such in accord with the circumstances. These autosymbolical phenomena constitute fatigue phenomena and a regression from a difficult mode of thought to an easier, more primitive type. This process, which is called according to Freudian terminology, "regression," denotes a displacement from an abstract form of thought to a pictorial form and from the apperceptive train of thought to the associative." †

This regression can also be called reversion. In the fully conscious waking state, stimuli proceed from the object to the organ of perception, join subconscious mental activities and lead to motor discharges. In the hallucinatory dream, according to Freud, the excitation takes a regressive course, spreading out over the sensory part of the apparatus instead of the motor part, and finally ending in the system of perceptions.‡ Even the intentional memory has regressive characteristics, only it does not create like the dream, pictures animated in hallucinatory fashion. "We call it regression when the idea in the dream changes back into the sensual picture from which it has once proceeded." || That the infantile wishes are also thereby awakened in pictorial form in the sleeping-room of memory, has already been explained.

We find this functional regression in the dream, in the hal-

* Same, p. 87.
† Herbert Silberer, Phantasie u. Mythos. Jahrb. II, p. 605.
‡ Freud, Traumdeutung, p. 362.
|| Freud, Traumdeutung, p. 363. Witz, p. 138.

lucination, in the waking phantasy, while the regression of content takes place unconsciously all the time when certain conditions are fulfilled.

The necessity and biological significance of regression is shown in two directions. Causally: One can show that the repressed wishes of childhood remain preserved in the disposition and manifest themselves upon every opportunity. Teleologically: One may point out that the unity of the personality can remain intact only on condition that the libido continually goes back to the initial stage of life.* Finally: The interests of the present, the acute wishes and needs seek to derive hope and consolation from the memory of analogous experiences, long past, which had favorable terminations. Our childhood contains the deposits on which we draw when the present oppresses us. But hate which gets intoxicated in plans for revenge, envy and jealousy also draw their strength from the infantile stage. Childhood is no Garden of Eden, where only beautiful flowers and spicy fruits grow. It is a forest which harbors besides the strawberries, the deadly nightshade, besides the roe, the wolf. It is of immeasurable importance for a human life, whether the ever-recurring enforced retreat into the land of childhood presents friendly or hateful pictures for contemplation. Richard Wagner expresses this purpose of regression sharply and clearly in these words: "All our wishes and ardent inclinations, which, in truth, carry us over into the future, we seek to fashion from pictures of the past into sensual perceptibility in order to gain for ourselves the form which the modern present cannot furnish them." †

* G. F. Lipps rightly says: "Our consciousness gives us simultaneously with the perception of passing present events, memories of the past, and on a basis of such memories, puts much before our eyes which we expect only from the future. It is, however, also dependent on all that which we experience and have experienced, without our having emphasized it separately and been able to distinguish it from other material. Thus it gains a quality which characterizes our whole design in its unified existence and reveals itself as the feeling in which our personality, our ego, finds expression." (Das Problem der Willensfreiheit, p. 80.)

† O. Rank, Die Lohengrinsage, p. 134.

While the free individual experiences from his contact with his childhood no inhibition to his forward striving, the psychoneurotic remains stuck in the regression to the infantile. We could see this in particular where we penetrated to childhood. If we investigate a refractory person who seeks quarrels with all in authority, we find as root of the trouble, the regression to the attitude of defiance which the child assumed toward his father and the fixation in this fatal infantilism. One can call the psychoneurosis a regressive attachment or fixation in the regression.

The pedagogic problem which the analysis forces upon us, is therefore illuminated from a new standpoint: separation from the bonds of childhood, release from infantilism, so far as these influence the control of the present and conquest of the future, becomes a problem, on the mastery of which, much of happiness and value in life depends.

c. The Atavistic Regression

Freud recognized that in dreams and similar products of the mental life, structures recur which correspond both in content and origin to the mythological creations of primitive periods. He thinks it probable that myths correspond to the distorted wish phantasies of whole nations, the secular dreams of young humanity.* In the dream and in the neurosis, he again finds the savages, the primitive men with the peculiarities of their mode of thought and of their affect life. † Jung, in particular, perceived that in the delusional structures of dementia præcox, the old mythology and archaic philosophical speculation recurs. This agreement became so certain upon extended investigations that he ventured to interpret mythology from phenomena observed in patients and vice versa. The revivification, he considers not a material one but only a functional one, so that archaic traces of memory might yield their memories to those suited to them. The neurotic producing archaic

* Freud, Der Dichter u. d. Phantasieren. Kl. Schriften II, p. 205.
† Freud, Nachtrag zu d. autobiogr. beschrieb. Fall von Paranoia. Jahrbuch III, p. 590.

content is in a psychological constellation similar to that of the son of antiquity, hence he creates strikingly similar formations. These extraordinarily keen investigations, executed with great sharpness of vision and astounding scholarship, owe their origin to insight won by analysis.* But in this as in so many other questions which we seek to solve in this book, it turned out afterwards that superior students of humanity, especially poets and philosophers, had even earlier perceived the true state of affairs. Nietzsche had already formulated the statement: "In sleep and dream, we perform the whole task of early humanity" . . . "The dream brings us back again to the distant states of human culture and provides us a means for better understanding them." †

This problem, which the application of biogenetic basic principles to the mental development proposes, is not of sufficient pedagogic importance to warrant my devoting a detailed discussion to it.

Every neurosis is a manifestation of infantilism, not only because it constantly revives infantile phantasies but also because it represents an infantile form of functioning. Hence the task of healing the neuroses is the conquest of the infantilism, of the regression to childhood and the abolition of this anachronism.

6. *The Condensation*

If we apply the analytic basic principle (page 8) to a manifestation, we gain material which greatly exceeds that manifestation in extent. Often, an apparently incidental trait of the complex-product points to an important episode or phantasy. Therein, one and the same sign has for determinants a whole series of reminiscences or other ideas, so that behind the "manifest content," there lurks a number of "latent com-

---

* Jung lays weight on the circumstance that he did not construct his libido-theory from mythological studies but found in these studies, a confirmation of the insight into the processes of the libido gained empirically.

† Nietzsche, Menschliches, Allzumenschliches. Cited by Jung, Wandlungen u. Symbole der Libido. Jahrb. III, p. 142.

plex thoughts,'' unconscious motives, and hence also, many interpretations are necessary in order to reveal exhaustively the mental content of the manifestation. Such formations are called stratifications. One is often much surprised at what an extensive material may spring from a very simple complex-formation as sum of motives.

In every manifestation, a condensation work comes to expression. This is most striking to external observation when contents are imposed on one another which in reality do not belong together at all, it may be that one single figure is created from heterogenous characteristics (composite figure), it may be that one complete act is executed in unrelated, mutually inappropriate sections. Such condensation formations often appear downright comical. This ludicrous result of many a condensation cannot surprise us for one whole group of witticisms depends on condensation.

(a) THE COMPOSITE FORMATION

We have already seen examples of such mental action. I call to mind, for instance, the vision of the devil (page 38). My patient recognized in the devil, who was at first unfamiliar, the hair and rough hands of his enemy whom he had called a devil, then the nose of a girl concerning whom the evil fellow had maligned our hallucinating patient. In reality, the nose did not suit a strange face at all. As expression of the unconscious wish: ''May you carry with you in your face the mark of shame for your desire for calumny!'' it is in its right place.

Wherever in dream or other manifestations, there appears an unknown figure, a strange face, a phantastic object, a senseless word-formation or the like, there is almost always condensation. In general, the analysis succeeds wherever it is applied in dissolving these false structures into well-known memories and the phantastic elaboration of these. An internal connection between the characteristics apparently thrown together so senselessly, will never be lacking in such cases.

Freud made the discovery that those portions of the manifestations which appear most persistently, do not betray the places behind which the strongest masses of affect lurk, but that in which the most concentrated condensation-work occurred.*

The pupil mentioned on page 67, who frankly admitted her hatred of her parents and brothers, suffered, every evening, from severe anxiety. Frequently, she hallucinated a man who disappeared behind her bed. She could not describe him clearly but had the impression that she did not know him. The eyes were exactly like those of a boy three years older than herself, who, eight years before, had seduced her, and in company with her brother and one of his school comrades had repeatedly misused her sexually. Other features, especially beard and stature, belonged to a man of forty years with whom she had become acquainted not long before, still others to her grandfather and the analyst. The patient was fond of masochistic and sadistic dreams: she is undressed by her naked father, tormented on the table and whipped. In the first weeks of the treatment, she brought the analyst into her phantasies in astonishingly numerous and clever devices. For the past two years, she has observed almost every night the sexual intercourse of her parents, to which the mother interposed vigorous objection. On these occasions, the girl displayed a rage at her father and a strong orgasm which she was accustomed to call forth voluntarily by day.

Also in waking life, she condensed constantly: Father, grandfather, teacher and analyst plainly have for her the eyes of her seducer, even though they differ according to the testimony of the girl, in color, size and position from those of that person. The reason for this condensation consisted in the fact that for the young catatonic patient, being looked at is toned with the strongest sexual emotions, corresponding to her unfortunate past. All the persons united in the composite figure belong together as libido-objects and form a unit for her. A longer analysis would certainly have traced back still other characteristics of the hallucination to their real origin in the

* Freud, Traumdeutung, p. 260,

longed-for men. But the case was far too serious to allow psychological curiosity to dwell on the phenomenon too long. There was also a condensation in the circumstance that for years the patient could only think of men as having erect penises: She combined the pictures of the young seducer, some exhibitionists whom she wished to have seen and of her father with those of other male persons. Jesus alone formed an exception: He was the only man who did not come into consideration as a sexual being.

When, after some months, the hallucinations recurred, simultaneously with the anxiety, religious phantasies began to be formed which bore almost visionary distinctness. The girl saw God whom she could not endure, standing in the air while she was most glad to pray to the Savior. His facial features changed from hour to hour or even during the consultation, so that for a time, the analysis was almost entirely spent in deciphering these astonishingly condensed features which were extraordinarily productive in religious psychological meanings.

I can give only a few sketches. At first, God appeared as human-like figure, some two meters in height, standing above a forest. His features were similar to those of an "old" (fifty years) cousin on her father's side, a stingy, bigoted pietist whom she hated even more than most other men. He contributed to the God-picture the dark features, the brown skin, the eyes and particularly the eyebrows. But the mother also contributed: the flabby face musculature of the phantasy figure came from her. The beard belonged to a St. Nicholas and to old Pastor J. The eyebrows pointed somewhat to the younger Pastor C. The nose was entirely that of the analyst.

In explanation, it may be added: The patient knows of God, who was always described to her as "father," only unpleasant things: He changed Lot's wife, who had only turned around quickly, into a pillar of salt. He sent a plague of locusts. Both narratives the girl has extensively elaborated: She herself like Lot's wife had turned around in unallowed manner in order to observe her parents. The pillar of salt resembled an iron maiden in which men were killed. In this phantasy was reflected the truly demoniacal hatred of the child for the masculine world. The plague of locusts reminded the little patient of how such insects jumped under her skirt and clung to her legs, of which she was violently afraid. The girl called God mean in full consciousness because he left her burning desire for sexual pleasure unsatisfied. The child, who for the rest seemed to be a model of propriety and innocence, told me soon after the beginning of the analysis that she had firmly decided a long time ago to yield herself sexually to the first boy or man that came along. Only after elimination of the anxiety, could the gross desire of the girl, who deep down was good-natured but corrupted by sexual brutality in childhood and misdirected pedagogy of her parents, be directed to higher paths.

Behind the stingy cousin, naturally lurked the likewise supposedly miserly, but in reality often financially embarrassed father, who constantly preached morality (and for the rest, was a very virtuous, upright man).

The flabby cheeks of God, plainly marked by a wrinkle, reminded her of how the mother in a severe illness, five years before, seemed to die. St. Nicholas was not long taken earnestly. Soon, he became only a comic figure. The old Pastor J. was a tiresome, infirm man who probably had not long to live. The young Pastor C. was hated because of his strictness. The analyst showed the sign of the so-called "negative transference" (see below), that is, he had to bear the hatred which is really thought against the persons mentioned in the analysis. Plainly, he should, like the father, mother, cousin, St. Nicholas and the two pastors, come to God and be taken away from earth. Again the hypocritically pious wish which we found in the vision of the angel (37). For what better can anyone wish a person than that he should be with God?

After this exploration, for some days, the phantom appeared blasphemous with funny face but this grimace was also easily removed by analysis. There followed a picture of God which took the sun as subject. The body had disappeared, the hairs stood out like a halo. The face was totally different. Its expression recalled that of a bird of prey, then further that of Pastor L. and still further those of Calvin and Bonnivard. The beardlessness corresponded with that of her grandfather and that of a Mormon she knew. The eyes were those of the avaricious Itzig in Freytag's "Soll und Haben."

The aspect of this new God was plainly entirely new. His psychic content has remained about the same as of old. The halo was associated with the hair of a little devil or of Peter Scrubby. Thus, scorn for God still prevails.

Pastor L. is a prominent preacher but a fanatic and enemy of enlightenment like Calvin who also proclaimed a gloomy God. Bonnivard lived for years as a prisoner chained to a pillar. The patient wished this fate upon all figures who were banished in the God phantasy. The pastor was likewise old like her father and cousin. The mother greatly revered him. Before he was associated with God's picture, he had been very ill and became helpless. Helpless also was the grandfather represented in the picture of God, who was always glad to admonish and preach. The Mormon was a rough peasant who had a pious countenance, did unbelievable things and spoke of being in love with canary birds but wished to entice quite different birds. The grandfather also spoke of being in love with the caged bird. The avaricious Itzig again emphasized a prominent trait of the old cousin.

Again there was crammed into the idea of God, fanaticism, gloomy nature, nagging, tiresome moralizing, avarice and to that a mean opinion. As punishment, helplessness appeared and again perhaps death. Hatred toward other people was thus set free on God.

I pass over the subsequent transformations. After some further attempts to save the blasphemous phantasies, these disappeared completely. The healing, however, came to pass only later.

Plain condensation work was executed by the unconscious, as we have mentioned, in a category of witticisms which we call "condensation witticisms." From the great collection of Freud's I will select an example from Heine: The proud assertion of the Jewish chiropodist and lottery collector, Hyacinth, that he had been treated by Baron Rotschild "ganz famillionär." The poor little Jew, under whose figure, Heine portrays himself,* intends to say: The Baron met me familiarly (familiär) as far as a millionaire may—a thought which certainly often passed through the mind of the poet in the house of his distinguished relative.

A witticism similarly composed appears in the third chapter of the same writing by Heine: Upon remembering his little stepfatherland, the little Jew sighed: "What is man? One walking satisfied from the Altonaer gate to the Hamburg mountain and there seeing the sights, the lions, the birds, the 'Papagoyim,' the monkeys, the noted men . . . ." "Papagoyim" is composed by amalgamation of "Papageien" and "goyim," heathen, contemptuous Jewish word for stranger. The word "Papa" is thus wittily joined with "goy." Behind lurks again Heine's distinguished father-substitute, the uncle, who would have preferred to behave as a stranger toward the poorly clad poet but could not, because he was a relative. Under the "Papageien" may further have been understood the elegant cousins whom Heine now denies as strangers (goyim) to him. Thus the composite word contains a sneer at the cold comfort of his relatives and at his near relations to these people created by his birth, and his distant relations created by psychological factors.

Leo Spitzer has pointed out the condensation as important speech-forming phenomenon in his investigations concerning "Die Wortbildung als stilistisches Mittel" (Word Formation as Means of Style), particularly in "Rabelais." †

* Freud, Witz, p. 119. To Freud's examples, I will add another: Chapter 6, Heine seizes the foot of the beautiful Franzeska; chapter 8, Hyacinth speaks of the pleasure of holding in his hands the little white foot of the beautiful lady. Thus Heine identifies himself with his comic hero.

† Leo Spitzer, Die Wortbildung als stilistisches Mittel. Exemplified in Rabelais. Halle, 1910. (Compare H. Sachs, Zbl. I, 240).

(β) THE SUPERIMPOSED MATERIAL

A chain of repressed ideas can be brought to common expression in a manifestation when they agree, either wholly or in some peculiarity, or when a common speech relation exists among them.

A lady of some thirty years afflicted with melancholia and victim of an unhappy marriage, has suffered since the beginning of her married life, sixteen years ago, from automatic contraction of the vagina (vaginismus). Sexual intercourse has therefore been almost entirely denied her, from which circumstance both she and her husband suffer severely. The symptom dated from a number of unconscious motives: When three and a half years old, she was carried by a man on his back with his hand placed in an improper position.* A few years later, a brother allowed himself improper manipulations which hurt severely. As adult, she experienced a similar treatment from another relative who told her he wished a woman as tightly built as possible. Further, she feared her husband might suffer an accident from her (penis captivus). Further, she wished to make herself attractive to him, remain young as long as possible and force him to strongest aggression. The contraction disappeared completely, the attitude toward life became fairly normal. The analysis was prematurely interrupted by the patient's going on a journey and yet soon after, complete health appeared without further treatment.

That even apparently totally different trains of thought can be superimposed on one another, is shown by the following dream of a woman, aged thirty-one years, who suffered from spinal syphilis:

"I was drinking water from a beautiful fountain, my hands

* The trauma seems to have been provoked. The patient remembers that she previously said to the man that she would lie down and sleep because she hoped that he would do something to her. Compare Abraham, Das Erleiden sexueller Jugendtraumen als Form infantiler Sexualbetätigk. Zbl. f. Nervenheilkunde u. Psychiatrie 1907. Nov. 2d. Number.

serving as cups. The water was clear but shining fish and mussels moved in it. The fountain reservoir looked like a gondola. Suddenly I stood in it and swept a wall in a church-like, vaulted building, although it was not dirty. In this reservoir, I climbed higher and higher. In so doing, I was afraid of falling down and held on to the wall. My husband stood there. I asked myself why he did not help me. When I finally reached the top in great anxiety, it cleared up beautifully. The wall went still higher. I was on a platform, however. The wall disappeared and I in great anxiety was in an evil-smelling tunnel. At one time, I had reached the top when Pastor P. stood by me and consolingly sought to allay my anxiety although it was evident that he had it too. He traveled with me in the depths whereupon I felt air. He blinked his eyes a little but also trembled as if he was afraid. Then the darkness was dissipated. A lattice extended to the knees and I thought: There I have absolutely no footing. We got along well, however. Below lay a beautiful garden which I saw when halfway down, somewhat like the hill on which I live. Below stood my husband laughing.''

A real analysis was impossible since the woman was finishing a mercurial treatment for the spinal trouble. I guarded myself well from telling the patient the meaning of the dream which was told to me without my asking as something beautiful. I cautiously obtained a few associations. Much was known to me.

The reservoir resembled my pulpit but also the fountain in front of my church. On Sunday before the dream, I had preached from the words of Jesus as given in John iv., 14: ''Whosoever drinketh of the water that I shall give him shall never thirst.'' This sermon made a strong impression on the dreamer, so she said. The hands held as cups express in the one-time Catholic, the attitude of prayer.

The religious phantasy is spun out further. Standing in the pulpit and sweeping the wall like a true servant, the dreamer felt herself lifted heavenward which gives a good religious meaning. Further, the anxiety over falling corresponds to the well-known fear of many religious persons of falling from grace. Her husband, when anxiety over her future came upon her, could not quiet her by religious conversation. The platform reminded her of a lookout on an elevated place. The fear of new darkness appeared: A terrible tunnel took the dreamer down. Still the pastor consoled and conducted the anxious one back to the light. To the one with wavering faith, he afforded sure help. A Garden of Eden, the longed-for Paradise, received her and her husband.

This much I could tell the woman. More would have robbed her of the harmless joy in her poem and disquieted her mind. The reader will probably have already guessed the gross erotic sense. It betrays itself already in the fishes and mussels of the fountain which plainly represent masculine and feminine symbols.

The sweeping of the church wall points definitely to masturbation since the church building is a typical representation of the female, usually maternal body. The church recalls that which the patient as a child was accustomed to visit (infantile masturbation). To "reservoir," the dreamer associated besides "gondola" and "pulpit" also "bed." The husband did not help her out of the anxiety because she forbids him intercourse or because he is impotent. At all events, the husband intimated to me that intimate relations with his wife did not exist.

The dreamer wishes to free herself autoerotically, which does not, however, gratify her (anxiety). Suddenly she sticks in the foul-smelling tunnel. From the analysis of women who are ungratified by their husbands, who are overcome in tunnels with severe anxiety, as well as from many dreams, we know that the tunnel is the symbol of the vagina. Our dreamer formerly suffered from syphilis, from which disease probably, tabes dorsalis has steadily developed. The memory of this critical state of affairs disturbs the unfortunate woman. Then she daringly allows the pastor to enter, who nevertheless, is only a cover-figure for another man: It is the seducer who impregnated and infected her at the same time; as immune, therefore, from her disease, he has nothing to fear. By chance, he had the same forename as the pastor. Her own sexual excitement is accordingly wished upon this man. Still, a scruple is aroused: "I have no support." But at the same time, a lattice reaching to the knees is noticed. In reality, the patient is without sensation as far as the knees because of destruction of the spinal cord. Her trouble serves the former prostitute as protective measure against the fear of infection for now there is nothing more to corrupt. In the dream, she carries out the adultery but suffers no injury therefrom.

Thus, the superimposition has not succeeded badly even though certain parts of the dream cannot be assigned equally well to the religious and erotic connections.

The condensation succeeded by the aid of a symbolism which gave various meanings to the same idea. The "being lifted," "mounting," "flying," could be considered in the religious as well as in the erotic sense, likewise the "reservoir" (gondola, bed), the tunnel, the falling, the lattice, the garden.

Often the similarity of the name suffices ("word-bridges," here for example, "being lifted") or another relation to a common third factor, to condense two quite distinct ideas.*

The condensation belongs to the most efficient means of the unconscious for guarding its secret and still affording its inclinations a certain, even though limited, realization.

7. The Disjection

I designate as disjection that activity contrasted to condensation, whereby a real quantity is represented in the manifestation by a number of separate ideas.

Freud has already pointed out that often in a dream, besides the self, other persons are present who turn out in the analysis to be representations of the person himself.† Freud shows in beautiful examples that wit also utilizes this mechanism.‡ After a too modern performance of "Antigone," the

---

* Freud, Traumdeutung, p. 235.
† Freud, Traumdeutung, p. 254.
‡ Freud, Witz, p. 19 ff.

Berliner Witz criticized: "Antik! O nee!", To the jesting question: "What is the best in the examination (examen)," the disjection answers "Ex amen!"

This dissection of a person is often found in art. In different pictures by Lukas Cranach, the Christ, for example, is expressed simultaneously in several figures, as crucified one, as risen one, serpent, lamb. In each figure, the hero is characterized according to one particular aspect.

Poetry also makes extensive use of disjection. It creates a new person from the ribs of a man. Thus Goethe appears simultaneously in Tasso and Antonio, in Faust and Mephistopheles.

Not less does religion like splittings: for example, Mary is divided by Catholic people into countless distinct personalities, a Mary of Einsiedeln, Mary of the Snow (Rigi), Mary of the Statue (Canton of St. Gallen), etc.

Even phantasies are broken up into various separate ideas when they are elaborated as result of changed relations in the repression. One of my analytic patients, for example, who revoked and remodeled the sadistic phantasies which had been created under the reign of hatred, produced the following result: Formerly, he pictured the analyst as an idiotic auctioneer standing on a high tower, opening his mouth without making a sound, degrading himself for a foolish thing and had him die; now from this picture, two day-dreams developed: The pastor appeared as an intellectual, forceful speaker and as an aeronaut who sacrifices himself for science.*

c. THE PRINCIPAL TENDENCIES

Even before the repression, one observes two principal tendencies in which the mental life exerts itself: a centrifugal and a centipetal. Diametrically opposite to the endeavor which is directed toward reality and which devotes its full interest and love to this reality, stands the endeavor to separate itself entirely from reality and to make its own gratifica-

* Pfister, Analyt. Unters, ü.˙ d. Psycholog. d. Hasses u. d. Versöhnung, Leipzig and Vienna, 1910, p. 38.

tion and enhancement the goal of all action and thought. Ethics long ago spoke of egoists and altruists, the philosophy of a-priorists and empiricists, and psychology recognized the difference between the shut-in natures, those turned inward, and the communicative natures which gladly unfold to the outer world and embrace it in love. Neither the centrifugal nor the centripetal tendency ever appears entirely by itself. The seemingly centripetal perception often depends on selfish, egocentric wishes which have selected from the totality of possible perceptions just those which enriched the given characteristics with other, not given ones and interpreted the incomplete picture in a particular manner, so that in the supposed perceptive picture, many unseen features were projected into it, etc. Conversely, the world-renouncing mystic constantly betrays his consideration for his environment; in its favor, he spins his delusion of grandeur and ideas of persecution, as he also gets his material for his ideas.

Thus every person takes part in both movements and that indeed in every movement of his action and experience. Still there exist great differences in the distribution of the tendencies. Many persons throw their emotions and interests into the outer world very easily. In this, it often happens that only the surface of the mental life follows this path, the depths remaining unmoved. Such persons frequently display strong love-emotions, but the glow of the conscious emotions is no proof of their genuineness, for on the morrow, they may perhaps have flown. This peculiarity marks the hysterical individual in particular. Conversely, one meets people who apparently have neither interest nor love for their surroundings and yet are capable of great kindness, indeed of considerable sacrifice for it. Likewise, a person who was happy in his childhood, may, as a result of certain inhibitions, be forced violently back into his inmost self. Hence one must proceed with great caution in assigning individuals to this or that category and in many, probably in most cases, guard against such classification. Extreme cases occur and may then, as we shall see, be forced into illness when one endeavor or some other obstacle presents itself against the opposite tendency. But among patients also, both tendencies often, probably usually, appear simultaneously so that the introverted individuals for example, that is, people with predominant centripetal tendency, can have many symptoms which usually prevail in hysterical individuals, thus, those people with whom the emotions press violently outward, and, conversely, hysterical individuals show in many symptoms, for example, twilight states, that renunciation of reality which constitutes the most prominent characteristic of introverted individuals.

CHAPTER XI

THE CONTENT OF THE MANIFESTATIONS

1. REMINISCENCES

WHEN we find a memory in a dream, hysterical phenomenon or other phenomenon, which we have to consider as reaction of an unconscious motive, this means: Something in the present situation agrees with something in the past or should agree with it. The same rule holds good when upon closer consideration, a manifestation turns out to be a reminiscence.

Heine's "Lorelei" affords a fine example. First, a picture producing a peculiar effect by its tone:

"I know not what it can mean that I am so sad." The continuation appears exactly as if the poet had instituted a little autoanalysis and deciphered his sadness.   .

"A legend from the olden times which will not leave my mind." The legend which follows plainly accords with the sadness because it conceals its relation to the poet's affairs. Otherwise it would leave him unmoved. It is characteristic that the sadness precedes and is felt at first as mysterious. The ballad represents, as is plainly evident from many analogies, the poet's death-wish created by unhappy love, as fulfilled, in the same manner as Goethe executes on his hero in the suffering young Werther, his suicidal impulse occasioned by the same motive.

Every dream when it contains no memories as such, leads immediately upon exploration to reminiscences. Frequently, the interpretation is an assured fact when the dream fragment has been inserted into its original connection as experienced. A young girl dreamed, for instance, in winter that she was sitting in a public garden. The analysis gained the following associations: "Last summer, I sat in such a garden with my parents and a friend. As a child of one year, I was often taken by our beloved servant maid into a public garden; there she played constantly. Afterwards, the vain young thing put on Mamma's best clothes and looked at herself in the mirror. Once when the parents were away traveling, she slept in Mamma's bed.'' Later, they often playfully reproached the child for being so frequently in the public garden while still so small. The memory of that maid's putting herself in the mother's place is closely joined to the previous visit to the garden. The clinical symptoms of the dreamer plainly disclose that she unconsciously identifies herself with the maid and likewise puts herself in the mother's place. This is shown for example in the following hallucination: At night, she sees her mother in night dress go to the chest to open it with the key. She calls to her to prevent her from doing what she intended. To her astonishment, the mother sleeping in the bed beside her daughter, asks what is the matter and why she calls. Somewhat later, the girl sees the mother go from wardrobe to window and sit on the windowsill, ''perhaps to throw herself out of the window.''

To ''chest,'' she associated: ''She wishes to get a handkerchief or bandage. One binds up wounds in cases of emergency with handkerchiefs. Once when I cut my finger, I fainted. The same happened when I was a very small child at the dentist's. On the vacation where I was, during the hallucination, the menstrual flow was always absent.''

The girl suffered from anxiety over blood and from excessive menstruation which always assumed the plain character of a birth pantomime.

Chest and key are to be understood as female and male symbols. The dreamer envies her mother her position in wedlock since she herself has an incestuous fixation upon the father. The mother should make away with herself in order to make room for the daughter.

We often stumble on reminiscences when we endeavor to get to the bottom of neurotic phenomena. I will add a few examples: In the first hours of the analysis, it struck me that the woman patient, of about thirty years, suddenly twitched slightly. Upon being questioned, she said that she suffered from sudden pain in the back and had some weeks before, put herself under medical treatment for this trouble. The physician thought the kidneys were out of order although the urine showed no anomalies. The pain often ran to the right hip. [This pain.] "When sixteen years old, I was grasped about the waist by a young man, right at the point that is painful now. He asked for a kiss. This I refused, of which fact, I was later very proud. When I was already secretly engaged to my husband, his friend and rival likewise demanded a kiss, at the same time seizing me there." The lady had previously told of her partiality for a physician who allowed her to love him (positive transference). Now she wishes that I should pay her court even if only that she may show her blameless mind. We shall see later that the analyst or any other educator cannot avoid such bestowal of emotion. Our case teaches us that the reproduction of an earlier experience can represent the wish for its repetition. This connection is always to be found.

At the beginning of the analytic investigation, the reminiscences were designated as a kind of foreign body which lies under the threshold of consciousness and asserts itself from time to time. To-day, we know that there is no such pure reproduction of an existing, disturbing content but that revivification corresponds to certain needs and fulfills a teleological mission. Before we present the proof for this assertion, we will collect a number of new facts.

2. IDENTIFICATION AND PROJECTION

Even in normal life we put ourselves countless times in other people's places, often without realizing it, or even in places of lifeless objects. The esthetic effects, the reactions of the moral consciousness depend in great part upon such substitutions or identifications.

I will first select an example from the field of poetry: "The Falling Leaf," by K. F. Meyer:

"To-day, an axe sounded the whole morning long
And continued till evening. The master is building
Only a shack, still I would like to see
Is it growing, is it beginning!"

The fatally sick knight who speaks these words is glad of the beginning because he feels his own forces failing and puts himself in the place of that which is growing.

"There was a carpenter who worked nobly
And squarely hewed his timber.
In good faith the man endeavored
Until the water from his brow did run.
At evening the master carpenter came,
A good-natured old man with long curly beard,
He touched the workman who never wished to rest
Upon the shoulder, saying: "Good man, rest now!"
Now the place became empty; I, however, slipped in
And seated myself on the beam.
Contemplating the hewn fir-stick
I pondered over my own day's work."

Here the comparison of his own life with the timber is plain: Both have been carved out with infinite exertion and lie there incomplete; from both, the active workman has been called away against his will. The timber consoles in so far that it attains its purpose the following day. To this revery, the hope is easily joined that the life-work may also be completed.

"I was staring down, lost in thought,
When a falling leaf struck my shoulder.
I shuddered when I spied the leaf
As if the master's hand had touched me,
And I thought: Enough! The sun is low,
Go in, thou workman, to the rest of thy Lord!"

The cottage is identified with the carpenter, the fallen leaf on his shoulder with the hand of the master and so the cessation of work is interpreted as a kind of hopeful invitation to a time of rest.

Thus all characteristics of a process which primarily has

no direct relation to the knight, gain by sympathy, identification or whatever we may name the psychological process, an intimate relation. The building artisan, the tireless workman who hates to leave his work unfinished, the shack, the touched shoulder, the hewn fir-stick, they are all representations of the cottage itself and more exactly the embodiment of inhibited endeavors of high valence, the so-called libido-symbols. Indeed the old man who calls to rest from work and the warning leaf expressing a wish which slumbers beside the preceding ones in the depths of the soul, are also libido-symbols in which the hero finds himself again.

We are dealing here, not only with an ''Einfühlung,'' * to use Volkelt's expression, but with a more or less clear thought process in which one compares himself with some object on a basis of certain similarities and puts himself in its place to appropriate to himself the advantages which accrue from the comparison. The similarity which is present is utilized to gain pleasant prospects for the undecided things in the person's life, which are solved in favorable manner in the object of comparison. In this substitution or self-installation in the place of an object, thinking, feeling and willing have a share.

In the ethical field, sympathy is the same kind of an activity. Unfortunately, in our representation, we cannot support ourselves by a recognized psychological theory but must ourselves seek out our conception. Schopenhauer, as we know, believes that sympathy is founded on the knowledge that the person cherishing sympathy is identified with the one pitied, on the ''Tat twam asi'' (This, you are). Adam Smith holds as a presupposition of sympathy that we put ourselves in the place of the other: ''We think ourselves over into his body, we become in some measure he himself and accordingly build for ourselves a concept of his emotions, indeed we feel something similar to his emotions although in much weaker intensity.''

This theory arouses an opponent in Störring who says: ''Such a confusion of our standpoint with that of the sufferer does not occur in sympathy: In the case of sympathy with

* No exact English equivalent, something like sympathetic insight.

a man, we do not at all imagine what we would feel if we were
in his place.   The situation is rather: When we see anyone
suffer, the perception of the physical phenomena which accompany suffering or of the causes of the same brings about
the reproduction of emotional conditions which have arisen
with us ourselves from similar causes or which were present
under similar physical concomitant phenomena.   This reproduction of emotional states on a basis of perceptions in a person does not presuppose, as may be seen, the idea that we
endure the pains of the sufferer but only the perception of
the accompanying phenomena of the pain or of the causes by
which the pain was produced.   The emotions reproduced in
us are then thought into the sufferer; we do not, however,
"think ourselves over into his body." *

This theory leaves the principal thing unexplained: If I
mentally transfer to another the emotions produced in me
from symptoms perceived in the other, why does there so often
remain with me such severe grief? Why does sympathy assume such highly varied degrees of intensity according as it
concerns a savage of the stone age or a beloved relative?

In sympathy, I treat the sorrows and joys, the intellectual,
esthetic and ethical preferences of another as things highly
important to me.   It must be admitted with Störring that a
clearly conscious "putting one's self in place of another" is
not necessarily present in sympathy, although sympathy often
receives a reinforcement when one construes this idea.   But
it may be asserted just as surely that dimly consciously or unconsciously, the substitution pointed out by Smith prevails in
general.

In substantiation of this opinion, I proceed from analytic
results.

A young merchant developed passionate fondness for Napoleon.   He not only studied with boundless industry a mass
of works on the great emperor but he allowed his whole outlook on the world to be determined by the Corsican.   In spite
of all ridicule by comrades, he was all the time turning the

* G. Störring, Moralphilos. Streitfragen I, p. 17.

conversation to his hero and seemed absolutely inaccessible to other matters. The young man is an hysterical individual. For some years, he has suffered from difficulties in swallowing. At the beginning of the analysis he could not in general swallow solid food. The exploration showed in a few minutes that the patient cannot and will not swallow all kinds of demands of his father, whereupon the disturbance in his throat disappeared for good.* On the other hand, the admiration for Napoleon rather increased. Its chief motives were as follows:

(1) The emperor is a substitute for the detested father.

(2) Napoleon was small of stature; his admirer is the same.

(3) The great conqueror triumphed over his enemies; our patient is filled with hatred for all comrades and mankind in general, his ambition knows no bounds.

(4) The profile of the young fanatic bears an unmistakable resemblance to that of his model. These motives worked for the most part unconsciously. That a comparison existed, is not to be denied.

Hate and love often depend on unconscious transpositions in the sense of projection of the ego upon the people in question. An example of this kind of origin for a passionate love for a nurse, I have already given (207). That hatred can arise similarly, I shall show later.

Ferenczi formulates the statement: "The neurotic individual is constantly searching for objects with which to identify himself, upon which he may transfer his emotions." † I do not think that this statement applies to all psychoneurotics. For the hysterical type, it is certainly correct. Another mode of identification exists in dementia praecox. Maeder mentions the exteriorization by which the patient thinks he can perceive his separate organs in the reality. For example, the

---

* This recovery also occurred too quickly, since it made further analysis seem superfluous to the neurotic individual. The youth suffered from his attachment to his father afterwards as before, so that his attitude toward life was entirely false. Goethe noted in his diary on May 27, 1811: "Psychic cure of hiccup in a youth." Cited by Stekel, Nerv. Angstzustände, p. 7.

† S. Ferenczi, Introjektion u. Übertragung. Jahrb. I, p. 429.

manipulations of the gas and water pipes is for one of Maeder's analytic patients an irritation of his nerves and vessels.* But this takes us to projection.

One can also be so closely united with a work, unconsciously, that we can almost speak of a substitution.

Under the influence of unconscious mental impulses, the normal individual also countless times identifies persons or other parts of his environment with one another. One individual is sympathetic to us at first glance without our being able to assign any reason for the fact. If we analyze, perhaps the likeness to a beloved person becomes conscious, of whom we did not think before. Thus we begin a transposition of persons.

As a matter of fact, the analyst is easily identified, unconsciously or from unconscious motives, with other persons. Amusing externalities aid the substitution. We met one example in the case of the patient who saw in her teacher as well as in other persons, the eyes of her seducer, although those organs looked quite different in color, size and position (246). In such cases, the real reason lies deeper: The patient wishes a renewal of the earlier experiences.

The young catatonic patient, who was pathologically ashamed of his nose (122) repeatedly said to me: "I see distinctly in you the physician who operated on me for phimosis; I know perfectly well that you are another man but for me you are that physician."

How fateful may be the outcome of such identifications, I may show in a case cured by analysis. It concerned a boy of seventeen years whom I had cured of three nervous tics in four consultations, a year previously. At that time, only the relation to boys was discussed. For three years, the boy had blinked his eyes every few seconds, turned up his nose and pulled the corners of his mouth upward. Three physicians and Christian Science were unable to help him. From his

* Maeder, Psycholog. Unters. an Dementia præcox-Kranken. Jahrbuch II, p. 241. Maeder. Zur Entst. d. Symbolik im Traum, in der Dementia præcox, etc. Zbl. I, p. 383.

dreams, it was revealed that he had fallen out with his comrades since they refused him on account of alleged scandal. It made him especially angry that they kept sexual enlightenment from him. His twitching said: "I don't want to see you and despise your obscenity." Naturally, I did not consider the youth fully freed after the little analysis of symptoms but had no occasion to urge him to continue the pedagogic course.

The course of the second treatment was much more tedious. The youth said that he could not concentrate himself and that he hated his parents. Melancholia was also mentioned. Some days before, the young introverted individual had retired from a course in dancing because the big, strapping fellow, in spite of eager desire, could not bring himself to overcome his bashfulness and speak a word to a girl. For two or three years, he had been a victim of bashfulness. Also with a young and pretty lady boarder, with whom he was in love, he never spoke a word and pretended indifference toward her. If he passed a girl, tears came to his eyes and he felt ashamed. This painful inhibition in speech even extended to a comrade who had two sisters. With the other boys, he had been on good terms since the earlier fragmentary analysis.

One of his first dreams was: "I was with a crazy old man whom I led by the arm, in front of a cemetery, the gate of which formed an obstacle. Suddenly we were in the cemetery, how it happened I do not know; you came from a side alley and took the old man into custody; I left you alone."

[The old man.] "A comic figure in the 'Fliegenden Blättern.' A stout man who wished to dine with a count and then also sup with him. The father of our lady boarder was also stout, his oval face and his beard resembled those of the dream figure. He was our guest a month ago. On the other hand, the color of his face was sallow like my mother's. Further, the nervous movements and the constant talking did not belong to the boarder's father." [Nervous movements, much talking.] "That agrees exactly with my father."

In explanation, I will borrow from the chapter which gives

us information concerning the meaning of manifestations (Chapter XIII) : The dream represents a secret (unconscious, latent) wish as fulfilled. The dreamer paints his father as a crazy, helpless old man in the cemetery where I am also kindly provided for. The same fate befalls the hated mother and the innocent guest. Why the latter? As father of the beloved girl, he is the father's double (father-in-law).

It is not determined that the hard-hearted son really wishes his father dead. As we have noticed and found confirmed repeatedly the father is only an image (Imago). The neurotic wishes to set free his libido which is joined to the father by making him the object of caricature. He seeks therefore, to bury a bit of his own bondage.

Whence, however, has come the hatred for the father who is a good-natured, generous, mild-mannered man without any austerity? I exerted myself to find the reason but could ascertain nothing except jealousy over the mother. The boy slept during his first eight years in the same rooms with his parents. Because of his sickliness, he was pampered by his mother who was decidedly hysterical. He was continually taken into bed with her. To the mother, he paid the compliment when quite small: "You are the prettiest woman in the whole world." And to this judgment, he still held, although the mother is distinguished rather by lack of good looks.

It soon became evident from the dreams that the bashful youth identified the girls who had impressed him, with his mother or saw the latter in the girls. Hence the girls bore traits of the mother picture, for example, the aprons of the mother.

As chief determinant of the alienation, I found a sexual phantasy which was long kept silent. Finally the youth revealed his secret. For a long time previously, he had known that he suffered much from masturbation. I had endeavored to help him with the usual assurances and advice but unfortunately without result. Finally, the analysis attained the goal here too. It showed that an obsessional idea underneath the onanism which naturally brought to naught all good resolutions: In phantasy, the boy lay beside a girl (usually clothed) in bed and clung to her. This scene immediately called up the memory of the almost daily morning visits which the child had made to his mother. The sexuality of the youth was thus anchored fast to the infantile desires and its normal development had been interrupted. He was ashamed in the presence of girls because in his phantasies he misused them (really the boarder) and saw in them the sexually-desired mother.

Also, improper wishes were directed toward his sister which wishes had derived their form from infantile bath scenes. Of the sexual life, the youth held the most disgusting ideas. The explanation exerted a saving influence on him.

The treatment took five months and proceeded with great difficulty since the not particularly intelligent youth revealed only very unwillingly the identification of the father and analyst and at first produced very few associations. Now, he is on excellent terms with his parents and behaves gallantly toward young ladies. His capacity for work has become entirely normal.

A typical example which illuminates many life histories, is the following: A widow of thirty-seven years, subnormal intelligence, begged me for consolation for severe anxiety conditions and religious depressions. She suffered from fear that God did not care about her, perhaps He did not exist at all. Accordingly, her religion was in profound need. The Sunday religious service she considered the finest hour of the week. Since she seemed too unintelligent for analysis, I endeavored to aid her with advice and friendly encouragement. The result was unsuccessful. I therefore investigated her life history which was only slightly known to me.

The widow had lost her husband five years before, a drunkard, about twenty-two years older than she, who did not trouble himself about her inter copulam. Since then, she has exercised an extreme grave cult and clung passionately to the man who had always treated her badly. She refused all courtships and lived only in her sorrow. On account of pains in her pelvis, she had both ovaries extirpated but experienced—like so many hystericals who have been operated on—no diminution in her suffering. The infantile experiences solved the riddle. The patient had a drunken father who bothered himself little about his family. He was somewhat taller than she with black hair and beard. The girl could not bear her mother and therefore transferred so much the more love to the father who left so much to be desired in other things. A sister, eleven years her elder, she loved, according to her own phrase, "abnormally fervently." To her, she confided everything and found complete understanding. Then the mother-substitute became tuberculous and passed quickly away.

When she was face to face with death, our hysterical patient became engaged in passionate devotion to her future husband who strikingly resembled in stature, hair, beard and other characteristics the father who had now been dead nine years and who had the same faults of character. Thus one sees: The love inhibited by the threatened departure of the mother-substitute, turns to the father-substitute. The girl was a female Œdipus like so many others.

A part of her love was directed toward God. After the death of her husband, strong sexual needs asserted themselves. Hence anxiety. Her religion could not afford her sufficient father-love and the sexual demands stilled by the father-substitute craved for more than piety. Thus the bounds of capacity for sublimation were plainly transcended.

One often meets similar identifications. A student of philosophy, aged twenty-three, fell in love with a teacher aged forty. He perceived the unsuitableness of this love but could not free himself from it. The conversation took the following course: [Is your mother still living?] "Yes." [Then you are probably not on good terms with her.] "Yes. How did you know that?" [Because you seek her love in a mother-substitute.] The youth saw his identification at once.

One might ask whether the expression, "identification," is altogether happy for the process described. If I unconsciously unite two persons in one figure, I do not wish to express their absolute identity but only their comparison in this or that regard. Perhaps the name substitution or interchange would be preferable. But these terms also have their defects, since often a substitute for the object indicated in the manifestation in question, is not present in the new figure because that first object retains its importance. Therefore, I keep the name "identification" in spite of its deficiencies but use the other expressions as well.

The motives of the substitution may be of different kinds. Frequently, the wish finds expression: "O were I such an one." I knew a student who successively imitated in striking manner the teachers he admired. From one, he borrowed the habit of constantly carrying a key in his hand on the street, from another, old-fashioned collars, the procuring of which must have given him not a little trouble, the third, he copied so in accent, use of eyes and manner of speech that the two men were mistaken for each other. One hysterical girl assumed with all its peculiarities the migraine of her mother, in whose place, she would have liked to be.

In other cases, the substitution of one's own person is explained by sympathy, in which the literal and the figurative significance of the expression work together beautifully. Sympathy as inclination leads to sympathy = to suffer with the beloved. Here, a powerful "Einfühlung" * occurs.

In this manner, the mystic, Margaretha Ebner † (1291–1351) identified herself with Jesus very plainly in a number of hysterical symptoms, as appears from her phantasies. She suffered from inability to stand and to walk, from pains in head and teeth, from hoarseness, stitch in the heart and in the hands, from the sensation of having all her limbs broken, intolerance against being touched ("Noli me tangere"), from the feeling of suspense, from death-marks on the hands, from the utterance of cries and other imitations.

A young student whose brother had died from subcostal

* See foot-note on page 262.
† Pfister, Hysterie u. Mystik bei Marg Ebner. Zbl. I, pp. 468–485.

abscess, was stricken on the funeral day with an obstinate pain in the same region. An analysis was not made.

I have already described a swelling of the tongue which a son imitated from his mother, the mother from a friend of her youth (177). Probably substitution existed there also.

An hysterical boy of sixteen with introversion phenomena, was seized during the analysis with a loud snapping or cracking in the joint of the lower jaw. The trouble which was plainly audible even at some distance when he opened his mouth, became so unpleasant that mastication was almost impossible. It occurred to the boy that his pretty aunt, aged thirty-five, had been subject to exactly the same trouble and likewise only on one side. This aunt, he loved very much and regretted that his father had not married her. That did not exclude his having considerable strife with her. After I had made a visit to his family, the cracking suddenly stopped until he came to my house, pretendedly from fear that I would disclose something of his inclination to his mother and aunt. As closer determination, I found: The pretty aunt liked to eat nuts; the nephew admired a comrade who could crack nuts in his teeth. (The father often hid the nut-cracker.) The grandfather forbade this practice since it might lead to blindness. The cracking in the joint realized among other things the wish to crack nuts for his aunt in order to gain her favor. The patient had, however, other nuts to crack: He had no pleasant relations to school and comrades, parents and brothers and sisters. He did not know what would become of him. The aunt frequently used the expression: "I must always crack nuts for others," which meant: "to submit, suffer, remove difficulties for others." The nephew said the same of himself. Immediately before the outbreak of the disturbance, the aunt had related that when young she had to live in a crowded attic and suffer injustice from her sister. Both things applied to the nephew also, particularly the strife with the sister. Finally, the cracking recalled the memory of a game that he often played with his sister: The two children wound a long thread about a spool which they rubbed and twirled while they held the plaything in front of the ear on the joint of the jaw. Then one heard a cracking "as of cannons." Now, the youth consoled himself: The war (Krieg) with the sister is, in spite of its noise only like the cracking (Krach) in the jaw caused by the noise of the plaything. Following these conclusions reached in four consultations, the symptom remained away for good.

In this case, I cannot possibly assume that the nephew found something worthy of imitation in the situation of his aunt.

Freud describes a third type of hysterical identification: "One patient has her attack to-day; directly it is known to the others that a letter from home, reviving the love trouble and the like, is the cause of it. Their sympathy is aroused, it is carried out in the following conclusion which does not enter consciousness: If one can have such attacks from such causes, so I too can have such attacks for I have these occasions." * I confess that I have never ferreted out this unconscious reflection and do not consider an uninterested conclusion from analogy as sufficient motive for symptom formation. According to Freud's opinion, there must certainly be instinctive impulses present as we demonstrate them in the covetous and sympathetic identification.

Of the *projections,* one case is especially important: The transpositions of wishfulfillments which one cherishes, upon other people. It is present most frequently in paranoia and its chief forms, the delusions of grandeur and persecution. A patient feels herself persecuted because all the gentlemen in the trolley car speak only of her bad conduct. She wishes so to live but does not dare. The gentlemen express what she herself must deny. The normal individual also often sees others as he wishes them. He thinks to read in their minds and yet only projects himself into them.

* Freud, Traumdeutung, p. 109.

3. SYMBOLISM

From the beginning, Freud insisted upon the assertion that the repressed material now and then procures symbolical expression. A beautiful example is that of the lady who had suffered for fifteen years from facial neuralgia. All external means of treatment failed: electric cauterization, alkaline waters, elimination methods, teeth extraction. Finally, the trauma was revealed in an illness of her husband's, in the narration of which, the sufferer seized himself by the cheek, cried out with pain and said: "That was to me like a blow in the face." Over this repression, which naturally formed neither the first link in the pathological chain nor the real cause of the disease, but only the exciting and form-giving occasion, other repressions had been superimposed. The same hysterical patient suffered from pains in the feet which rendered walking impossible for her. These pains had appeared at the moment when the house-physician offered her his arm and she was overcome by the fear whether she could "appear correctly" in strange society.* (One notices the word-bridges: "blow in the face" and "appear.")

Such processes, Freud terms "symbolizations by means of verbal expression." We have found them substantiated in a very considerable number of analytic results. I mention the dumbness, dimness of vision, astasia, tactile hallucination on the breast, as manifestation of the thoughts: "I can no longer speak, everything is dark before me, I hang only by a thread" (31). I mention further the hysterical crown of thorns (36), the obsession for washing (68), the aversion for cleansing work (78), the finger movements under the nose (78), the anxiety for the legs of doves and children besides shame on account of the nose (122), the anesthetic toe (176), the obsessional movement upon extending the hand (177), the fatigue (180), St. Vitus' dance movements (185), sleepiness (197), anxiety for the offending bedside table (211), tearing of skin on the thumb, ravenous hunger for carrots,

* Freud, Studien über Hysterie, p. 157 f.

violin playing (213f), overlooking the waning moon (220) dream of a person with spinal syphilis (251).

I ask that provisionally the expression "symbol" be allowed to apply to all events in which a symbol represents the pictorial representation of an idea related by content but still aiming at something else, to put it briefly: under symbol, I understand provisionally the veiled, masked expression of a thought in a phantastic form which contains an analogy. Concerning the speech usage, I will speak later.

(A) PSYCHOLOGY OF THE SYMBOL IN CUSTOMARY SPEECH USAGE

The Freudian theory of symbols has stirred up much dust. Many persons were very indignant that the psychoanalyst should make the unconscious use a varying speech of double meaning where it would be much nicer and prettier if it used a scientific, logically correct manner of expression. But does the symbolizing activity not belong to the most universal and most important functions of the mental life?

I shall introduce some evidence. Speech constantly makes use of the metaphor as is well known. Its words have developed from visual ideas, even the abstract expressions which are now construed figuratively. In the statement just made for example, the words "ideas" (Vorstellungen), "developed" (hervorgegangen), "abstract" (abstrakt), "expressions" (Ausdrücke), "figuratively" (bildlich), "construed" (gefasst) embrace sensual processes and objects but denote facts of the inner, mental world as well. The terms Pneuma (Greek), Rauch (Hebrew), spiritus, signify really breath (Hauch), then, also soul (mind), the actual prepositions all go back originally to relations of space.* According to Max Müller, in a certain stage of development of speech, all thoughts which went beyond the narrow horizon of every-day life were expressed in metaphors.† Indeed, the highest terms of phi-

* Höffding, Psych. p. 3. According to Wundt, Logik, 2d ed. I, 150 ff., this applies only to the majority of prepositions (Messmer).
† P. 209.

losophy, as "substance," "cause" and the like, are in a certain sense, symbols.

Poetry also rests in part on symbolism. One needs only to mention some titles like "The Wild Duck," "The Sunken Bell," to illustrate this. Especially in folk legends is there a symbolism of which Riklin has given us valuable proof.*

Painting symbolizes industriously. One thinks of Segantini's "Two Mothers," Steinhausen's "Representation of Sorrow," that picture in which beside the discouraged peasant sitting before his broken plow, there is a withered little tree, while over his believing wife, a blooming tree is seen.

The symbol is particularly frequent in religion. Schleiermacher even considers religion the product of symbolizing activity.† F. A. Lange attributes high value to religion so far as its truths are considered only as symbols.‡ Recent religious philosophers esteemed the symbol formation scarcely less important even though they also thought at times that they could strip off the figurative character without endangering the religious nucleus. Rauwenhoff says: "Nothing is clearer than that the circle of ideas which the religious man has formed regarding that transcendental force which he has made an object of veneration, has constantly been the production of his poetic phantasy." ‖ Lipsius asserts: Every religious emotion is accompanied by an act of formative phantasy; the intuitive picture created thereby is "unconscious symbol" of a transcendental one.¶ Siebeck distinguishes a "more unconscious" and a conscious mode of symbolization.§ Sabatier names as

* F. Riklin, Wunscherfüllung u. Symbolik im Märchen, Leipzig and Vienna, 1908.

† G. Runze, Katechismus der Religionsphilosophie 273, 278. In dogmatic theology, Schleiermacher denied "sensual selfconsciousness." Der christl. Glaube, Berlin, 1884, I, p. 30.

‡ F. A. Lange, Gesch. d. Materialismus, Iserlohn, 1877, II, p. 494 ff.

‖ W. E. Rauwenhoff, Religionsphilosophie, Braunschweig, 1894, p. 428. Likewise pp. 445, 449.

¶ R. A. Lipsius, Lehrbuch d. ev.-prot. Dogmatik, Braunschweig, 1893, p. 53.

§ H. Siebeck, Lehrbuch der Religionsphilosophie, Freiburg, 1893, p. 282.

one of the characteristics of religious knowledge that it is symbolical.* Eucken finds that religion only gains an effective result on human life when its truths gain illuminating colors by phantasy and become impressive symbolic figures; † the highest religion also requires the symbol ‡ even though one must hold the symbolical character of all human modes of expression for the present, in order to combat anthropomorphism.‖ Finally, Höffding teaches: "Religious symbolism is distinguished (considered epistomologically) from the metaphysical only by the fact that its pictures are more concrete, of richer colors and fuller of expression"; ¶ "if the religious ideas have any kind of significance, it can only be that they serve for the symbolical expression of the mood, the aspiration and the wishes of men during the life struggle." §

The images of God are symbols, the Apis bull of the Egyptians as well as Ishtar, the goddess of love of the Babylonians who was given the attributes of the panther and the morning-star. Most of the ritualistic acts are of symbolical nature, the taurobolium of Attis—where to-day, St. Peter's of Rome glistens, the pious individual allowed himself to be covered with blood from the sacrificial animal and greedily lapped it up with his mouth—not less than the noble celebration of the Christian Lord's Supper. The central idea of Christianity is expressed in the symbol of the cross as that of Buddhism is in the lotus flower which lies motionless on the pond allowing the rain to trickle off it, and at night withdrawing under the surface of the water.

Less known are the individual symbolical acts with which the Old Testament for example is filled. Jeremiah, for instance, smashed a pitcher on the place where the children were sacri-

---

* A. Sabatier, Religionsphilosophie auf gesch. Grundlage. German by Baur, Freiburg 1898, p. 307.
† R. Eucken, Der Wahrheitsgehalt der Religion, Leipzig, 1901, p. 340.
‡ P. 376.
‖ P. 425.
¶ H. Höffding, Religionsphil., Leipzig, 1901, p. 70.
§ P. 83.

ficed, in order to express the approaching destruction *; he placed cords and yokes on his neck to signify the approaching slavery.†

Folk superstitions are filled with symbolisms which are often no longer understood. In order to render teething easier for children, they laid on the gums, the prepared claws of a field mouse (arvicola amphibius L.). "As the mouse which digs in the earth breaks through the earth crust and works upward to the surface, so shall the sprouting tooth break through the gum." ‡ The ordinary forms of daily life also have in great part figurative value, the uncovering of the head, the bow, the shake of the head, etc. There are also symbols artificially formed. Riklin recalls the fact that on time-tables, a post-horn refers to the postal communication present.‖ He also calls attention that to the concept of symbol, the characteristic of secret or mysterious is usually joined.¶ Thus, for example, only the initiated could understand the runic writing.

How and why were symbols formed? Why is not the clear, definite scientific term preferred? One reason lies in the easily grasped distinctness of the picture, while on the other hand, the concept requires far greater effort of thought. In the symbol, one speaks of facts which are expressed on a basis of analogies by a pictorial idea easily comprehended at a glance. Even in science, we think in symbols as a rule. When we have perceived that "sweet" and "white" are sensations which are present only in a subject equipped with a sense apparatus but never in the outer world itself, for example, in a piece of sugar, still we think in our deliberations of the sugar as white and sweet, qualities to which the sugar never attains. Wundt

* Jeremiah, xix.
† Jeremiah, xxvii. Numerous examples in C. Kautzsch, Biblische Theologie des Alten und Neuen Testamentes. Tübingen 1911, pp.208 ff, 212, 319.
‡ O. Stoll, Zur Erkenntnis des Zauberglaubens, der Folksmagie und Folksmedizin in der Schweiz, Zürich, 1909, p. 74.
‖ F. Riklin, Wunscherfüllung u. Symbolik im Märchen, Leipzig and Vienna, 1908, p. 30.
¶ P. 31.

says quite correctly: "After the whole sensory content of ideas, as result of the development of the perception of knowledge, is withdrawn into the subject, the ideas, from then on, can apply only as subjective symbols of objective significance, by the elaboration of which symbols, a knowledge of the outer world is to be gained only in conceptual way." * "Not images, but symbols of reality, constitute science." † For the strictly scientific mode of thought, the symbol is not sufficient; this thought must go on to abstract formulations. But of these, too, Dürr rightly says: "Abstractions comprehend concrete objects by means of symbolizing conceptions." ‡

In the symbol, there usually exists, even when it is unadorned, an esthetic stimulus, which precise terms lack. In this point, it is surpassed by the artistically interested allegory.

Further, the symbol possesses a richness which the concept lacks. The picture is not exhausted by one interpretation or indeed by several. One is never quite certain when a symbol is exhausted in all its possibilities (for example, the cross). In this sense, the symbol exceeds the concept in extent.

The symbol includes not only reality as it is. It embraces besides all possible characteristic elements borrowed from reality, also such as correspond to our wishes. On a basis of analogies existing in reality, the symbol makes a comparison in which the traits which are undecided in reality, are decided according to the wish. Thus, the symbol is real and unreal at the same time and so suffices in certain relations for the reality-principle and the pleasure-principle of our mind, of which we shall have to speak. It expresses hope and creates a hopeful presentiment. Just here, lies an especial attraction which Mallarmé describes in these words: "To name an object, is to suppress three fourths of the pleasure of the poem which consists of the pleasure of divining little by little." ‖

Many symbols would declare and conceal simultaneously,

* Wundt, System d. Phil. p. 146.
† E. Dürr, Erkenntnistheorie, Leipzig, 1910, p. 147. Compare p. 278.
‡ Same, p. 51.
‖ Cited by Hamann, Der Impressionismus in Kunst u. Leben, p. 108.

thus, the secret rites, the names of certain secret societies, the pentagram, etc.

It is an error to think that the symbolical always expresses an abstract idea. When a boy expresses something improper with his fingers, his comrade understands that an entirely concrete wish is thereby communicated.

Reality can also become a symbol. Hamann remarks: ''It (the stimulating excitation) is truest and finest where the symbols do not belong to a richer, strange and beautiful world but where apparently every-day words and experiences are full of mysterious references and hidden meanings.''*

Besides the concepts of symbol given above, there is yet another still more extended meaning. In antiquity, ὀύμβολον signified in addition to sensual representation of an idea, as much as characteristic, mark or token, such for example as those carried by the judges or participants in the mysteries, then further, an agreed-upon sign, for instance, the soldier's watchword. In church history, symbols mean also the formulæ or books by which a religious sect stated its beliefs in order to distinguish themselves from other groups, sects or churches. The characteristics of figurative distinctness, esthetic reality, secret wisdom are thereby lost.

So far as the symbols in ordinary speech usage are concerned, their origin in brevity, distinctness, easy comprehension, esthetic acceptableness, fulness of content, suggestive promise, discrete disguise is well founded and justified. The symbol appears therefore, not only as Silberer says, wherever the thought cannot manifest itself in consciousness in its ''real'' form from any reason whatever.† It is indeed correct that even a scientific thought may be anticipated symbolically —one thinks of Kekulé's benzol ring (240)—but a symbol may occasionally be preferred in the presence of the full intellectual mastery of the material.

---

* Hamann, p. 108.
† H. Silberer, über Symbolbildung, Jahrb. III, p. 664.

(B) SYMBOL FORMATION AS MANIFESTATION

(1)   *Psychological Remarks*

The neurotic and dream symbols agree in most characteristics with those of ordinary mental life. They also express one idea by another, whereby this symbolic idea often expresses only a characteristic, a related object or an analogous process. It makes use of allusion. In the plain simplicity (which represents a condensation), the expressiveness, the excitation to foreboding expectations, the conscious and unconscious symbols are a unit.

The fundamental difference between the two kinds of symbols lies in the fact that the conscious symbol serves the purpose of communication to other persons, thus, is a social function, while the automatic symbol is of autistic nature (see below). Paul says in one place: "He that speaketh in an unknown tongue edifieth himself" (not for other men) I Cor. xiv, 4. This holds true of all manifestations.* The manifestation must be incomprehensible for its producer. It is as we saw, even an attempt to overcome the resistance by distortion. The pent-up instinct, inhibited from open activity, utilizes metaphorical automatism to gratify itself at least to as high a degree as possible.

A distinct difference may not be disputed here. But should the name "symbol" be withheld from the manifestation on this account? No. Not only do the psychological and logical characteristics of both symbolisms agree, aside from the social teleology, but also the history of language, which considers the symbol simply as sign, completely justifies the psychoanalytic speech usage. For the rest, no one is forbidden to give a new sense to a scientific term where no confusion threatens. All terms undergo a change in meaning.

How closely related both kinds of symbolisms are, is seen

---

* There are also manifestations with social aims, for example, fainting as a demand for tenderness. But there too, the content of the symptom is still asocial (flight from reality).

particularly in those formations which can appear just as well automatically as on a basis of conscious deliberation. For example, we heard on page 68 of a patient who had to wash himself continually in obsessional manner. As cause for this obsession, we found the unconscious wish to free himself from the reproach of self-pollution. I found the same motive in some other youths. A woman patient in the middle thirties, who had to perform her astoundingly complicated washing ceremony under severest mental anguish, three to six hours every day and could never wear the same linen two days, so fastened both arms every night with safety-pins that they could not touch her body and in addition, the nightdress had to be pinned tightly together below. The formative determination of this obsessional neurosis is plain enough.

The discovery of this connection was made by Freud by means of analysis. Then, however, he found that a great poet had already discovered the state of affairs by intuition *— as in general, analysis has found scarcely one important fact which profound students of humanity had not already perceived more or less clearly. Shakespeare describes in his "Macbeth" (V-1) the Lady walking in her sleep after the murder of the king:

Doctor: What is it she does now? Look how she rubs her hands.
Waiting-woman: It is an accustomed action with her, to seem thus washing her hands; I have known her continue in this a quarter of an hour.

Lady Macbeth: Yet here's a spot . . . Out, damned spot! Out, I say! . . . Yet who would have thought the old man to have had so much blood in him? . . . What, will these hands ne'er be clean?   ·
Doctor: Foul whisperings are abroad: unnatural deeds
Do breed unnatural troubles: infected minds
To their deaf pillows will discharge their secrets:
More needs she the divine than the physician." †

The connection, as Shakespeare represents it here, can be shown in individuals who are readily analyzable, often with

---

* Freud, Obsessions et phobies. Kl. Schriften I, p. 90.
† Theory of abreaction!

the greatest ease and clearness.   Error seems to me absolutely excluded.   It should be emphasized that the patient himself does not once suspect the cause of his obsession.   Is this symbolism so uncommon?   Have we not already found it a hundred times?   We find washing among many peoples as a symbolical act which is meant to express the wish for purification of the soul from guilt.   The Old Testament affords a multitude of examples: for instance, Isaiah i, 15, 16: "Your hands are full of blood. Wash you, make you clean." Jeremiah ii, 22: "For though thou wash thee with nitre, and take thee much soap, yet thine iniquity is marked before me, saith the Lord God."*   At the time of Jesus, the proselytes probably had to undergo an immersion in order to be received into membership in the Jewish religion.†   Primitive Christianity understood, with John the Baptist, baptism to be a purification ceremony.   (I Cor. vi, 11; Eph. v, 26, etc.)

The difference between unconscious washing symbolism conditioned by complexes and conscious washing symbolism is slight.   The former is not understood by the person using the ceremonial, the latter is well understood.   The difference becomes even smaller yet: The religious baptismal ceremony became an incomprehensible, magic-working mystery which was executed more or less obsessionally with secret fear.‡

(2) *The Meaning of the Symbols*

A. POSSIBILITY OF INTERPRETING SYMBOLS

Many persons will not dispute the fact of symbols conditioned by complexes but deny the possibility of a reliable interpretation and, like Isserlin, accuse the analysts, who nevertheless venture an explanation, of "grotesque statements." ||

* E. Kautzsch, Die H. Schrift des Alten Testaments, Tübingen, 1909, Vol. I.   Further examples in Exodus xxxvi, 25, Psalm li., 4 and 9.

† H. Guthe, Kurzes Bibelwörterbuch, Tübingen and Leipzig, 1903, p. 653.

‡ Freud, Zwangshandlungen u. Religionsübung. Kl. Schriften II, pp. 122–131.

|| M. Isserlin, Über Jungs "Psychologie der Dementia præcox" und

It is to be admitted that in Freud's writings, the proofs for particular interpretations are not given in satisfactory fulness—volumes would have been necessary to do this. But Freud did not write for scholars who would take counsel and advice only from books, he turned to investigators who were willing and capable of opening the book of reality.

The interpretation of many symbols does not really demand much acuity of vision. It has been a subject of jest that the Zeppelin airship in dreams was considered a masculine symbol. The following little fragment of dream analysis will give the uninitiated person ground for deciding whether that exegesis was so very artificial.

The patient with obsessional neurosis, aged sixteen, to whom I referred on page 72, dreamed: "I saw a Zeppelin airship and went after it. It landed in H. on a meadow. Then there was something with maps in the car or somewhere else. Then I went off and was finally in C. near the station there. I asked for directions how to get home and was led to a house. There were various dried fish and thick green seaweed, out of which, a white worm came. Then, I finally came home. Everything was full of laundry in great disorder. Then the Zeppelin flew directly over our house and made a kind of salt hail. Then someone said to me, that is a trial of a method by which it could destroy all crops in case of war."

[What comes to mind in connection with the dream?] "It reminds me of the white body of the flounder which was so significant for me.

[The airship.] My oldest anxiety-dream dealt with a dragon which flew over my bed. His tail reminded me of the worm-shaped organ of the flounder.

[The meadow.] In its neighborhood, was the river in which in the previous dream, I fished for cladophora which in reality were not there at the time. One showed a long thin bent stalk at the end of which, many threads separated clockwise, the

die Anwendung Freudscher Maximen in der Psychopathologie. Zbl. f. Nervenheilkunde u. Psychiatrie 1907, 329–343 (p. 336).

other looked like frog-spawn. The meadow also resembled that on which I actually saw the Zeppelin balloon.

[Maps.]   The region of Paris.   The key to the signs was disagreeable to me.

[The engineer.]   He showed me the maps.

[C.]   In a little street by the station, I inquired the way. There I saw rays in a show window.

[The house with the fish.]   The table is that of my room. The seaweed was an ulva, a structure in reality about a foot long.   The white worm did not really exist; it reminded me, I think, even in the dream of flounder and dragon's tail.

[Dirty linen.]   As when I go in my room too early before it has been put in order.   I felt uncomfortable.

[Did something happen to the linen that night?]   At the end of the dream, I had a pollution.

[The salt hail.]   I read that such a thing happened in 1870 when the wind drove seawater upon the land.   Otherwise nothing.   The salt looked in the air like flakes, only on the earth like salt.

[Crops (grain).]   I saw something black in the grain that I took for a mushroom.   It was only pitch however.   I was angry at being so stupid.   I eat much rye-bread.''

We will not interpret everything in this dream.   Our interest concerns first the airship.   It resembles the organ which the dreamer considered a member, further the dragon tail which aroused anxiety.   "Map" is the vulgar term used by young people for pollution stains.   Further, the phantastic cladophora taken beside the meadow have sexual significance as the sketch made by the dreamer immediately betrays.   Paris comes into consideration as city of immorality.   The engineer is the analyst who had given his anxious youth quieting assurance concerning the harmlessness of the pollution.*   The street in C., the disordered linen, the ulva touch the same

---

* In very many cases of too frequent pollutions, the mere calming assurance without analysis suffices.   Concerning severe cases, compare chapter XXVII, section 6.

sexual theme. The flake-like salt hail over the house refers to the cause of the malady, the incest with the sister. To my question: "Does not salt serve for sterilization of land?" he answered: "I do not think that this is the case here." Naturally he is right. Salt is here, as in folklore, symbol of creation and fruitfulness, to which Schleiden referred in 1875, in his book, "Das Salz. Seine Geschicht, seine Symbolik, und seine Bedeutung in Menschenleben." (Salt. Its history, its symbolism and significance in human life.)* Ernest Jones gives a mass of ethnographical proof for the sperma symbolism of salt in an exhaustive article.

How one can deny the sexual significance of the airship in this pollution-dream is inconceivable to me.

In a later pollution-dream, the youth saw Count Zeppelin standing there, in a still later one, he caught sight of him only on a medallion. Timid minds who take offence at the discussion of such objects should notice that the analysis eliminated not only the extremely complicated obsessional neurosis but also improved in most gratifying manner the moral dignity of the youth who had caused his parents great concern.

Space is lacking to give many analyses of symbols. The reader will be able to make such for himself very easily if he studies this book.

A symbol can express different thoughts at the same time. The cross is the emblem of the Christian religion but also expression of the idea that by the greatest sacrifice, the highest victory must be purchased, or that even death can afford no check to heroic love, or that injustice may befall even the holiest. So also can the symbol conditioned on complexes lay claim to many interpretations in order to be fully understood. In the dream of the patient with spinal syphilis (251f), most of the ideas, for instance, water, gondola, being lifted, pastor, etc. had a religious and an erotic meaning. Freud's dictum: Behind one dream interpretation may always lurk another,

* Compare E. Jones, Die Bedeutung des Salzes in Sitte und Brauch der Völker. Imago I, p. 367.

so that one is really never sure of having completely interpreted a dream,* is true also of the symbol.

The question whether every symbol can be interpreted, I think should be answered in the negative. Naturally, one can find some kind of sense in all. But the deeper an interpretation is, just so much the more important it is. Since not every dream can be interpreted,† and is often condensed into a symbol of the dream content, so one need not feel bound to decipher every symbol. Nevertheless the connection with other dreams and manifestations yields the correct meaning.

B. TYPICAL SYMBOLS

One can very well understand that the assertion that certain dream ideas signify, always or almost always, such and such real objects, should have occasioned violent indignation. By this theory, the danger is incurred of wanting to interpret the dream mechanically by the aid of a lexicon. This stupid method repels one. Stekel, although he has deciphered many symbols with great ingenuity, has published others as typical with too little motivation and too hasty generalization and later recalled them. But he himself emphasizes the artistic factor in the dream interpretation.‡

On the other hand, the fact of typical symbols, if they exist, facilitates the work of patient and analyst to a considerable extent. Let us bow, therefore, to the force of reality.

That there are typical symbols, I will show first in a neat example: the picture of the serpent. The phallic significance of the serpent runs through wide stretches of religious history: Dieterich relates that in Greece on certain feasts, a phallus or a serpent was placed in a chest.‖ The serpent cult of the negroes of Haiti and Louisiana bears a phallic character.¶

* Freud, Traumdeutung, pp. 109, 223.
† Same, p. 350.
‡ Stekel, Die Sprache des Traumes, p. 533.
‖ Dieterich, Eine Mithrasliturgie, 1910.
¶ P. D. Chantepie de la Saussaye, Lehrbuch d. Religionsgesch.

Among the Arrhetophorians, pastry in the form of phalli and serpents was thrown into the chasm during the Thesmophoria in order to obtain fruitfulness in children and harvests.* The serpent, besides other objects known to the analyst as sexual symbols, is the symbol of Hecate Aphrodisias.†

The mother of Augustus dreamed that she was impregnated by Apollo changed into the form of a serpent and has borne since then the figure of a serpent on her thigh.

The legend also makes use of the serpent symbolism. In Bechstein's "Oda und die Schlange," the serpent taken into bed by the girl changes into a prince.‡

Art often replaces the phallus by a serpent. Möricke speaks plainly enough in his "Ersten Liebeslied eines Mädchens" (First love song of a maiden):

> "What is in the net? Just look
> But I am afraid;
> Do I grasp a sweet eel?
> Do I grasp a serpent?
> It slips through my hands.
> O, woe! O, joy!
> With twisting and turning
> It slides to my breast.
> It bites, O, wonder!
> Me right through the skin,
> Shoots down to the heart.
> O love, I shudder!
> I must be poisoned!
> Here it sneaks around
> Blissfully buries itself
> And puts me to death." ‖

Freiburg and Leipzig, 2d ed. 1897, I, p. 25. Maeder gives further ethnographic evidence in "Die Symbolik in den Legenden, Märchen, Gebräuchen und Träumen. Psychiatrisch-neurol. Wochenschrift, Year X, Nos. 6 and 7. Also Riklin, Wunscherfüllung u. Symbolik im Märchen, pp. 40–44.

* Jung, Wandlungen u. Symbole der Libido. Jahrb. IV, p. 372.
† Same, p. 397.
‡ Riklin, Wunscherfüllung, p. 41.
‖ E. Möricke, Sämtl. W. W., Stuttgart and Leipzig, p. 8. Jung, Jahrbuch IV, p. 126.

If we wished to give the whole poem, we could show with ease from a mass of analogies what "bite," "heart," "poison," "bury," "put to death" (umbringen), mean.

Lessing points out in Laocoön (Section II) that the mothers of Aristomenes, Ariotodoma, Alexander the Great, Scipio, Augustus, and Valerius dreamed during their pregnancies that they had to do with a serpent.

Goethe uses the serpent symbol in the same sense. In the 12th Roman elegy, he describes the person being initiated into the Elysian mysteries.

> "Strangely wandered the novice through circles
> Of rare figures; in dream, he seemed to ramble; for here
> Serpents squirmed about on the ground, locked caskets
> Richly crowned with spikes, girls here bore by,
> Only after many tests and trials, was to him revealed,
> What the sacred circle strangely hid in pictures.
> And what was the secret, except that Demeter the Great,
> Once obligingly submitted to a hero,
> As she once to Jaoon, the valiant King of Crete,
> Granted the gracious secrets of her immortal body." *

It is not necessary to tell more clearly what serpent and casket signify.

We too have met the serpent as phallus-representative several times: In the obsessional neurotic patient, who, after a bath with the father, could no longer hold his hands in water for fear of a serpent (72), and in the patient with anxiety hysteria who saw hallucinated serpents crawling over her feet but which could no longer bite (66), etc.

I could easily present a number of dreams which give serpents the same representation. Only two examples:

"I went with some girls to a meadow beside the flowing brooks. In these, lay serpents, small ones about fifteen centimeters long, and large ones which were about six paces long. We wanted to jump away but always fell on the serpents. I could not jump because of anxiety and called after the others. They came and took me home with them. There we made

* Goethe, Röm. Elegien XII. Zbl. II, p. 291 f.

serpents in sardine-boxes (sic). We cut up the serpents with knives, afterwards, put oil on them, no, only water, and ate the serpents.''

On that meadow, the dreamer, a twelve year old girl whom we met on page 185, had really gone. With her girl friends, she had looked at a picture-book in which there were serpents. Further associations did not come. I therefore said outright: ''Tell quite frankly what really happened.'' The little one reported amid tears that one of her friends had just that morning explained, she was so tired. Then she had confessed that she had practiced sexual intercourse with a boy, which agitated the hearer. The latter, when five years old, had been improperly handled by a boy. The box corresponded, like the chest of the Greek feast and the casket in Goethe's elegy, to the female organ. Freud calls attention that πνξις, English box, has this special meaning. The cutting up of the serpent corresponds to the sadistic poem, in which, of the children crawling in the body, one is dead, one blind and one with a hole in its head. The eating of the serpent is that process which Freud calls displacement from below upwards.*

The other dream comes from a fourteen year old hysterical girl whom we met on page 212, and abbreviated runs as follows: _

''I went away from my parents and met many serpents who said to me that I should immediately turn around or a great misfortune would befall me. I ran, however, filled with anxiety, farther among the serpents. Then I came to a hole which was quite black with serpents. They crawled upon me, ever closer and closer so that I could scarcely breathe. I called: 'Help! Help!' Then my mother and a girl comrade

---

* Jung interprets the cutting-up of the serpent as symbolical expression of rebirth. The regressive libido is cut up and sacrificed to the purpose of the rebirth. He recalls Dionysos who, in the form of a serpent under the name of Zagreus, was cut up and whose heart, Zeus with the aim of rebirth, swallowed, further he recalls the Orphic sacred feast dedicated to Dionysos Zagreus in which the cut-up serpent was eaten. A mass of other historical observations also compel him to this interpretation of the serpent-symbol.

came quickly and cut the serpents apart with knives.   Then I awoke and was free again.''

The similarity to the preceding dream stands out plainly. Again we are dealing with an anxiety dream which with the strong pent-up sexual desire of both girls, cannot be wondered at.   Again the serpent is cut in pieces.

[The serpents.] ''They lay in a ditch beside the road.   I really saw an adder once, lying so.   (The symbolism of the ditch is not difficult to decipher in this and the preceding dream.)   At a fair, I saw a woman who wore a snake about her neck.   The smaller serpents were about 0.5 meter, the larger, some 5 meters long.''   (As in previous dream; exaggerated representation of various conditions.)

[The warning of the serpents.] ''Serpents cannot speak. Otherwise, nothing.''

[The hole.] ''In the garden of a pension for young men, there is such a hole.   Water dropped from above (stalactites, phallus-shaped).   The serpents gave out a white foamy liquid.''

[They crawled up.] ''On the legs, about the neck and head. It seemed very odd to me.   I thought, now it is ready, now I shall be bitten.''

[Help! Help!] ''My father once struck my mother. Then I called help, help!''

[Mother and comrade come to help.] ''They wore red aprons.   I too have one at home.   When my father saw it, he scolded because it was too expensive.   The comrade, I see often; she does not wish to know me longer but goes into school with me, nevertheless.''   [The cutting up of the serpents.] ''On my body.   Now it came to my mind how father struck mother and we scratched him.''

The anxiety itself betrays to everyone who has analyzed a few dozen anxiety-dreams, the suspected sexual situation.   The warning of the serpents shows the fear of sexuality.   In the garden grotto, the little one often saw young men even years before.   Behind the encircling serpents, in the first rank, stands the father; the little daughter identifies herself with her mother while the whole father becomes a serpent which is cut in pieces. One notices here besides the sexual desire, the sadistic hate. The cause of the dream is the sight of the parents united in wedlock after a separation of years, whose bed stood beside that of the child.*

I have now shown in sufficient observations that the serpent occurs principally as a masculine symbol. I could show that the fish of related shape appears typically in similar application. As proof, I mention only the habit of a normal boy of taking fish in the aquarium in his hands, whereupon, a high degree of sensual pleasure appeared. Further, the Chinese dragon which makes itself now small, now large, could be introduced with its myths. But the serpent symbol is not yet disposed of.

The serpent appears also as feminine symbol. The serpent in paradise is often pictured as a female being.† The woman plays a rôle as serpent also in folk sayings.

Further, the serpent is the being into which the soul after leaving the body changes.‡ Jung indeed reads from the picture of Priapus who was castrated by a serpent and from a man pictured by Rubens as in the flood, to whom the same thing happens, as well as many other monuments that the serpent may be the own (repressed) will to die.‖

Conversely, we recognize the serpent again as personification of Æsculapius, as genius of mineral spa, incarnate earth- and fire-god, etc. Jung remarks: "Whatever else the symbolism of the serpent may relate to, its interpretation is very dependent on age and circumstances of life. To youth, repressed

---

* Jung interprets this dream also asexually: The serpents are death-symbols (compare Wandlungen, Jahrb. IV, 462), the flight into caves means withdrawal from life. The meaning would then be: Wish for the overcoming of the anxiety over rebirth. The anxiety says: You should be anxious concerning sexuality, otherwise you will fall into the bottomless pit.

† Jung, Wandlungen, Jahrb. III, p. 212.

‡ Riklin, Wunscherfüllung, p. 43.

‖ Jung, Wandlungen, Jahrb. IV, p. 472.

sexuality is symbolized in the serpent, for the advent of sexuality brings an end to childhood. To age, on the other hand, the serpent signifies repressed death thoughts." *

Finally, Jung finds in the dragon which fights the mythological hero, "the repressed libido of the son striving for the mother, thus as you might say, the son himself." †

At all events, the simple symbol of the serpent is in general of many meanings and it is awkward and stupid to identify the serpent every time with the phallus.‡ I have also found the serpent atypically as allusion to the pretendedly poisonous tongue of the wife.

The discussion of one particular typical symbol has detained us for some time. I would gladly introduce a number of others but we would lose too much time. Enough that there are typical symbols in great number. It is also certain that their typical interpretation possesses only high probability, nevertheless, it often renders possible a positively correct explanation of the connection of the majority of such complex structures. He who does not like to publish his intimate secrets, should guard against relating to an analyst his dreams and phantasies. How often have I had the experience of having someone, in spite of warning, persist against this advice and blushingly have to acknowledge the interpretation of the analyst who read from it impotence or some other discrete intimacy!

Merely as examples of frequent meanings of typical symbols, not as infallible translations, a few especially frequent ones may be mentioned.

As symbol of masculine sexuality appear:

(a) Objects of similar shape, as pistols, guns, needles, knives, daggers, lances, pencils, paper-cutters, umbrellas, towers.

(b) Male animals: bull,‖ elephant, usually with upraised trunk, tiger, lion.

* Jung, Wandlungen, Jahrb. IV, p. 462.
† P. 395.
‡ The same is true of the fish.
‖ According to Jung, this appears also as feminine symbol, as also the fish (Jahrb. IV, p. 242).

As feminine symbols are recognized: chests, boxes, pockets, books, butterflies, shoes, holes, churches.

Masculine or feminine may be: bird, dog, cat, mouse, horse, tree,* plum, foot, sun (father or mother).

Sexual activity is expressed by striking, biting, riding, eating, fighting, swimming, flying.

In the following sections, we shall see whether these sexual interpretations must be replaced by a deeper asexual explanation as Adler and Jung assume.

How does the knowledge of the most frequent meanings of symbols help us in the manifold meanings of symbols? Were it not better that one knew nothing of these meanings and sought for himself? Certainly it is desirable that one should find as much for himself as possible. But I admit that here and there I could not solve a dream but when I put in an interpretation of Freud's, Jung's or Stekel's, it yielded good sense which also fitted excellently in the mental condition as it was disclosed by other phenomena. He who denies typical symbols as a matter of principle may quietly investigate and analyze as if they did not exist. He will soon perceive his error. Freud emphasizes † that typical symbols occasionally occur atypically and Stekel, who according to his confession, often errs in this respect, recommends taking familiar symbols into consideration only as possible solutions.‡

Freud says expressly that many typical clinical phenomena, after their true meaning has become known, will some day disappear, since the neurosis does not hold its secret before the window.‖

C. MATERIAL AND FUNCTIONAL SYMBOLISM
(THE LIBIDO-SYMBOL)

Herbert Silberer performed no small service in demonstrating the fact that many symbols express objective thoughts,

---

* Jung, Wandlungen, Jahrb. IV, p. 262 (feminine), p. 264 (masculine).
† Freud, Traumdeutung, p. 210.
‡ Stekel, Fortschritte d. Traumdeutung, Zbl. III, p. 158.
‖ Freud, Die zukünftigen Chancen d. Psychoan. Therapie. Zbl. I, p. 7 f.

others, on the other hand, subjective performances.* The investigations from which his distinctions proceed, are primarily of synthetic nature. Meditating on a problem in a sleep-like state, he suddenly saw a dream picture before him which represented the theme in symbolical form. He was thinking, for example, of his scheme for improving a rough place in an article, and saw himself planing a piece of wood smooth. Or he wishes to warn another from executing a dangerous decision since it threatens misfortune and he sees three frightful looking horsemen on black steeds charging along over a barren field. The analysis of these phantasies would yield refined details of the position and solution of the problem of symbols. In contrast to these two material phenomena, we put two functional ones: Silberer wishes to recapitulate an association in order not to forget it; he sees an obliging lackey before him. He loses the thread in his train of thought; a piece of composition appears to him, the last lines of which have fallen out. Unfortunately, the keen-witted author omits the exact analysis, probably because it would disclose too much intimate material. It is evident that in the symbolical representation and solution of problems, manifestations of personal complexes would be interwoven. As often as I have employed the interesting method of Silberer's, this union of material and personal interests was shown, for the dream is, as a matter of fact, always egocentric, indeed, Freud goes so far as to say, egoistic.†

We now go a step farther than Silberer. Previously, we showed that the material phenomena did not mean what they expressed but had reference only to an image of reality (146). He who suffers from a negative father-complex actually hates, not the real father, but the father present in his phantasy. If one investigates this psychological state of affairs closer, one finds that in it besides the conscious grudge, an unconscious attachment is fixed by the idea of the bad father, as a result of

* Herbert Silberer, Bericht ü. e. Methode, Gewisse symbolische Halluzinations-Erscheinungen hervorzurufen und zu beobachten. Jahrb. I, p. 516 f. The third group, that of somatic phenomena, is less important for us here.
† Freud, Traumdeutung, p. 254.

which, the attitude to other men and to the tasks of life is determined thus and so. Or he who dreams of incestuous relation to the mother, betrays thereby that his instinct strives toward her picture. Thus in the symbols which we have to consider as manifestations, there lurks not only a material but also a functional disclosure. The symbol gives hints concerning the condition of the subject's own person. Therefore, its recognition is of the highest importance for the healing of the sick and the exercise of pedagogic influence.

Also in poetry, an historical figure is often not to be understood as such. K. F. Meyer said that his Dante in his novel, "Die Hochzeit des Mönches" (Wedding of the Monk) did not stand for the poet but for the spirit of the Middle Ages.

A young girl who suffered from disagreement with her parents and loss of affection for her fiancé, as well as hallucinations, anxiety ideas and melancholia, dreamed: "On the Etzelberg, stand two high towers, one of which I climb. I am given a sleeping-potion." [Etzel.] "I was there yesterday." [Tower.] "The colosseum in Rome; there I climbed around. The tower in the dream was much higher." [Sleeping-potion.] "I do not know who gave it. The drink had the same color as the sleeping-potion my mother had to take when she was sick and could not sleep. I find it sad that one should be in this condition."

[The other tower.] "It is empty. I think there of a passionate admirer and a beloved friend who experienced great difficulties in their passions and are unhappy. The former does not come into consideration for a marriage, the latter suffers from loss of her love."

The dreamer identifies herself with her mother: She takes her sleeping-potion. The old high tower probably denotes the father. The girl does not climb the empty tower on which she thinks of people unhappy in love, she does not wish to love her fiancé in earnest, but allows herself quietly to assume the rôle of the sick, sleep-desirous mother.* Her life-force remains at-

* Jung explains: One tower is, as often, the mother (compare Maria as ivory tower), the other the father. The dreamer yields her-

tached to the infantile, chained to phantasies that have no outlook, passive. The bold step into reality, she will not undertake. The analysis nevertheless acted satisfactorily; after some weeks, the attitude toward the fiancé became correct. A sincere love replaced the faithless wavering between passionate devotion and icy coldness.

We can determine the meaning of the functional symbol somewhat closer still. In order not to create the impression that we are dealing with isolated instances, I beg to give still another dream. It concerned a man in the thirties, who had been married nine years, whose young, pretty and good-natured wife felt unhappy and directed her love passionately upon an old gentleman, a very plain substitute for her father. Her physically superior husband, she underestimated, called him terribly tiresome in spite of his culture, was angry at his rare courtesy and tenderness and wished either to get a divorce and marry the old sport or die. In such cases, it is necessary to analyze both husband and wife. The obsession of the desperate wife who had suffered severely ever since the beginning of her married life from her obsessional love for the father-substitute, was easy to eliminate. Still, the husband rendered difficult a complete regulation of the marital conditions since he treated his wife like a sister and was afraid of a child. The following dream shows the reason; it was brought out at the first consultation:

"I was on a balloon journey. In the neighborhood of Frauenfeld, we climbed out of the basket. For the passage, I had paid one hundred francs. Here, more was demanded since the trip took considerably longer than had been specified. I was afraid that it might be eight hundred or one thousand francs. It seemed as if I heard this price mentioned. I thought, how shall I get this sum. I asked myself how should I pay it since in neighboring H., at a rifle-match, I had shot away so much money and on account of bad weather, had hit little. My colleague M. was also on the trip and reviled me.

self to the mother and returns like Hölderlin in paradise-like condition of sleep (Jahrb. IV, p. 424 ff.).

In the basket, suddenly sits Engineer N., who would drive the balloon farther by making rocking motions with his body as in coasting. I awoke.''

I give only the most important associations. [Balloon journey.] ''It happened that I was looking at a flying balloon when someone told me of psychoanalysis for the first time. At that time, the conversation was about a gentleman who lived dissolutely, used much money and was to be won to no ideal.'' [Frauenfeld.] ''A friend is seeking a wife and finds none since he can never make a decision. He is bombastic. Tomato salad, for instance, he calls love's apple salad.'' [Frauenfeld.] ''The barracks there. The Confederation wished them in Wyl but the inhabitants of that town explained that they desired no Confederation brothel in their city. In Frauenfeld, lives an old relative who was unhappy in her love for an artist. She did not dare to marry the latter on account of his sister.'' [Basket.] ''Hencoop.'' (Hühnerkorb). (In Swiss German, ''hühnern'' is an indecent term.) ''I found that the money for the whole journey had been demanded previously and was embarrassed on account of the money to be raised. I thought it would be a disgrace if it were known that I had so little money in my purse.'' [The journey longer than presupposed.] ''The shooting-match in X. was dearer than supposed.''

[On account of bad weather.] ''My brother-in-law also hit nothing and was out of sorts. I suggested sharing a sleeping-room with him. My wife said they had demanded more from me in marriage than I could give; I have entered upon the marriage and have seen that they desire more from me. It seemed to me that the balloon trip was the wedding trip. After the sexual intercourse on this trip, we were both used up and found there was nothing in it, it was not worth the trouble.''

[Colleague M.] ''He is a gossip and faultfinder who does not, however, defend his idea. Otherwise he is not disagreeable, likes a drink, rides out in style. He was my school comrade. He is industrious. Now he possesses his own little house. He may have attained advancement by fraud.''

[Engineer N.] ''A roué, unreliable, who was attentive to

my wife at a ball. He had to marry a girl of doubtful reputation; I had disembarked when N. made his motions."

The meaning of the dream is clear. The balloon trip is the wedding trip as the dreamer himself interprets it. The intermediate landing at Frauenfeld discloses the present situation: The wife does not wish to stay in her marriage any longer. Much more is demanded of him than formerly: Money is true love, which so far is lacking, as the unsatisfactory intercourse shows. This expenditure of love he cannot make, it had been very costly to him without his having won anything worth while, as the memory of the rifle-match, to be understood as sexual symbolism, shows. The colleague shows traits of the dreamer himself: He also finds fault easily but nevertheless lacks strong arguments for his ideas; he also likes to live well, longs for his own villa, likes costly trips. To my question, why, after nine years of married life, he still does not want children, he replied that he would then have to give up house and travel. The wife, on the other hand, had longed for children from the beginning. Therein he is an egoist who is to blame in great part for his trouble, although he believes he is striving only for the good.

The following presentation shows he refused the proper marriage as immoral (hencoop, brothel, roué). It is indicated that he longs for his sister (the artist who remained attached to his sister; passing the night in the room of his sister's husband).

The meaning of the dream runs as follows: I will not pay the price of increased expenditure of love demanded of me for the continuation of my marriage and will leave such affairs to impure fellows. One understands that the overaffectionate relation only disguises the deficiency in real love and that the wife, whose unconscious naturally perceives the state of affairs and repays in like coin, could not feel herself gratified.

Thus, all the dream figures appearing here, embody the resistance. They are nothing else than resistance-symbols. They show why the dreamer does not give up his love: Basket (hencoop), Frauenfeld (literally, ladies' field), sums of money, shooting-match, colleague, engineer, coasting. This does not say that also in other dreams, every symbol declares resistance. In these resistance-symbols, we distinguish one tendency attracting the love (fixation on the sister) and another current repelling the freeing of the love from repression (pleasure seeking).

Which of the two is the more important? Or is one only a derivative of the other? We will consider these questions directly.

First, we will recall that Goethe also knew how often we have to understand other people really symbolically. In "Tasso," he remarks: "We seem to love the man and we love with him only the highest which we can love." Tell me whom you love and I will tell you how it is with your life-desires.

(3). *The Deeper Meaning of Symbols*

According to Freud, the fundamental basis of the neurosis lies in the repression of an incestuous relation to the parents. Every neurotic individual is an Œdipus who loves his mother and would like to kill his father out of jealousy. In this family-romance, lies the nuclear complex of all neuroses.

Jung, on the other hand, considers the mother only as libido-symbol. The incest prohibition is only the resistance set up against the libido; the symbol-bearer desires no real incest but regression to childhood, return to the mother's womb for the purpose of rebirth. "One of the simplest ways would be to impregnate the mother and to create himself identically again.* Against that, the incest prohibition protests. Religions seek to attain the rebirth, therefore, by spiritualizing the incest phantasy, for example, in Jesus' talk with Nicodemus †: "Verily, verily, I say unto you, if a man be not born of water and of the spirit, he cannot enter the Kingdom of Heaven." Jung interprets: "To be born of water always means only: to be born from the mother's womb. 'Of the spirit' means: 'from the fructifying breath of the wind' ‡ that is, impreg-

* Jung, Wandlungen, Jahrb. IV, p. 267.
† John iii, v. 3 ff.
‡ Jahrb. IV, p. 268.

nated by a spirit-being in extraordinary manner." Thus the person may think of birth from the mother (water), not however of copulation with her. In Jesus' command lies also, according to Jung, the command to consider the rebirth phantasy symbollically and thereby set free the incestuous libido. "Thus the libido which lies bound, inactive in incestuous wishes, suppressed and transformed into anxiety before the law and the avenging father-god, may be directed by the symbol of baptism (birth from the water) and the creation of the symbol of out-pouring of the Holy Ghost over into sublimation." *

It is first of all to be emphasized that Jung, although it does not appear in the passages cited, by no means always takes the mother-image in the sense of pure symbol, that without exception, only one phase (that is psychological conception) of rebirth with her is to be considered. Also he admits that the actual incest desire often actually prevails, even at the time when a present inhibition has brought about a regression to infantile desires. Herein, he is right, though I wish that I could contradict it.

What the symbolical interpretation of the longing for the mother's womb means, can obviously be decided, as Jung also admits, not by mythology but by observation on living subjects. The following conclusions seem to me certain: We find often with certainty a longing for return to the uterus without a trace of desire for rebirth. I analyzed one introverted individual who would have been passionately glad to live in a grave his life long as a Buddhist saint and who sat hours at a time before the insane asylum with voluptuous longing, meditating on how fine it would be to dream within that place the most grandiose phantasies until life ended. In his paintings,† were plainly seen the wishes for the sight of the undressed mother, for taking the father's place in regard to sexuality, for mutual rest with his sister in the mother's womb. Of rebirth thoughts, there was before this analysis no trace.

* Same, p. 270.
† Compare chapter XII, section 9.

That, in the talk with Nicodemus, a very deep-rooted mother-womb phantasy of incestuous character is disclosed and that the low, gross desires of people may be won for reality by sublimation, I consider a very important thought. The longing for rebirth runs through all secret religions, which, as is known, enjoyed an enormous vogue at the time of Jesus, especially the Osiris-, Attis- and Mithra-cults. Just as little is the frequency of the wish for return to the mother's womb to be doubted. Otherwise, whence would come the incredibly frequent mother-womb-phantasies? * That Jesus, in John's Gospel, gave to the gross, regressive, incestuous, mother-womb phantasy, an ethically purified religious idea which gained the highest mental powers for the noblest application as sublimation, is at least very probable.

That many symbols conceal incestuous wishes is therefore obvious and just as certain as the fact that many incestuous wishes themselves are to be understood only as compulsory regression and possess psychological reality only in the same sense as the insatiable girl hunger of Don Juan who is ever disappointed because unconsciously and fundamentally, he seeks only the mother (compare page 126).† Whether the incest is constantly the innermost nucleus of the symbols, as Freud assumes, or whether the incest-wish, even where it expresses an actual desire, is to be constantly solved as symbol, as Jung asserts, is for me undecided. As remarked before (165), I consider the incestuous wish to be the expression of an actual wish which bears witness to old inhibitions without including at the same time a sublimated impulse. That one can afterwards read in such an one, is obvious. Often, however, the incestuous phantasy already forms the transition required by the law of reference to a spiritualization of the incest.‡ Still

* Compare my article: Zur Psychologie d. künstler. Inspiration. Imago II.

† Freud, Beiträge zur Psycholog. d. Liebeslebens (1st article) Jahrb. II, p. 389 ff.

‡ Riklin leaves the question open whether the incest-prohibition in the manifestation has the same value everywhere. He conceives it now as real, now as symbolical, "now as sexual problem in the narrower

more remote from this discussion is Adler's theory which likewise considers the sexual manifestations as mere symbols, in which the tendency to assurance against the feeling of inferiority, the enhancement of the feeling of personality, comes to expression.*

4. THE PLEASURE PRINCIPLE OF THINKING AS CONTRASTED WITH THE REALITY PRINCIPLE; AUTISTIC THINKING

In his article, "Formulations concerning the Two Principles of Psychic Activity," † Freud develops the thought that the primary mental processes consist in the production of pleasurably toned phantasies, while the disillusion which appears therewith compels understanding reality so as to be able to draw an actual gain of pleasure therefrom. Thus the reality principle appears alongside the pleasure principle which originally prevailed alone.

We must consider this theory more closely. In the "Interpretation of Dreams," we found the following conclusions regarding the pleasure principle: If the child, after it has suffered from a need (for example, hunger) has experienced gratification by outside aid (for example, giving of nourishment), then when the need is renewed, that previous experience of gratification is considered in hallucinatory ‡ manner, to the end that pleasure is attained.|| Our night dreams and day phantasies are remains of this long past childish mental life.¶ Bleuler attacks this view. "I see no hallucinated gratification in the suckling but only one following actual reception of nourishment. Further, I do not see in the somewhat older child that it would prefer an imaginary apple to a real one." § In

sense, now as picture of human thought- and culture-development," according to the connection. (Ödipus u. Psa., Wissen u. Leben V (1912), p. 552.

* Adler, U. d. nervösen Charakter, pages 5, 101, 131, 162 f.
† Jahrb. III, pp. 1–8.
‡ Freud, Traumdeutung, p. 376.
|| Jahrb. III, p. 2.
¶ Traumdeutung, p. 377.
§ Bleuler, Das autistische Denken. Jahrb. IV, p. 26.

that, he is certainly right but he does not touch Freud for the latter has never asserted what Bleuler imputes to him. Freud does not say that the hallucination brings about complete gratification but he speaks in his statement, which is for the rest very carefully formulated, of a wish which discharges itself in an hallucination as the shortest way to wishfulfillment. I admit that I must accord Freud's assumption a high degree of probability, especially when one thinks how near to hallucination very vivid imaginations come. Who imagines so facilely as children? I disagree with Freud only in that he considers the unconscious processes controlled by the pleasure principle as the only original kind of mental processes.* Sensation must be considered as just as old, thus the reality principle is just as original as the other. The same simultaneousness of the two, we find in the beginning of conscious life. Hallucinations presuppose perceptions, thus reality functions.

Against the pleasure principle of Freud's, Bleuler sets up the autistic thinking.† It consists in a thinking which is characterized by "the predominance of the inner life with active turning away from the outer world."‡ In it, the affectivity predominates. "There are, therefore, no sharp boundaries between autistic and ordinary thinking since the autistic, that is, affective directions, very easily force themselves into the ordinary thought." || The autistic thinking is distinguished from Freud's application of the pleasure principle by two characteristics:

(1) By turning away from reality;

(2) By being conditioned not only by pleasure-hunger but by favorite affects.¶

This second distinction can have no very great importance. There is no emotion which does not contain contributions of pleasure or pain or both. Further, I can conceive of no affect

* Jahrb. III, p. 2.
† Bleuler, Das autistische Denken, Jahrb. IV, pp. 1–30.
‡ Same, p. 1.
|| Same, p. 4.
¶ Same, p. 6.

which does not serve the elimination of pain and gaining of pleasure, even where this acquirement is not conscious. When Bleuler refers to the delusion of littleness or delusion of grave offence "which may be brought into the pleasure principle only by long hypothetical by-ways," I cannot agree with him. I have frequently seen the pleasure of self-minimization and self-martyrdom, like other masochistic impulses, as conscious or unconscious motives and hence do not see why they should be withdrawn from the pleasure principle.

Whatever the first distinction, the characteristic of withdrawal from reality, means, Bleuler expresses clearly only what Freud has in mind. The latter will calmly concede to his opponents that thinking does not bother itself exclusively according to the pleasure principle about contradictions and the possibility or impossibility but simply believes what is pleasant.

The question whether the function of reality or its denial is to be understood as an activity of the libido alone, is affirmed by Abraham, denied by Bleuler and Jung.* Freud considers the question unsolvable at present.† We pedagogues are only indirectly concerned with the question at issue.

Jung differentiates thinking with directed attention ‡ or "directed thinking" which can also perhaps be called "grammatical thinking" ‖ from dreaming and phantasying,¶ from subjective thinking.§ For him, these are the two forms of thinking. "The first is intended for communication, has grammatical elements, is tiring and exhausting, the second, on the other hand, deals without tiring, as you might say, spontaneously, with reminiscences. The first creates new acquirements, adaptation, imitates reality and seeks also to influence the same. The second, on the other hand, turns away from reality, liberates subjective wishes and is entirely unproductive from the

* Jung, Wandlungen, Jahrb. IV, p. 182.
† Freud, Psychoanal. Bemerkungen ü. e. Fall v. Paranoia (Dementia paranoides). Jahrb. III, p. 65.
‡ Jahrb. III, p. 128.
‖ P. 134.
¶ P. 136.
§ P. 148.

standpoint of adaptation.* Directed thinking is entirely conscious, the phantastic, conscious only in part, but "at least as much occurs in half-shadow and a large indefinite amount in general in the unconscious and is therefore to be made accessible only indirectly." † "The conscious phantasies tell us of a mythical or other element of wish tendencies in the mind, which is either not yet recognized or no longer recognized," ‡ a fact which Jung shows in a beautiful example.

In these sentences the comparison is made of "reality-thinking" with the grammatical and the "directed" thinking. The dreamer also often clothes his phantasies with words as one may see in the monologues of sleeping individuals or impassioned poets.‖ Further, the phantasies are likewise directed, even though not by attention, still by complexes. Very important is the remark that the "subjective" thinking—this term also is open to criticism ¶—takes place simultaneously consciously and unconsciously. It seems to me that the two thought-processes cannot be so sharply separated as is customarily done. There is no "autistic" or "subjective" thinking which may not have taken its elements from the reality-thinking. There often appears in the midst of these phantasies the need for logical connection. Inversely, thinking according to the reality principle cannot deny being conditioned by conscious pleasure tendencies, not even strict philosophical thinking, which according to Fichte, plainly betrays what kind of a man one is. The most exaggerated position in this respect is that of pragmatism which, in its more radical form, makes the truth of a conception dependent not on its logical foundation, but on its practical value.§ But our reality-thinking is also biased in other ways by conscious or unconscious wishes and

* P. 136.
† P. 148.
‡ P. 151.
‖ Jung distinguishes with right between language (Sprache) and speech (Rede). But all speech is also language.
¶ There are also scientific opinions which do not deny their subjective origin.
§ Compare the sharpsighted criticism of Dürr in his "Erkenntnistheorie," p. 167–177.

its objectivity influenced. Ordinarily, therefore, I prefer
Freud's expression: "Thinking according to two principles."
Where one of the two is predominantly in the background, we
may still speak of "phantastic" or "autistic" thinking or of its
opposite, "reality-thinking."

For us who are here concerned only with the manifestations,
the phantastic principle comes into consideration only so far
as it is conditioned by the unconscious. For a beautiful example, Jung is indebted to Anatole France: *

The pious priest, Abbé Oegger, phantasied much over the
question whether Judas was really condemned to eternal torment of hell or, since he acted only as the tool of God, he would
be granted grace. He implored a sign that Judas was saved
and felt a heavenly touch on his shoulder. The next day, he
communicated to the archbishop that he would go into the
world and preach the gospel of boundless grace of God. Soon
after, he withdrew from the Catholic Church. Oegger himself
was the Judas who betrayed his lord, hence he had to be assured first of the grace of God. Jung justly remarks: "What
would Oegger have said if he had been confidentially informed
that he was preparing himself for the rôle of Judas?" † Thus
Judas became for the priest the symbol of his own unconscious
tendency.

A young teacher suddenly finds a girl pupil, who had already
been entrusted to his care for two years, enchanting and clever,
while previously she had not impressed him. Why? Only the
analysis revealed the reason: He has been in love with a girl
who was descended from a prominent poet but did not bear
his name. The pupil had the poet's name and the forename of
the beloved. After some months, the pupil receded to the
every-day level, the teacher treated her coolly. It happened at
the time that the loved-one began to become indifferent to
him.

Many a teacher cannot easily bring himself to judge according to the reality principle the performances of pupils who are

* Jung, Wandlungen, Jahrb. III, p. 149 ff.
† P. 151.

extremely sympathetic to him. An educator influenced by complexes can commit the most enormous injustices without having only the slightest suspicion of it. Yet the analysis has already opened the eyes of one and another to his reprehensible conduct. Our scientific judgments are also influenced, times without number, by the pleasure principle. We judge a new theory only all too often according to our sympathy or antipathy for those who put it forth, according to the advantages or disadvantages which its diffusion will promote for us, etc. The struggle against such weakness is easier for us when the pleasure factor is conscious. If this factor remains below the threshold of consciousness, we fall victims to it in spite of the most honest intention, it may be that we escape the unpleasant truth by avoiding or forgetting it.

It is certain that the autistic thinking can bring about a great spiritualization and deepening of the emotional life in a good sense. But it is equally certain that in the overemphasis of this phantasticism, which would offer a substitute for a deficiency in reality, an immense amount of noble strength is lost to reality.

Bleuler says: "It is so pretty to spend one's sympathy on the phantasied Gretchen that costs nothing but a theatre ticket. When, however, the Gretchen in life approaches the Faust devotée, she finds stony hearts and closed purses and a Pharisaic kick." * It is seductive, year by year, to sing her unfortunate love in sweet verses but to construct a new and healthy life with the aid of reality, costs self-control. Many a person robs himself unmercifully by spending his lifetime in satisfying himself with phantasies and dreaming of white deer, while noble quarry rushes by him. But so we are. Jung justly remarks: "He who observes himself attentively and relentlessly, knows that a being dwells within him who gladly disguises and covers up everything difficult and questionable in life in order to carve for himself a free and easy path." † "The world of the poet is the world of solved problems. Real-

---

* Bleuler, Das autistische Denken. Jahrb. IV, p. 25.
† Jung, Der Inhalt d. Psychose, p. 25.

ity is the unsolved problem."* From these considerations, serious tasks develop for the educator.

With the neurotic, the rôle of the wish-phantasy is much greater than with the normal individual. He puts his whole life-force into it. He solves the problems which life imposes on him by a phantasy, for every neurotic phenomenon is only the automatic realization of an autistic phantasy. It is therefore quite correct for him to esteem an unallowed phantasy as highly as an act. To many, the autistic activity is so dear that they would rather endure the severest suffering than part with it.†

Grillparzer describes in his poem, "Der Bann" (The Ban) with psychological skill and truth, the automatism which devastates life:

> "Farewell, beloved! I must go!
> It drives me forth in fear and woe
> Forth from the dwellings of my friends
> Forth from the woman of my choice.
>
> For know, when you embrace me,
> You embrace no freeman;
> The idol whom you adore
> Is covered with grief and woe.
>
> The princess to whom the world belongs,‡
> Whom all adore, who therein live,
> Before whom all beings bow,
> In madness, I have resisted.
>
> With her sister ‖ infatuated,
> Who without home and without house,
> Through earth and sky and water wanders,
> I did in mad chase ride.
>
> In moonbeam, on careless feet,
> I joined with her the spectral host,
> And every honest pleasure renounced
> To gain the vain mirage.

* Jung, Der Inhalt d. Psychose, p. 16.
† Stekel, Fortschritte der Traumdeutung, Zbl. III, p. 157 f.
‡ Reality.
‖ Phantasy.

Then spake the princess, in anger glowing,
'Disdain thou so what I did bid thee?
So shalt thou ever be condemned
To be bird-free e'en unto death.

From wish to wish in endless sequence
And restless as thou art, so shalt remain!
For thee, no home, no place,
No friend, no brother and no wife!

A companion though is given thee,
Thee will he never leave,
He'll whip thee endlessly through life
The savage demon, phantasy.

He'll urge thee on to seize upon
With eager greed, all that which earthly beauty hast;
Yet hold, thou must hate all this
And see the flaw in every joy!

Condemned the shadows to pursue,
Lover still of the moment's kiss,
Thou lackest the power to renounce,
And self-control in pleasure.

Thy speech I'll change,
Thy hearer shall misunderstand;
Misfortune shall thy acts pursue
And ever two be head and hand!

Fly from her who loves thee;
She whom thou longest for shall recoil from thee in horror,
Tell her that if she granted
Thy passion, it would kill her.

And that the last consolation be denied,
Perpetual wrath and sorrow be,
So doubteth he to whom thou complainest
The reality of thy misery!

Go on, betrayed in all thy luck,
And court my sister's favor,
See if what the life denies
The art can recompense to thee!"

Then fared I forth with the powers of night
And truth it was which she had spoken;
The heart in my bosom broken
And the inner driver awake.

Since then, I wander, banished, alone,
Betraying others like myself;
Thou, however, poor woman, weep for
The one thou lost eternally!"

The autistic thinking can then become a burden when it makes the reality thinking fall short of full development. This is the case with many pupils who spin out their phantasies with immense demand upon the emotions, for hours at a time, or carry their complexes in the material afforded by these phantasies in order to continue the automatism. The passion for reading of many children is to be judged from this standpoint. This phenomenon always occurs only in children whose demands for love, mastery or execution are too little gratified in reality. From the kind of reading preferred, a skilled educator can at once say what kind of an unsatisfied longing exists in the young book-worm: whether love-hunger or hate, sadism (detective novels) or desire for recognition. Even plans for invention often form a bit of automatism. Behind the aviatistic endeavors of boys, there often exists that sexual desire which also manifests itself with extreme frequency in dreams of flying. If one forbids such automatisms without providing something better, one blocks up a harmless, indeed under certain circumstances, useful outlet and easily strengthens the father-complex, while by means of analysis, the condition is often easily corrected and fundamentally improved. Excessive smoking, sport and other youthful pleasures are often to be considered automatisms. Obviously they are to be interfered with analytically only when they endanger the mental and social position of the individual.

The task of the analyst consists, therefore, very often in guiding back the pleasure-seeking automatist from his "private theatre," his "cloud-land," and gaining his life-energy for humanity and productive ends.

5. SUBLIMATION

(A) ITS PSYCHOLOGICAL PHENOMENA

In every manifestation, an instinct which has been inhibited from direct activity seeks to create an indirect expression. Among substitute formations, we found many pathological conditions: the whole array of neuroses and psychoses, as for example, physical (hysterical) disturbances, anxiety and obsessional phenomena, delusions of reference (of grandeur and of persecution), etc.

There is also, however, a useful application of the libido deprived of its primary or direct function. It consists "in the erection of a higher goal which is no longer a sexual one, for the particular impulses, in place of the unsuitable one." * "To the contributions of energy gained in such manner for our mental performances, we are probably indebted for the highest cultural attainments. A premature appearance of the repression excludes the sublimation of the repressed instinct; after the elimination of the repression, the way to sublimation becomes open again." †

In formal aspect, the sublimation, the great importance of which for education is easy to perceive, puts before us no new phenomena. That the complex creates for itself new ideas (analogies, cover phantasies, composite formations, symbols), we have shown (pages 224f, 245f, 273f). We likewise spoke of transposition of emotion (page 209). To the concept of sublimation, belongs nevertheless, the fact that the pent-up instinct is expended not only at the mental level but also that this instinctive activity is recognized as superior and of high ethical value.

Thus it is no sublimation when Margaretha Ebner stills her passion in her phantasies of the figure of the Savior or when Zinzendorf satisfies his perverse sexual desires, his sadism, his homosexuality, on the figure of the heavenly bridegroom plainly

* Freud, über Psychoanalyse, p. 61.
† Same.

endowed with masculine and feminine sex characteristics, to which end, he changed himself in his foolish phantasies into a woman. Such unrefined, unpurified eroticism which gives rein to its ardor in religious phantasies of extraordinary emotional intensity, does not deserve the name of sublimation. I have proposed the name "elevation" for it.* History shows us that this autistic love-delirium is intimately associated with moral incapacity. Viewed from the esthetic standpoint, it is usually ugly—one of the most beautiful exceptions is formed by Mechthild of Magdeburg—in religious ethical aspect, it belongs to the most deplorable phenomena. The worship of Baal by the Canaanites with its orgies and Islam with its sensual hope in the future belong here, while the great Israelitish prophetic writers transport the libido into powerful social impulse and an ethically important piety, thereby winning true sublimation. Base elevations meet us in the inquisitors who indulged their sadistic desires in the name of religion in order to do it with calm conscience.

The sublimation can turn chiefly to emotional expressions, for example, love of nature, art and poetry. It also travels very often, however, with great success the paths of the volitional activity and leads to general usefulness, social work, humanitarian enthusiasm. Finally, it changes the manner of thinking and becomes philosophy, mathematics or astronomy.

Examples of the artistic and religious sublimation, we shall demonstrate later. At present, only some cases of intellectual and social higher directing of the life-energy will be introduced. Freud recalls that Rousseau in sexual embarrassment received from a woman the advice to leave the women and study mathematics.†

Wherever I found passionate devotion to astronomy or postage stamps among married women, there was always the need of love in the background as I showed on page 207.

In a student aged twenty-four, I found great preference for Plato and Kant proceeding from the wish for gratification of

* Pfister, Marg. Ebner. Zbl. I, p. 483.
† Freud, Gradiva, p. 29.

sexual need. Both philosophers, as is well known, deny sensuality and admire the strongest preference for the intellect. One young lady showed very prettily the humanitarian sublimation: As trained nurse, she hoped to be trusted with the care of her new-born nephew. The jealous sister-in-law declined her aid and engaged a stranger who by bad conduct brought the child into mortal danger. The disdained deaconess founded a child's nursery and thus turned her life-force to the use of the community.

Similar ethical transpositions are described by Ibsen at the end of his "Klein Eyolf," by Björnson in his novel, "Der Vater."

(B) THE PSYCHOLOGICAL PROCESS

The sublimation appears to be a very simple process. The man about town who has his desires gratified, has no other interest, no strength for cultural achievements. The primarily unsatisfied life-instinct soars to a higher level as the damned up flood rises.

But the comparison limps. The sublimation product is in no way merely a function of pent-up instinct. It would be nonsense to wish to consider the derivation of the law of tangents or the calculation of a fixed star by a starving married woman as a sexual function and it would be just as senseless to consider religion or art or morality merely as a performance of repressed instincts, as for instance, inhibited love, hunger, ambition, etc. Let us not forget that the reality-thinking also has its share in all high works of culture, even in the logic of genuine art and that the inhibition of the life-force in one instinct may stimulate other instincts. Freud speaks in the place cited only of mental performances which receive investments of energy (from the unconscious) in the sublimation. It is also obvious that logical, musical or architectonic emotions appear without being derived from complexes.

How the higher movement of the instinct actually proceeds, is not easy to see. Dürr defines sublimation "as the utilization of sensual dispositions in the service of ideas and thoughts more valuable to the organic resonance and in particular also ideas and thoughts motivating valuable acts."* "The sensuality, that is, the totality of the dispositions related to the sensations of special sense, the emotions joined to these and the instinctive acts thereby conditioned, forms the basis of the human mental life, from which, no one who will remain active mentally or physically can tear himself loose, just as little as one can succeed in jumping over one's own shadow." "The sensations produce, by ideas and thoughts centrally conditioned and excited indirectly over motor nerve paths, the resonance so important for all mental life.† By inhibitions of sensuality and especially of that part of the same belonging to the sexual sphere, energies are dammed up which benefit valuable functions by appearing in the service of their organic resonance.

If we consider Dürr's "energies" as dynamic expression of the libido, which I think correct, then I do not know what objection we would have to offer from the psychoanalytic side against these theories and we can only rejoice over the fact that so distinguished a psychologist agrees with Freud on one of the most important points. Only I cannot understand the expression, "resonance" clearly enough and think that we are in a position to describe the sublimation process more exactly by the aid of the theory of the paths of the complexes described by us, especially the theory of memories, symbols, condensations, transpositions and counter-reactions (still to be considered).

According to these theories, the life-force turns from primary functions chiefly to such higher activities as realize those functions symbolically, that is, those that afford the maximal conversion of the original tendency.

(c) CAPACITY FOR WORK AND BARRIERS TO SUBLIMATION

The neurotic fixation hinders the sublimation and therein shows itself to be the enemy of the higher civilization. It binds the instinct in harmful chains. The sublimation, on the con-

---

* Ebbinghaus, Grundz. d. Psych., 3rd ed. revised by E. Dürr, II (1913), p. 585.
† P. 584 f.

trary, creates life conditions for the instinct which, under favorable circumstances, affords a higher degree of happiness and ethical efficiency. There are people who in full health find a rich life interest in art, science, philanthropy, and religion but are extraordinarily reserved in relation to sensual pleasures (in broadest sense).

Not all people possess the capacity for this transformation, however. The "mobility and capacity for transformation of the libido," which according to Jung,* forms the secret of culture, varies greatly in different individuals. Many persons have no trouble in making the sacrifice which exists in every sublimation, the renunciation of certain lower desires. Others, however, cannot give up such demands. Freud finds: "A certain part of repressed libidinous impulses has a just claim to direct gratification and should find this in life. Our cultural demands make life too hard for most human organizations, compelling thereby the renunciation of reality and the originating of the neuroses, without attaining a surplus of cultural gain by this excess of sexual repression." † It is a thought similar to that of Luther's who took the field against the monastic sublimation practice. Pure elevation of instinct which goes beyond the power of the individual, often leads to fanaticism, narrow-mindedness, narrowing of the horizon. The danger of immorality often lies nearer to forced, inwardly constrained sublimation than one thinks. The ascetics who have renounced all worldly pleasure are most strongly exposed to temptation. It is not just to consider zealots for morality who had fallen, as hypocrites. Schiller says well and truly: "The fire which the Heavenly Venus enkindles, is turned to account by the earthly and the natural instinct often avenges itself for its long neglect by a mastery just so much the more unbridled." ‡

A certain amount of primary application of instinct seems for many persons to be a presupposition for sublimation of at least a part of the instinct. I know an official who had fallen

* Jung, Wandlungen, Jahrb. III, p. 134.
† Freud, Über Psychoanalyse, p. 61.
‡ Schiller, Ü. Anmut u. Würde (Abschnitt "Würde").

out with his wife and was a slave to drink, who maltreated his wife and child, so long as his demand for love remained unsatisfied. He fell in love with a widow and carried on an intimate relation with her. From that hour, his morals left nothing to be desired. After more than a year, his legal wife wrote the widow a warm letter of thanks for having changed the supporter of the family into a noble man and begged her not to give up the relation from moral considerations. In some similar cases, which were likewise outside my pastorate, I saw alcoholism disappear in the presence of love and immediately return after erotic inhibition.

The Protestant morality with its affirmation of the primary instinctive life, so far as it serves the moral idea, is thus substantiated by psychoanalysis.

Of extraordinary pedagogical importance are the cases in which a sublimation is built up on neurotic repression. The housewife who can give her husband no love, seeks to afford a compensation by passionate devotion to fulfiling her household duties; the merchant flees from his sexual obligations into business, the pupil occasionally into his tasks. This work performed by force (of will) absorbs an enormous amount of strength and easily leads to severe states of exhaustion. Such people suffer from inner inhibitions and grievous, unconfessed self-accusations; they must exert powerful effort to repress their need, to overcome their feelings of deficiency, to attain properly their repression and sublimation. From this struggle, which, as we know, is a contest with illusions and ghosts, only the conscious compromise with reality saves.

Of the many factors which can destroy the sublimation and have always been familiar to the educator, I may mention only one, since psychoanalysis shares in regard to its important theories: alcohol. Different authors (O. Gross,* Abraham,†

* O. Gross, Das Freud'sche Ideogenitätsmoment u. s. Bedeutung im manisch-depressiven Irrsinn Kraepelins, Leipzig, 1907.
† C. Abraham, D. psychol. Beziehgen. zw. Sexualität u. Alkoholism. Zschr. f. Sexualwiss. 1908, No. 8.

Freud,* Juliusberger,† Ferenczi‡ and others), have recognized that alcoholism in many cases is to be considered as the result of complexes, as neurotic compulsion. I consider this fact as proven. Even if we knew nothing of the effect of alcohol in deadening, in causing amnesia and freeing primary tendencies, we would have to expect a priori, neurotic compulsion to alcoholism. Experience confirms this surmise. Also we know something of the causal connection between alcoholism and the complex, even though not everything, and I am surprised that Bleuler disputes this finding. Further, I consider Freud's dictum that alcohol releases the (ethical) inhibitions and renders sublimations regressive ‖ to be proven empirically. Bleuler disputes this opinion and remarks: "What kind of sublimations would become inversely manifest under the influence of alcohol at a patriotic celebration or some other kind of moral festival, everyone knows who knows how to observe." ¶ The objection does not apply. Bleuler will probably only assert ironically that alcohol creates sublimations. The moral disposition at patriotic celebrations is already present before the alcoholic pleasure. If this disposition is inflamed by alcohol, then this can form a counter-reaction to immoral impulses or—what I consider improbable—can signify a better performance analogous to the intellectual ones which appear immediately after the taking of alcohol. That the large consumption of alcohol very soon frees the human brute from the prison of the moral control, Bleuler knows as well as Tolstoi or any other student of humanity.

Does it follow now, however, from the fact that alcoholism often, naturally not always, figures as manifestation and as such, as we shall hear, possesses a certain function as protection

* Freud, Psa. Bemerkungen ü. e. Fall v. Paranoia. Jahrb. III, p. 56 f.

† O. Juliusberger, Beitrag zur Psychol, der sog. Dipsomanie. Zbl. II, pp. 551–557, Zur Psychol. d. Alkoholismus, Zbl. III, pp. 1–16.

‡ Ferenczi, Ü. d. Rolle d. Homosexualität i. d. Pathogenese d. Paranoia. Jahrb. III, p. 106 f.

‖ Freud, Paranoia, p. 56.

¶ Bleuler, Alkohol u. Neurosen. Jahrb. III, p. 852.

or relief valve, that we should fight against it less energetically? Ferenczi said on a basis of statistics, the reliability of which he himself impugned, and still more on the basis of his own observations: "The destruction of alcoholism is thus an apparent improvement in hygiene. For the mind from which alcohol is withdrawn, there are numerous other ways at hand for flight into illness. And if the psychoneurotic, instead of falling into alcoholism, comes to anxiety-hysteria or dementia præcox, one regrets the enormous expenditure of energy which was put in motion against alcoholism at the wrong place." *

I cannot accept this reasoning. If Ferenczi admits that the powerful alcoholic desire of the neurotic leading to debauchery, destroys the sublimations and is "an unconscious attempt at palliative self-treatment by poisoning the censor," then he must fight sincerely against the enemy. The proof for the belief that the enjoyment of alcohol provides a defence against dementia præcox or anxiety-hysteria, he has not attempted to offer. He too knows plenty of neurotics and psychotics among alcoholics. In addition, as Jung reproaches him, he leaves out of consideration the social aspect.

Certainly, I admit that many alcoholics can be cured only by psychoanalysis. I substantiate indeed that many one-time drinkers can attain by analysis the power to enjoy alcohol without injury. Since this, however, is not by far the case with all victims of alcohol, since a mass of psychological, hygienic and politico-economical facts prove the collective effect of alcohol to be enormously injurious and standing in no perceptible relation to its advantages, since further, psychoanalysis is to-day and perhaps always will be inaccessible to many endangered by alcohol, I would greatly regret with Bleuler if one attempted to apply psychoanalysis against the abstinence movement.

It may estrange some individuals that psychoanalysis should find sexual energies in the highest achievements. Therefore, it should be remembered that keen observers of the human mind have already recognized this fact before. Schiller writes: "If the sensual nature in moral affairs were always only the

* Ferenczi, Jahrb. III, p. 107.

suppressed party and never the coactive, how could it yield the whole fire of its emotion to a triumph which is celebrated over itself? How could the sensual nature be so lively a participant in the guilty self-consciousness of the pure spirit if it could not finally join the spirit so intimately that even the analytic reason cannot separate one from the other without violence?"* And Nietzsche testifies: "The degree and nature of the sexuality of a person extends even to the highest point of his mind." † Another time, he says: "Therewith the possibility should not in the least be excluded that that particular sweetness and fullness which is suited to the esthetic condition, may take its origin from the ingredient "sensuality" (as from the same source, that "idealism" arises which is suited to the marriageable girl),—that therewith, the sensuality is not eliminated upon the entrance of the esthetic condition as Schopenhauer thinks, but is only transfigured and no longer appears in consciousness as sexual stimulus." ‡ Nietzsche puts forward the thesis: "Almost everything which we call "higher culture" rests on the spiritualization and deepening of cruelty—this is my hypothesis; that savage beast has not been killed at all, it lives, it flourishes, only it has deified itself. That which constitutes the painful pleasure of the tragedy is cruelty; that which works agreeably in so-called tragic sympathy, indeed in all sublime even to the highest and tenderest thrill of metaphysics, gets its sweetness entirely from the intermingled ingredient of cruelty. That which the Romans enjoyed in the arena, Christ in the ecstasies of the cross . . . these are the spiced drinks of the great Circe, cruelty." ‖ How sad that Nietzsche spoiled correct insight by exaggeration.

6. THE REACTION-FORMATION

Among the sublimations, under which name I understand the products of the sublimation process, there is a group which

---

* Schiller, Ü. Anmut u. Würde.
† Nietzsche, Jenseits von Gut und Böse. Aphorismus 75.
‡ Nietzsche, Zur Genealogie der Moral, 3rd Article, section 8.
‖ Nietzsche, Jenseits, III Part, p. 229.

proceeds from the repression of a counteracting impulse. This group is called that of the reaction-formations.

Even in the simplest manifestations of the dream and neurotic symptom, we often find that an idea to be expressed, is denoted by its opposite. This inversion, Freud calls indeed "one of the favorite means of representation capable of the most many-sided application in the dream work." * I myself have not met the condition so often. In some cases, the representation by opposite was also conditioned by a positive motive. If, for example, according to Spielrein,† the sexual activity is expressed by death symbolism, then I would trace this incontestable phenomenon back not only with her to the negative mechanism but also and chiefly to the disappearance of the senses in the ecstasy. Or when Jung, at that time still assistant physician, is dreamed of as a little man with beard and no longer young,‡ so there again, a positive basis may be coactive: the jeer at him by the comparison with a superior who showed the characteristics named.

Still, as mentioned, I admit representation by opposite. The normal life shows the same process: irony and contradictory meaning of primitive words.‖ Freud discusses the latter in his article on a work of Karl Abel who shows that in the Egyptian, a considerable number of words denote a thing and its opposite. "To command" means also "to obey," "strong" means also "weak," etc. The Latin "altus" means "high" and "deep." Language also shows another favorite inversion

* Freud, Traumdeutung, p. 238.
† S. Spielrein, Ü. d. psycholog. Inhalt eines Falles von Schizophrenie. Jahrb. III, p. 400.
‡ Zbl. I, p. 267.
‖ Here the inversion is also to be mentioned. Among the ancients, one often finds mirror-writing, of which Leonardo da Vinci also frequently made use. The child too loves this old mannerism at a certain age, as speaking backwards. Bertha Mercator, in a little novel, has an old professor say to a young nurse: "You old boy? Do you not understand? This is a circumlocution. Just when it is clear to me that you are a pretty, very young girl, then I must call you 'old boy' else I would become sentimental which is disgusting to me."

found in automatic secret speech and hysteria, for example, "Topf" is called pot in English, Balken: klobe, club.*

In the reaction-formation, the life-force which belongs to a repressed, thus unconscious, instinctive activity, applies itself to a manifestation which pursues the opposite direction, either on the same level or a higher one. Bleuler calls the instincts appearing in contrasting pairs or the ideas accompanied simultaneously by positive and negative emotions, ambivalent.† We meet an ambivalence of a higher order in the reaction-formation.

A lady of thirty-seven years suffered from fanaticism over purification and truth. She washed herself daily for many hours and daily put on fresh underwear. Because for reasons of affection, she concealed from her husband that though full of admiration for him, she did not love him as dearly as she wished, she suffered unspeakably but did not dare to make him unhappy. As a child, she was extremely unclean, wetting her bed until her tenth year. In school, she experienced a scene which troubles her even to-day: She declared a circle to be drawn free-hand, but the teacher discovered the hole made by the point of the compass.

The fanatical adherent of nature-cures, who makes a tremendous cult of health, proves without exception in cases analyzed by me, to be a neurotic, who would drown out the consciousness of illness. In so doing, many fall into the most unnatural activities.

The man who is horrified at the nude, who goes into a rage over a harmless clay model, regularly discloses in the analysis a mass of dirty wishes which are held in check only with difficulty. Fanaticism over morality is often merely a refuge for weak voluptuaries who are afraid of sinking in the mire of wickedness.

The flatterer conceals by his cringing nature his evil mind. He cannot disclose how he feels because he would betray himself. His reaction-conduct looks forced, insincere.

---

* Freud, ü. d. Gegensinn der Urworte. Jahrb. II, pp. 179–184.
† Bleuler, Das autistische Denken, Jahrb. IV, p. 20.

One whose harmless joys of childhood were embittered by over-austere parents, turns to a gloomy Puritanism which is far separated from liberal charity.* The gushing harlequin and joke-maker is uncommonly often, certainly in a majority of instances, an unhappy person who wishes to get a double value from the moment, for behind him lurks dire misery.

We have already discussed the fact that the desire, torn from an erotic object and repressed, often turns to a contrasting substitute, a person who possesses the opposite characteristics. Wherever an expression of will appears very extreme, fanatical, strikingly one-sided, the suspicion is aroused that we are dealing with a reaction-formation.

The importance of the subject causes me to add a few additional examples: A girl, aged fifteen, loves the mother as passionately as she hates the drunken step-father. If the former does not come home at the minute expected, the child suffers a severe anxiety attack and runs weeping through the streets seeking for her. In her dreams, she regularly sees the mother dead. Some time before, she was in the habit of wandering at night and at that time went to an umbrella-stand in the dark hall, from which she could not free herself, so that she awoke with loud cries of anxiety, whereupon the parents ran to her aid. Asked for her associations to that place, the girl said at once that she was afraid a man would step forth there. This man, she described with the characteristics of her step-father who put his umbrella (typical sexual symbol) in that stand. The repressed sexual desire corresponded to the conscious hate—the man is too coarse to allow of love being mentioned—as jealous hatred lay at bottom of the unnaturally strong love for the mother (female Œdipus-complex).

A widower, aged thirty-eight, complained to me that his longing for his wife who had been dead five years, was constantly increasing. He could never marry another, no matter how necessary she might be to him and his children. His marriage

* E. Jones, Psycho-Analysis and Education. Journal of Educational Psychology, Nov. 1910, pp. 497–520.

had been "wonderfully harmonious," "really ideal," it was "absolutely out of the question that he could ever find a similarly perfect happiness." The forced expressions struck me as odd. I made inquiries therefore, whether there had never really been a disturbance of the marital relation. The widower reported that some months before the wife's death, something happened, but he guarded well against looking squarely at it. In case something had happened, he has pardoned it. Really, when his wife was staying for treatment at a sea bathing place, the director of the hotel where she lived wrote him that the patient was excited by a love-affair, the husband might straighten it out. The wife declared herself innocent; an investigation cleared the way for her husband. It turned out further that sexual intercourse had been discontinued long before. It came to light further that the wife, after she had clung to him in the first years of their wedded life, had taken sides against him in favor of her mother, while he had inwardly returned to his own mother. In short, the marriage had really been unsettled but the widower clung to an illusion which he had constructed out of the first part of his married life.

A dream revealed the true ground: he lies undressed in bed; his mother goes by the window and sees him. Analysis: The day before, a charming lady who was in love with him and whom he had courted for a year, had gone by. From the lady, he makes his mother to whom he loves to show himself in the manner of a love-hungry child. One understands now why the man, whose sexuality is fixed in the infantile exhibitionism in respect to the mother, incapable of love, glorified the earlier love.

I found quite similar motives in a man of some fifty years who, after the sudden death of his wife, suffered from a severe anxiety neurosis. He accused himself of having called too few physicians to the death-bed of his wife and thus to have been guilty of her death. His marriage had been of wonderful sincerity, there never lived two people so suited to each other, so devoted to all noble, public-spirited works, as he and his wife, etc. That sounded very fine but still I was not surprised when the morally vain man disclosed himself as syphilitic who had had no conjugal intercourse for years and had oppressed his wife with brutality. The undoubtedly very intimate love in consciousness was only the reverse side of a deep estrangement. Among the reaction-formations, two kinds are to be differentiated: some as additional affirmation, others as additional negation. The pastor's son, too strictly educated, can tend either to Catholicism or political absolutism and find a father-substitute with fanatical zeal in priest or sovereign, or he may become libertine, revolutionary or anarchist. He who has fallen out with the mother may easily fall passionately in love with an elderly lady or hate all girls.

The reaction-formations are in no way so good from the ethical standpoint as one is often tempted to believe. Freud says in one place: "He who has become overgood from violent suppression of a constitutional tendency to hard-heartedness and cruelty, will frequently expend so much energy in the effort that he will not execute everything which corresponds to his compensation-impulses, and on the whole, will accomplish rather less good than he would have brought about without suppression."* Therewith, it naturally would not. be recommended to yield the reins to cruelty but it indicates the necessity for a rational sublimation. Every unprejudiced individual will admit that the enemy to enlightenment whose narrow-minded strictness vexes youth, does less and can do less for charity than the individual who has grown in the light of a broad friendliness.†

7. THE RATIONALIZATION

If one gives to the suitable subject in hypnosis a command which is to be executed only after the subject's awakening, then the subject becomes obedient to the order, the origin of which is entirely hidden from him. If he gives himself or others

* Freud, Die "kulturelle" Sexualmoral und die moderne Nervosität. Kl. Schriften II, p. 196.

† We shall see that in the place of the counter-reaction in the manifestation, dependent on unconscious instinctive impulses, the clearly elucidated reaction based on control of instinct should appear.

justification for his action, he devises instead of the real ground for action, some kind of excuse or other, as plausible as possible. Forel gives two simple examples: He says to a hypnotized person: "After you awaken, the idea will come to you to put the chair there, on the table. . . ." The one commanded, obeys. Asked for his motive, he says the chair was in his way. The suggestion that he will take a hand towel and wipe his face, he likewise executed; as reason for the action, the assertion that he has perspired so freely, serves.* Such an argumentation which wishes to give a rational reason for an action (often a thought process) which proceeds from unconscious motives, is called, in accordance with Jones' proposal, rationalization.

This process plays a rôle in daily life which is scarcely to be overestimated so that the educator must be thoroughly familiar with it. All feelings and actions are rooted in good part in the unconscious and so far as they rest on rational motives, it is a rationalization.

Someone would submit to an analysis which he has recognized as beneficial. But he finds a thousand objections which he himself believes: His parents will be compromised by his confession, the educator might have been guilty of an indiscretion, he would lose his independence. Or, during the analysis, the explorer is now too cool, now too cordial, his face is unsympathetic, his voice sounds hypocritical, he is capricious, ambitious, etc. And yet the motive lies in resistances against rendering conscious of unpleasant occurrences supposedly overcome, and against the new-canalization of the instinct, against the revelation of infantile wishes and against the mastery of reality. Or transference processes take part, which we will discuss later.

A young analytic patient feels every morning a dislike for her fiancé who at evening is entirely sympathetic to her. She thinks she knows the exact reason for this: The youth is not so very handsome. The fact that this ground for antipathy must also have held at evening, the otherwise intelligent girl has not noticed. In reality, the young hysterical suffers from

* Forel, Der Hypnotismus, p. 32 f.

a distaste for sexual life grounded in the unconscious: One morning, she had surprised her parents and experienced an unconquerable fear which she repressed. This connection she found herself, whereupon the erotic disturbance ceased.

The choice of a vocation is also often rationalized. The patient with obsessional neurosis mentioned on page 73, in whose life, noli me tangere, crabs, jumping bugs, flounders, etc., played a great rôle, had to study natural science. He sought fundamentally, as almost all his dreams showed, the sexual secret. Instead of this motive, he gave quite other ones.

A young man who married the mother of his friend, gave as motive: His wife could cook so well, sew and keep the house in order. That young girls are also skilled at these tasks, he had to admit. His attachment to his mother, he did not recognize. The student, aged twenty-three, of whom we spoke on page 269, did not bring a rationalization for a long time. He informed me that he was inextricably in love with a lady of forty, although he considered a union with her foolish.

Especially in the religious life, does the rationalization frequently appear. It does absolutely no good to try biblical science, church history or dogmatism on persons held by strong complexes, who have taken refuge in bizarre forms of religion. In a whole series of cases in which young Protestants wished to become Catholics, I easily discovered the root of this inner necessity and overcame the impulse. Some simple examples, I have described elsewhere. I will add a plain case. A cultured student, aged nineteen, informed me of his decision to become a Catholic, since he had been convinced by Catholics of the superiority of their confession. [Did this happen from several Catholics or only one?] "From one." [Or perhaps a Catholic girl?] "That is also true." [I am surprised that a lady has exercised so much influence on a man of your education. She is probably older than you?] "Yes, some years." [Then I assume that you love the girl and suffer from a conflict with your mother.] "That I must also admit."

It was an easy task to explain to the youth the concept of

the substitute for the mother. Discussing the special religious determinants proved to be entirely unnecessary.

One should not judge such a victim of an illusion scornfully. How much imposing dogmatism, what high-sounding philosophy is exactly the same: a keen sighted subtraction from a theory which in reality rests on totally different pillars, namely unconscious ones, and with these pillars, it must fall.

Finally, I refer to a case which is extraordinarily important for the educator. We struggle against ambition with beautiful exhortation but often accomplish precious little in so doing. With people who ruin their careers by disgusting place-hunting, one often finds an enormous deficiency-complex (Adler). One such unfortunate person who was consumed by ambition, said in the analysis that he was the illegitimate son of a distinguished man, was constantly goaded by the thought of chastising the father because he scorned such a wonderful son. Another suffered from poverty and legal punishment of the parents. Both, however, gave ideal motives for their actions in good faith.

CHAPTER XII

THE FORMS OF THE MANIFESTATIONS

1. Dispositions and Moods

I do not intend to describe systematically the whole of the creations of complexes. With the aid of the tests conducted here, it should not be difficult to detect other phenomena of related nature.

Pedagogically valuable is the psychological understanding of the dispositions and moods which, without analytic subliminal psychology, form a barren enigma.

One example begun analytically but not completed, we recognized in Heine's "Lorelei" (258).

A gentleman, aged thirty-five, was asked to be chivalrous to a young lady who was visiting. Although he esteemed the looks and culture of the girl very highly, he evaded the request and behaved anything but gallantly. Scarcely had the guest departed than a highly disagreeable mood seized the ungracious cavalier, who meanwhile did not think of a connection between his disposition and the visit. Finally, exasperated with himself, he asked an analytic physician friend for information. Asked for associations to the mood, he recalled a scene from his fifth year: He was playing with his little sister in the garden and was enjoying himself very much when his elder brother came along, took his playmate for himself and left the little fellow alone. The young girl was now introduced to him by an elder friend, the older one had claims upon her. Our patient with the bad mood transferred himself, entirely unconsciously, upon accepting his commission, to that scene of his childhood in which the girl friend was taken from him. He would like to be friendly with the young lady but was afraid as a burnt child fears the fire. Into consciousness came only the end-effect of the ill-humor. The overdeterminants I do not know.

A word may be devoted to the foreboding or presentiment. The clever Mme. de Stael saw the connection with the unconscious when she said: "Quand on est capable de se connaître, on se trompe rarement sur son sort, et les pressentiments ne sont le plus souvent qu'un jugement sur soi-même, qu'on ne s'est pas encore tout-à-fait avoué." (Hebbel cites this saying in agreement.) *

2. Love

It is characteristic of the distressed condition of the traditional psychology that it knows as much as nothing of the chief forms of love, the prime importance of which must be known to it, and the same is true of the origin and conditions of change in eroticism. Psychoanalysis here opens for us promising paths as has been repeatedly shown.

From the multitude of types, I may mention only three which are important from the moral pedagogic standpoint: the Don Juan, the division of eroticism into immoral and ascetic love, and those incapable of love.

(A) THE DON JUAN

The Don Juan is far from being in all cases a heartless voluptuary, even though there certainly are morally depraved persons who get girls into trouble with pleasure and without remorse. In my educational activities, I have repeatedly met Don Juans who suffered grievously from their instincts without being able to give them up.

The seventeen year old peasant boy, described on page 126, wished to defend himself against his unfaithfulness by severe pains but this did not succeed. Perhaps his symptoms had also the meaning of a self-punishment.

The longing for the mother is considered by the majority of analysts as the motive for Don Juanism.

* E. Kuh, Biographie Friedrich Hebbels. Vol. II (1907), p. 127.

(B) THE POLARIZATION OF THE EROTICISM INTO EARTHLY OR VULGAR AND HEAVENLY

Twice, I have met youths who loved with equal fervor girls of high moral character and prostitutes. By the former, they wished to be saved, the latter, they sought to save, which did not at all exclude the possibility of their indulging in dissolute practices with them. Only the youth mentioned on page 68 came into my pastoral care. He had been engaged innumerable times but only a single time did he remain captivated, this time by a penniless girl who had vaginismus (automatic contraction of the vagina) and who was therefore considered by him as a constant virgin. With this girl, the young and well-to-do youth eloped and married her but kept his preference for prostitutes and laid snares for virgins with the same assiduity. As soon as it developed that a girl already had a lover, he lost all interest in her. Every street-walker, he loved momentarily to the point of madness.

In the virginal love-object, I recognized without trouble a substitute for the mother, but on the other hand, allowed myself to be misled in tracing the love for prostitutes back to an early affair with a girl, whom he asserted, fell to the streets on his account. This explanation is incorrect, however. The youth knew quite well that the girl had been a prostitute previously. On account of my inexperience, I did not succeed in detecting Don Juanism in him while I banished an extraordinarily long chain of phobias, obsessional acts and hysterical symptoms.

Freud first opened my eyes—too late for the young man—the prostitutes also represent the mother and indeed as sexual being.*

(C) INCAPACITY FOR LOVE

When we discussed deficiency in emotion, the incapacity for love was shown and explained (193). Further, the theory of

---

* Freud, Beiträge zur Psychologie des Liebeslebens, I, Jahrb. III, p. 394 f.

identification and projection gave us the reason for incapacity for love (265).

The life-desires in such persons as are incapable of conjugal and philanthropic love can be driven into thousands of channels: incest phantasies, perversities, sport, science, reaction-formations, pathological phenomena, such as anxiety, melancholia, world-weariness, physical defects, etc. There are no persons with primary incapacity for love.

Since only a very few cases of the very frequently occurring perversities have been presented (analeroticism 201, homosexuality 203), a very plain case may be added.

An hysterical young man, aged twenty-three, was hindered from loving a girl. A few times in the presence of young ladies who impressed him, he had attacks of perspiring but to love, he never came. Instead, he had an unbelievably passionate fondness for ladies' clothes. Not only did he choose his vocation according to this tendency but he spent his pocket-money almost entirely for fashion journals. A beautiful gown put him into ecstasy, while its wearer left him cool. Often he traveled by night in a gondola and hallucinated nixies who teasingly theatened to put out the lanterns. Their veils were wonderful to behold, their bodies did not interest him in the least. Whence came this fetichism?

When eleven years old, he spent his vacations with relatives in the country. The careless peasant people allowed him to sleep for four weeks in the same bed with his girl cousin aged thirteen or fourteen. Naturally, this led to mutual inspections. When twelve years old, he was often shown by comrades in school obscene pictures which excited him. In his sixteenth year, he heard the minister preach earnestly on the sin of eye-lust. The boy frequently phantasied in sleep at that time, female figures and had pollutions. Now when the minister discussed eye-lust, a terrible anxiety came over the boy, first in the form of a feeling of guilt, for he said, if he had not looked at the pictures, the pollutions would not have occurred. He sublimated religiously and after conversion, passed into passionate adoration of Jesus—God as father, he could not endure, like his own father, he wished to know nothing of him—and somewhat later into fetichism for clothes.

The connection between philanthropy and affection toward the nearest relatives, thus between love for those nearest and love for those farthest away, may be shown very prettily by analysis.

3. HATE

All hate arises from an inhibition of the life-will, it may be from envy, revenge, jealousy or unpleasant identification. Love alone is primary.* Here I am speaking of hate only as far as it represents a manifestation of latent, unconscious impulses.

Hate as unhappy love was shown to us by the boy who awoke his brother every morning by sticking his finger in the brother's mouth (159). This common case, fortunately usually built on nobler desires, affords the analysis the best chance for success. The wrangling between brothers and sisters is frequently a healthy effect of the incest barrier and deserves to be preferred to an unfortunately frequent concord, behind which a pernicious fixation lurks. Of course, the wrangling should be and can be replaced, by tactful analytic education, by more rational guidance of instinct.

The hate arose from unconscious identification in a girl of sixteen, about to be confirmed, who told me that she hated her neighbor although the latter was a good girl and certainly did not deserve her antipathy. Asked to associate to this girl, the patient remembered that the girl had a bad opinion of her teacher while outwardly she accepted his friendship. Further, the neighbor had a habit of moving her mouth in a manner

* Inversely Stekel considers hatred as the primary thing and basis of all mental phenomena, even the altruistic impulses (Sprache des Traumes, p. 536). I consider this conception as erroneous. As support for his hypothesis, he adds that among criminals and anarchists, there are so many illegitimate children; "these apostles of hate have not been through the school of love in their youth." But have these not perhaps first learned hate as a result of their loveless education? Stekel remarks further that hate often makes its appearance in children. But has not love appeared still earlier?

which reminded of kissing. Further associations revealed that the patient acted toward the teacher exactly like the hated one: she flattered him and ridiculed him. Also, in former years, she had had a tic of the mouth like her comrade and kisses are distasteful to her. Thus she hates in the other only unpleasant traits of her own person.*

Sadism also often has a share. Tasso remarks to the point: "Nothing can take from me the pleasure of thinking worse and worse of him (the enemy)." † How cleverly hate knows how to adapt to itself all material which is heard and seen and revel in murderous phantasies without incriminating itself, was shown in my article: "Analytic Investigations on the Psychology of Hate and Reconciliation." ‡

4. THE ASSOCIATION-EXPERIMENT AND THE "PHENOMENA OF REPRODUCTION"

(A) DEFINITION OF THE ASSOCIATION-EXPERIMENT

An essential contribution was made to the psychoanalytic investigation by Jung's association studies.‖ I will devote a few pages to discussing and testing these results. Psychology usually calls the experiment which Jung with the earlier psychology denominates "association-experiment," by the term "reproduction-experiment." This harmonizes with the thought that if one calls a word to the subject of the experiment, an idea will be brought to consciousness in the latter, which idea was once before joined to the idea denoted by the word given. "The mind does not take up much from the material temporarily pressing in upon it; but that which gets through by favor of the circumstances, the mind spins out and interweaves with its own past.¶ That is to say, the mental pictures appearing in consciousness, themselves occasion this completion

---

* I described an analogous example in my article: "Kryptographie, Kryptolalie u. unbed. Vexierbild bei Normalen." Jahrb. V, p. 134 f.

† Goethe, Tasso, IV, p. 2.

‡ Jahrb. II, also separately from Deuticke, Vienna, 1910.

‖ Diagnostische Assoziationsstudien, Leipzig, Barth, Vol. I, 1906, Vol. II, 1910.

¶ Compare p. 230 f., the theory of the regression.

by the past and therein comes about the effect which they unfold.''* It is noticed further that ideas and thoughts which are not the same as those entertained previously but only resemble these, may arouse mental pictures which were formerly joined to these similar ones,† only at that time they were clearer and more diversified.‡ As the only constant basis for the process, one assumes ''a capability or disposition of the nervous elements to be aroused later, always easier in the same groupings in which they have previously been arranged, and to radiate their excitations reciprocally when these are once aroused from the periphery by a part of the functional complex belonging to them.'' ‖ Under association, one understands with Offner the ''disposition to further conduction of psycho-physical excitation from one group of ideas to another group of ideas.'' ‖

Wundt, on the other hand, uses the term association to cover successive associated memories,§ though he emphasizes that real associative processes can never consist in an addition of elements.** He lays great stress on ''simultaneous associations,'' for example, the blending of sensations, in which one element gains the mastery over the others (e. g. the fundamental tone over the over-tone).†† Thus there exists in the association a creative agency.

In the analytic experiments established by Jung, we are dealing with the gaining of a new idea by the giving of a preceding idea, of a ''reaction-word'' by a ''stimulus-word.'' We shall see, however, that of mere ''reproductions'' there are none, since between the two words, an unconscious thought process may lie which leads by a really productive operation creating new psychic values, to a new idea.‡‡ On this point, as we shall

---

* Ebbinhaus-Dürr, Grundz. d. Psychol. I, p. 634.
† P. 635.
‡ P. 636.
‖ P. 712.
¶ Offner, D. Gedächtnis, p. 21.
§ Wundt, Grundz. d. phys. Psych. III, p. 544.
** P. 522.
†† P. 527.
‡‡ This subliminal new-creation, the "disposition-psychology" over-

see, Wundt would be correct, except that he drew much too narrow bounds for this creative activity.

(B) THE SCHEMATIC ASSOCIATION-EXPERIMENT

It would take us too far afield to derive inductively the association-experiment cleverly developed by Jung. We shall limit ourselves to the most important results.

The method consists in instructing the subject of the experiment to respond to the word which is called out to him with the first word that comes to his mind, and to do this as quickly as possible and entirely without consideration of the content of the word. The time elapsing between the calling of the word by the analyst and the reply by the subject (reaction-time) is accurately measured by a stop-watch in fifths of seconds, the reaction-word written down as quickly as possible and the next word in the list given. When one has gone through the whole list of words prepared beforehand, say one hundred words, he then immediately starts at the beginning again with the command to give the same reaction-word as before. If this is done successfully, one speaks of successful reproductions, otherwise of false reproductions.

Not always, by far, is a conscious or unconscious complex stirred by the stimulus word. From thousands of reactions, certain symptoms for the manifestation-significance of a succeeding association were found. I shall attempt to arrange these systematically.

System of Complex Indicators.

A. *External stigmata.*

1. Conversion (physical manifestation) ; hesitation, stuttering, expressive movement before or after the reaction, twitch-

---

looks. It conceives the unconscious as potential energy to which a psychic correlation may be coordinated. But the tremendous change between repression and manifestation, this often grandiose, creative, poetic transformation, proves that very much kinetic energy has been exerted, consistently with which, an unconscious thought- and will-process, succeeding to new values, is coordinated.

ing, secretion of tears, sighing, psychogalvanic phenomena, changes in the pulse, etc.

2. Immediate correction of the reaction or its beginning (mistakes in speech).

3. Prolonged reaction-time. We speak of this when the "probable reaction-time" is exceeded. One gains the latter not by means of arithmetic but by the following method: The reaction-times are arranged in a series according to their value. The average of these numbers is called the probable reaction-time. The arithmetical mean is worthless because reactions are often absent altogether, though one waits twenty, fifty or one hundred seconds. Jung does not wait more than twenty seconds; I have repeatedly obtained valuable associations, however, after a longer period.

B. *Characteristics according to Content.*

(*a*) **Previous to the reaction:** False understanding of the stimulus-word. Herein applies the rule: The complex seeks to interpret everything heard in the sense of its gratification.

(*β*) **During the reaction:**

1. Diversions: (a') To an object of the surroundings, e. g. inkwell, window.

(b') Translation into foreign tongue.

2. Superficial reactions:

(a') Repetition of the stimulus-word or previous reactions.

(b') Insignificant change of the stimulus-word, e. g. sicksickly.

(c') Slang associations, e. g. puns.

(d') Banal definitions (Imbeciles present enormous numbers of definitions).*

(e') Stilted reactions (pompous expressions).

(*γ*) **After the reaction:**

(a') Perseverations: An idea may act so strongly on the subject that the content of the next following stimulus-word is not noticed and the reaction is joined to the previous stimulus-word. The perseveration can persist for two or three stimulus-

* K. Wehrlin, ü. die Assoz. v. Imbezillen u. Idioten. 2d Beitr. d diagnost. Ass.-Studien.

words. Often, one reaction follows quickly but the idea still rules the following associations.

(b') Disturbances of reproduction: The subject can no longer give his earlier reaction or unwittingly gives another.

It is very easy to perceive that exactly the same complex-indicators may also appear in ordinary speech. Even the opponents of psychoanalysis, like Isserlin, must admit this in essentials so far as they recognize it.* It is not well to analyze all reactions. It is sufficient to test those that are most strongly stigmatized. I will select some tests which will bring the poetic production of the unconscious plainly to expression.

Stimulus-word: long. Reaction: long street. Time: 7.6 sec. Association: "I saw a picture which represented a long street converging in perspective. On both sides, stood houses. Poor peasant people who were going along in a wagon thought they could not get by that narrow end of the street. 'Love as long as you can.' Thus sang a mother by the cradle of her boy. The mother died, the son sang it ever after. The song made an impression on me although it is sentimental." As the pupil produced no further associations for a long time, I unwisely put the direct question: Are you thinking of your mother? Answer: "No." Following stimulus-word: Boat. Reaction: Port. Time 4.2 seconds. Association: "Sagt Mutter, 's ist Uve!" (O. Ernst). "I have often thought it would be beautiful if I stood by my mother as others do by theirs. But it cannot be. At my house, no one says a kind word to another."

It is plain that the boy, although he did not perceive it, was referring to his position to his mother in the two melancholy songs. I might have brought this out psychoanalytically without the following reaction and could have shown that "no" of the overconsciousness included a deception.

The association of the picture, I understood at once. In order not to disturb the analysis, however, I kept silent and seven days later, again gave the stimulus-word. The reaction was the same. "What is probably lurking behind the picture?" Answer: "I do not know and cannot think." "De-

* Isserlin, p. 338.

scribe the peasant." "He is rather simple but true and noble, perhaps also somewhat stubborn. He has a crafty facial expression. He holds the bridle in his hands. The whip, he has stuck beside him." I repeated: "Rather simple, true and noble, somewhat-stubborn, crafty, bridle in hands. Now?"— The youth, greatly astonished: "That may perhaps be I!" Then he realized at once that the street end was the narrow gate of conversion, of which I had spoken to him before. He thought he could not pass this gate; the association draws the fear into the laughable (simple peasant). The whip has sexual symbolical meaning. The boy struggled desperately against onanism. Now the ugly masturbation phantasy is interpreted according to the law of complex-recasting into the opposite sense: The hand holds the whip in order to direct.

[To plow.] "Scarcely" (kaum). Time: 13.2 seconds. "I thought at the same time of sharp (kühn). [Scarcely.] "Scarcely has one plowed than comes the seed. Perhaps thus with me, so that I would not detect the result of my bad habit. To "keen" there occurs to mind a picture by Albrecht Dürer: "Knight, Death and Devil." The knight is not particularly keen, he presents a quiet, half-scornful smile. Thus one gets on best. I am ashamed in front of the picture because of my sin. To the word, "plow," immediately occurred to me also the place M. (a region about three kilometers from his residence). Recently, I met some young girls and went as far as M. with them in the hope of getting up an acquaintance. I did not succeed however. To 'plow,' to 'dig' comes into my mind: it means: digging after something."

Let us seek the explanation. The enormous reaction-time betrays strong resistance. The stimulus-word, plow, is understood in a double sense: First as preparation for sowing; to this is joined the reaction "scarcely," which expresses the hope for quick reward for giving up onanism. The pupil seeks a compensation for the pleasure given up. Of what this reward shall consist, the other associations show: plow-dig, to seek something. For what does one dig? Naturally for a "treasure" and that the young fellow also seeks such an one, of course in transposed sense, is shown by the reaction "sharp," as allusion to a little adventure which an acquaintance with girls would bring about. The word "sharp" refers, however, not only to the boldness shown therein but also as the reference to Dürer's knight shows, to the wished-for boldness in the struggle with the vice.

The word "plow" would thereby be understood without doubt sexually symbolically, as is well known in folk-lore which is accustomed to use plowing as symbolizing the sexual act. The badly educated boy of doubtful morals wishes to change from autoeroticism to normal intercourse and this as soon as possible.

In this conception, we see the three simultaneous, mutually dependent associations, "scarcely," "sharp," "M.," explained. The third stimulus-word following was:

[Table.] "Flower." Time 24.8 seconds. "I looked to the side and perhaps imagined a flower table." [It really stands there.] "The 'scarcely' from before started up again. Then I saw almost as if written, the word 'nose.' I really liked to pick my nose and found great pleasure in so doing, further, I enjoyed polishing my dirty finger-nails and derived a feeling of great pleasure from the process. I registered these too among my bad habits in my diary but it did not help, I always succumbed again. Then I let it stand." [Once more: table-flower.] "I keep thinking only of the 'scarcely.'" [Thus a girl affair again? Does "flower" stand for girl?] "I have already thought that."

The interpretation is not at all artificial. The flower-table beside the boy awakened the association of "flower" to "table," which expression immediately received strong affective emphasis because it was perceived in the vulgar speech usage as term for a girl. At once, the previous girl phantasy was continued: "scarcely" and "picking, digging" again emerged, this time the latter word plainly in new sexual symbolic meaning. The picking of the nose corresponds to the earlier plowing. It is a dirty and yet in a certain sense, hygienically commendable, and allowable act. The finger has here the same meaning as in nail-polishing and previously given cases (finger under nose, 78, anxiety on stretching a glove finger, 160, compare the anesthetic toe, 176).

One sees plainly that in the moment of uttering the reactions, an important, newly fashioned work, of which consciousness knows nothing, has been performed. The scheme carefully worked out by Jung shows the following stimulus words:

1. head	29. lamp	57. pencil
2. green	30. rich	58. sad
3. water	31. tree	59. plum
4. stick	32. sing	60. meet
5. angel	33. pity	61. law
6. long	34. yellow	62. love
7. boat	35. mountain	63. glass
8. plow	36. play	64. fight
9. wool	37. salt	65. traits
10. friendly	38. new	66. great
11. table	39. custom	67. potato
12. ask	40. ride	68. paint
13. state	41. wall	69. part
14. defiant	42. stupid	70. old
15. stalk	43. handle	71. flower
16. dance	44. despise	72. strike
17. sea	45. tooth	73. chest
18. sick	46. right	74. savage
19. pride	47. folk	75. family
20. cook	48. stink	76. wash
21. ink	49. book	77. cow
22. bad	50. unjust	78. strange
23. needle	51. frog	79. luck
24. swim	52. divide	80. tell
25. journey	53. hunger	81. decorum
26. blue	54. white	82. narrow
27. bread	55. ox	83. brother
28. threaten	56. attend	84. injury

85. stork	91. door	97. month
86. false	92. choose	98. colored
87. decorum	93. hay	99. dog
88. kiss	94. steep	100. speak
89. fire	95. derision	
90. dirty	96. sleep	

Even without analysis, one can draw important conclusions from the associations. For instance, if a person prefers in high degree adjectives of value, then she discloses that she has much free floating life-force, thus that she is badly situated in relation to life and love. Emma Fürst found in an extensive material that in women over forty-one, this "value predicate type" predominates, while of the men, only those past sixty-one go over to this subjective type. Betraying are the reactions to the scattered group of four words: "water," "boat," "sea," "swim." If all four are strongly marked, one can conclude with probability upon suicidal intentions. The girl mentioned on page 179, who had denied such an intention, confessed when she saw how she betrayed herself that as a fact she had attempted suicide in her bath a week before. In general, liars are often discovered by the association-experiment. He who suppresses a word, betrays the fact by long reaction-time or other complex-indicators. Jung even unmasked a criminal by his method.*

A number of similar results may be derived by careful elaboration of the reactions. The skilled person may gain from them a summary diagnosis of his patient or normal subject of analysis.† For psychoanalysis, the method may be dispensed with and is to-day no longer much used in spite of the ease of its application, except where a quick diagnosis is wanted or where theoretical conclusions are sought. One critic expresses doubt, obviously without having made any experiments, on the diagnostic reliability of the reactions; I would strongly advise him not to trust his own associations to publication. He

---

* Jung, Z. psycholog. Tatbestandsdiagnostik. Zbl. f. Nervenheilkunde u. Psychiatrie, 1905, No. 200.

† Freud, über Psa., p. 32.

might reveal some very unpleasant experiences like some other doubters.

Important for pedagogues are the investigations of the previously mentioned physician (Emma Fürst) on the family resemblance in reaction type.* The basis is Jung's scheme of classification which in turn rests on the excellent works of Kraepelin and Aschaffenburg. The reactions were differentiated according to fifteen relations: Co-ordination, sub- and super-ordination, contrast-association, personal judgment, other predicates, subjective relation, objective relation, determination by time, place, means, etc., definition, coexistence, identity, motor-speech, union, word assimilation, complimentary words, slang associations, other groups (false, senseless, mediate association).†

One computes now how large a percentage of reactions fall into each group. If one wishes to compare the relation between reactions between two members of a family arithmetically, he computes the difference of the two percentages in each of the two groups, adds the sums of these differences and divides by fifteen. Then one knows how much the average or as it is usually expressed, ''the mean difference'' is.

The principal results in nine families containing thirty-seven members, persons of little culture, investigated, ranging in age from nine to seventy-four years, were as follows:

All children under sixteen years, had more internal associations than the mother, all children over sixteen (with one exception) more external.

The mean difference among related men was 4:1, that among related women, 3:8. Among persons not related, the difference is considerably higher. Relatives, therefore, possess a tendency to agreement in reaction-type,‡ and this agreement between mother and children (3:5) is greater than between father and children (4:2). Still, the reaction relationship between fathers and sons (3:1) is almost as great as that between

---

* Emma Fürst, 10th Beitr. d. diagn. Ass.-Studien.
† Same, p. 80.
‡ Same, p. 110.

mothers and daughters (3:0). The mean difference of fathers and daughters was 4:9, of mothers and daughters was 4:7. It follows therefore: "The best and most uniform agreement occurs between parents and their children of the same sex." *

(C) THE FREE ASSOCIATION CHAINS

Freud allowed apparently meaningless series of words to be formed and gained by aid of these series, glimpses of repressed mental content.† Jung too made use of the method ‡ and Stekel applied it with success.||

I give a short example from a previously published work ¶:

[Water.] Corpse. 4 Seconds. Boat, a drunken man. I looked on as a drunken man was drawn into a boat. [Name all the words which come into your mind now.] Bathing, swimming, bathing-establishment, bathing-attendant, ground, sea-weed, shark, earth, stone, spring-board, air, chain, beam, submarine boat, crew, no air, drowned, diver, diving-bell, gold, rope-ladder. [What comes into your mind now?] In the moving-picture theatre, I saw two divers who found gold. One cut the air-tube of the other, took the gold and ascended.

[Bathing.] Because my brother bathes much. I also like very much to bathe.

[Swimming.] My brother asserts that he has dived from the spring-board almost to the bottom. This made a deep impression on me. It rained a lot. I dove to the bottom once in a less deep place. Drowning comes to mind. I saw in a moving-picture theatre how one drowns.

[Sea-weed.] One may get caught in'it. This happened to me once.

[Earth.] The bottom of the water. Gloomy, black. The tomb in Busento. (Four days later) : therein is someone on a horse, large, robust, pale. It is my brother.

* Same, p. 111.
† Freud, Hysterie, p. 241.
‡ Jung, Ü. d. Psychol. d. Dem. præcox, p. 130.
|| Stekel, Nervöse Angstzustände, p. 67.
¶ Pfister, Analyt. Unters. ü. d. Psychol. des Hasses u. d. Versöhnung, p. 7 f.

[Chain.] Outside at the bathing establishment by the keg. Arno once went there into the depths and remained some ten meters under the surface of the water hanging by one finger. He said then he didn't care much for life and liked to do dangerous things as coasting on a bicycle.

[Submarine boat.] I saw in a picture how the crew of such a boat suffocated. (Four days later) : [Do you know anyone large, robust, pale?] It is again my brother, Arno.

[Diver.] The drowning diver in the moving-picture theatre. One sees the pale face through the glass. The man was large and dark. We received from a panopticon, a life-size wax mask which represented a dying king. The eyes were pointed upwards. Arno put this head on his shoulders once and draped a cloth around him. Then he looked like a ghost. I was greatly frightened. The dying diver reminded me of that wax model. (One sees clearly the work of the repression: the subject means the one who lurks in the wax mask, Arno, but does not allow this idea to come through.) [The murderer.] He was a smaller man. His face was not visible. He was greatly afraid of solitude and because he had killed the other.

[Make a series.] Pity, punishment, captain, search for the murderer, electric chair, the past, heaven, hell, last judgment, God, Abraham, Lazarus, the rich man, abyss, water, brothers, Lazarus at the foot-stool of God, the prayer of the rich man, the man who wished a palace in heaven, on whom Peter had pity, the man on tip-toe who looked through the knot-hole, the King-dom of God. (Four days later) : The murderer is small, agile, short-armed, half-sick, greedy, brutal. [Who is it?] Yes, I. I noticed that four days ago but thought it had no value. I am not brutal in ordinary life? [No, but you are what is so well termed two-faced. You harbor evil wishes and would carry them out. That has not completely succeeded. Hence your malice, your dark tendency to evil.]

The detailed analysis would take us too far. Here is the result: The murderer, Max, is executed in the electric chair, consoles himself nevertheless with the hope that he might not, like the rich man in the parable of Jesus', suffer eternal torment in hell but will, like the rich man in the beautiful tale of Volk-mann-Leanders, receive in hell a splendid castle full of gold, standing on tip-toe, one may see heaven through a knot-hole and finally be saved. In the man on tip-toes, the subject recognizes himself.

It is worthy of note that the boy while giving his words, had no suspicion that behind these words, murder phantasies against his brother were hidden. And yet it may be shown with certainty from the members of the chain of associations not reproduced here that they were present. Behind the two series of associations which were narrated in a few minutes, there existed phantasies which wished death upon the brother in sixteen ways, upon himself in three ways, upon other persons in six ways, besides a mass of other accidents and active crimes.

The value of such chains lies in the fact that the unconscious is outwitted. The painful thought can find expression in the disguise. The analysis seizes the criminal and unmasks him.

These chains are also always applied during the dream analysis as the free phantastic continuation of the dream and manifestations.

5. ACCIDENTAL ASSOCIATIONS

When an idea clings to us tenaciously even against our will, we are not wrong in the assumption that we are dealing with a manifestation.

(α) Word association.

An example of a word obsession was given on page 41 ("Pentakosiomedimnen").

(β) Obsessing melody.

Jung has discovered that the melodies which haunt us are to be explained in the same manner.* Another example may be added:

A young analyst was long haunted by the melody:

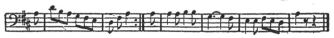

---

* Jung, Dem. præc., p. 62 f.

Finally he submitted to autoanalysis and found it was the melody of Beethoven to Goethe's verse: "Mit Männern sich geschlagen" (Fought with men). Then he remembered that he had fought an unpleasant duel with an opponent. Work pressed, a period of quiescence ensued. Then there began to run through his head:

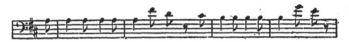

In vexation, he asked himself what was the matter now and wished to dislodge the disturber of the peace by denial and concentration. He had to analyze again. Then it was revealed: The melody was in the student song-book and belonged to the preceding text and ran: "With men have fought, with maidens got on well." Then it occurred to him that he had a conflict with his wife in which he yielded against his conviction, which he regretted immediately afterwards. For this, the song consoled further: "And more credit than money"—correct, this also occurred to the autoanalyst in a moment—"thus one goes through the world."

Thus the two melodies suited the situation nicely and contained excellent consolation for his repressed ideas. The song of Beethoven's begins: "Mit Mädels sich vertragen" (With maidens got on well). The error shows the influence of the repression.

(γ) Association of numbers.

(Analyses of associations of numbers and dreams of numbers occur as follows: Freud, Zur Psychopathologie des Alltagslebens, 109 ff.; Adler, Drei Psycho-Analysen von Zahleneinfällen und obsedierenden Zahlen, Psych-neur. Wochenschr., 1905, No. 28; Jung, Ein Beitrag zur Kenntnis des Zahlentraumes, Zentralblatt I, 567–572; Stekel, Die Sprache des Traumes, 410, 430; Marcinowsky, Drei Romane in Zahlen, Zentralblatt II, 619–638.)

Since I had plenty of dreams of numbers for this book but no associations of numbers to use, I asked a merchant of middle age to give me a little number analysis. He assented and named the number 24.

[24.] "Love, lip. 2×4. $4 \times 4 = 16$. As a boy, I cele-brated my birthday on Oct. 24 instead of 23. Upon admission to the technical school the birth certificate gave it as 23. The teacher registrar entered this date, against which I protested. Smiling, he noted down therefore Oct. 23/24. To-day, I feel as if new-born for I have received glad tidings from my dear girl. On my birthday I receive much love and many kisses. Love and lips belong together.

$2 \times 4 = 8$, $4 \times 4 = 16$ making together the number 24. 8 means "esteem," $4 \times 4 = 16$, "double esteem," 24 "triple esteem." My fiancée shall for the time know nothing of the fact that I love another more than her. I discovered a short time ago that I carelessly left a tell-tale slip of paper sticking in the pocket of my great-coat.

[$2 \times 4 = 8$.] Twice a four-in-hand team. Puss-in-Boots came in a four-horse wedding coach. I took part in the wed-ding of a friend whose bride was pretty but she is a bad, un-affectionate wife. I fear that it will be the same with my fiancée who already treats me coldly and imperiously. I wish for myself a second more pleasant wedding coach.

4 might be a 4-leaved clover leaf. At first, I was happy with my fiancée, now I long for better luck.

[4×4.] I dreamed of four boats, in one of which I went away. The name of this boat agreed with that of my present love.

"4" (vier) sounds like "Füür" = Feuer (fire). 2×4 means double fire, double love. The folk song is not right in its assertion, love blooms but once in a life-time (compare two wedding coaches).

$24 = 4$, fire, and 20. My friend wrote when 20 that she had to suffer much from burning desire and asked herself if Ellen Key were not right in her contention for free love. This dis-quieted me but on the other hand, the natural sensuality pleased me which differed pleasantly from the cold prudery of my fiancée.

[24.] The girl will be exactly 24 years old when I can marry her. Then her extravagant ideas of free love and exaggerated sensual demands will disappear spontaneously. When she is 24 years old, I will be born into a new life, then will be my birthday!"

Since this mathematics is unfamiliar to us, I offer for consideration a number dream.

". . . I hastened to the station in order to travel to Genf. Then it came into my mind that I had too little money in my purse. I consoled myself, however, that there might still be a gold piece there. The ticket cost eighteen francs, leaving me six francs over." [Genf.] "Some weeks before, I visited several acquaintances there. At a later day, I discovered to my vexation that a charming girl whom I knew, had stayed there without my knowing it." [18 francs, 6 left over.] (Immediately.) "$18 \times 6 = 108$, 18 must be the beginning of a count of centuries, I do not know how though. (Pause.) Ah, so! It might be the number of the year in which we went, $1800 + 108 = 1908$. When I named the year 1908, I did not yet know how it was related to the preceding numbers." [1908.] "When I was vexed because of the visit which I had missed, I consoled myself with the thought that I could go to Genf again soon. The dream confirmed: yes, in this very year!" [Do you know what the ticket to Genf costs?] "No. I think about 16 francs." (We looked up the amount and found to our astonishment, 18 francs, 65 rappen.)

"Now something else occurs to me. Yesterday before the dream, I told a mathematician that I had entirely forgotten all mathematics. The dream will plainly console me."

We will concede that the operation with 18 and 6 as multiplication and addition was carried out right cleverly.

The computation is not quite correct: It lacked 5 rappen.

Since mathematics in a dream may still seem strange, although it agrees most exactly with the dream logic, another example may be added. An acquaintance learned from his wife that he had called out in his sleep: "6 × 6 = 36, Schleswig-Holstein, meerumschlungen, meerumschlungen." He did not think any more about the dream. The analysis taught him: "Because 'meerumschlungen' (surrounded by the sea) was called out twice, there must be a duplication in the preceding material. (Who outside the dreamer would have arrived at this conclusion?) The halves of 36 are 18. Right! 18 placed before 2-6s gives 1866. Of this date, I spoke with my wife before the dream night. At that time, Schleswig-Holstein came to Prussia. I defended the Prussians, my wife the Danes. I stopped in order to avoid strife." The deeper meaning of the dream cannot be given here.

In the many number dreams which I have investigated, the associations have constantly yielded the same mathematics of the unconscious.

6. DREAM, HALLUCINATION AND WAKING-DREAM

(A) ESTIMATION OF THE DREAM

According to Freud, dream interpretation is the via regia to a knowledge of the unconscious.* Psychoanalysis is founded on dream interpretation.† So much the more do I regret that I cannot present here the whole dream investigation in all its refinements. For this purpose, a whole book would be needed; such a book, we possess in Freud's masterpiece.

The estimation of the dream in present day psychology is a most varied one. One experimental psychologist explains it most recently in his lectures as a negligible quantity from which no kind of conclusions regarding the mental activity of a person can be drawn and with which one would better not deal at all.

Such an opinion is in conflict with the everyday experience of healthy human reason, of poets and of those psychologists who consider more than that part of the mental life fathomable by physical instruments and expressable in mathematical formulæ as worthy of notice.

* Freud, Über Psa., p. 32.
† Freud, A note on the unconscious in Psycho-Analysis, p. 317.

Even the Bible relates of dream interpretations which every pedagogue without more ado must recognize as psychologically correct. Joseph dreamed that the sheaves of his brothers bowed down before his and the brothers reproached him: "Will you become king over us and rule over us?" The ambitious youth saw in sleep the sun, moon and eleven stars bow before him and had to receive his father's rebuke: "Shall I and thy mother and thy brethren indeed come to bow down ourselves before thee to the earth?" (Gen. xxxvii, 10). Everyone will admit that the narrator wishes to show the ambition of the boy by the report of his dreams and does he do this without psychological justification? When a boy dreams before Christmas of a cannon as high as a table jumping about his room, the educator will assume, unless he accidentally belongs to that skeptical experimental psychology, that the child would like to possess such an object. And when—this example also springs from reality—a boy who in jumping over a brook has broken his leg and can only tediously limp, joyfully jumps around in his dream, the pedagogue reaches the conclusion without scruples that the dream realizes a longed-for wish. Because a symbol is present in Joseph's dream, is the interpretation of his brothers and father so artificial?

Indeed the most important ideas in Freud's dream theory exist in outline in the Bible without his having known it. This happens in the interesting places, Dan. v, 25–28. The seer interprets the secret writing to Belshazzar: "Mene, tekel, upharsin." Verses 26 and following say: "The interpretation is this:—Mene: 'God hath numbered thy kingdom and finished it; tekel: Thou art weighed in the balances and art found wanting; upharsin: Thy kingdom is divided and given to the Medes and Persians.'" Mene means also "mine" a money term, tekel (= shekel) is about 1/50 mine, peres, a half-mine, singular of the plural form, p(h)arsin, Persian. The stem means "to divide." One sees in these terms a reference to the powerful Babylonian kingdom (mine), the deficient Median rule (shekel) which at the time of the dream lay in Belshazzar's hands, and refers to the Persian power appearing again more strongly but not attaining the Babylonian splendor. At all events, Daniel puts a deeper meaning under the money terms, he considers them as overdetermined and symbolical. The meaning which the Jewish seer derives from the secret writing (cryptography) contains also a thought most suitable to the Jewish wish-phantasy: the miserable Median rule shall be broken but not by a new world power resembling the Babylonian. Beyond this meaning, there is the double significance "Persians-divided," an allusion to the incapacity for life of the future heathen power.

Therewith, the author of the apocalyptical writings may have known something of the fundamental idea that behind the dream-content—here we are dealing with a cryptogram but the mechanism is the same—there lurks a quite different (latent) thought. He recognized the condensation, the plural meaning of the dream idea, the wishfulfillment in the manifestation.

Still more important is the passage, Daniel v, 12, where it is said of Daniel: "Interpreting of dreams, and shewing of hard sentences, and dissolving of doubts, were found in the same Daniel." Is not the expression "analysis" there anticipated in the plainest and most striking manner?

I would like to quote the sayings of some poets, for they, according to the confirmative judgment of psychologists, know not a little of the mind.

Richard Wagner puts these words in the mouth of Hans Sachs:

> "Just that is the poet's work
> That he may note and interpret dreams;
> Believe me, man's truest vision
> Is given him in dream.
> All poetic art and poetry
> Is nothing else than true interpretation of dreams." *

Johann Peter Uz (1720–96) rhymes:

> "Every one is like his dreams,
> In dream carouses Anacreon,

* Richard Wagner, Meistersinger. Reported by Robitsek, Die Analyse in Egmonts Traum. Jahrb. II, p. 464.

A poet exults in his rhymes
And flits across the Helicon.
For you, monad, fight with conclusions,
A lover of ontology;
And every maiden dreams of kisses
For what is more important for her?" *

Tolstoi has his hero, in whom he probably depicts himself, testify: "When I awake, I can well be deceived concerning myself, the dream on the other hand, gives me the correct measure for the stage of moral perfection which I have attained." †

Hebbel says in his distich "Der Traum als Prophet":

"What shall befall you, how can the dream tell you?
What you will do, that it shows you already."

The poet has his Judith narrate a dream and add: "I know that one should not despise such dreams. See, I think like this: When a man lies asleep, set free, no longer held together by consciousness of himself, then a feeling of the future represses all thoughts and pictures of the present and the things which shall come, flit as shadows through the mind, preparing, warning, consoling. Hence it comes about that anything true so seldom or never surprises us, that we long before confidently expected the good and involuntarily tremble before every evil." ‡ If this sounds somewhat unscientific, the diary explains: "Our suspicions, beliefs, presentiments, etc., we have until now brought into use only as proof of the existence of a world existing outside of us, still incomprehensible to us in its reality; to me they are more, they are to me like the pulse beats of a world still slumbering and locked within us." ||

That the poets know the meaning and psychological structure of the dream and attribute to it a great importance, is a fact familiar to every analyst.

---

* Zbl. II, p. 292.
† Zbl. II, p. 615, reported by Mira Gincburg.
‡ Hebbel, Judith, Act III.
|| Hebbel, Tagebücher, Berlin 1905, I, p. 146 (Zbl. III, p. 168).

Goethe describes Egmont's dream.* The man condemned to death longed for freedom and his beloved. Then the dream begins: Clara appears as freedom. The hero awakens strengthened. Robitsek sought to interpret with extraordinary sharp sightedness the particular relations but did not find undivided approval.†

Björnson describes in his novel, "Arne," the mother of the hero in concise terms: "She was the only child of her parents. In her eighteenth year, she remained sitting too long at a dancing festival." She danced with the violinist. "In this night, Margit dreamed of a great red cow which had stolen into the grain in the field. She ought to drive her away but though she strove hard to do so, could not move from her place; the cow remained standing quietly and ate until she became round and sleek." ‡ After this dream, in which the dreamer symbolized her life-desires and herself in a cow and expressed her most secret wish, we are not surprised at the fact that on the next Sunday, she sought the violinist again and was seduced by him. The poet gives us only a little data from a whole life history but among that a dream. This shows how great value he attributed to it as the indicator of the mind.

The finest work of art in relation to dream and delirium is Jensen's "Gradiva," on which Freud has written a monograph. A similar estimate of the dream, we find among numerous poets. I mention only Jeremia Gotthelf's "Anne Bäbi Jowäger," K. F. Meyer's "Glöcklein," Tolstoi's "Gebet," Wildenbruch's "Hexenlied," Andersen's "Mädchen mit den Schwefelhölzchen," Hauptmann's "Hannele," Ibsen's "Klein Eyolf." Painters also compose this way: I mention only Moritz von Schwind's "Gefangenen" (Prisoner) for whom the Brownies sawed through the trellis bars and to whom a kind angel brought refreshment.

The folk-song also knows the symbolic significance of the dream. A song in "Des Knaben Wunderhorn" runs as follows:

* Robitsek, pp. 451–464.
† Silberer, Vorläufer Freud'scher Gedanken. Zbl. I, p. 446.
‡ Björnsons ausgew. Werke (German by Lobedanz), Vol. II, p. 14.

"When I the whole day through
Have done my tasks
Still there is more to do.
At night when I should sleep
Oft am I awakened
By a dream with awful fear.

In sleep I see the ghost
Of my most beloved
With mighty bow
To which are many arrows drawn
Wherewith he will me lift
From out this grievous life.

Gazing at such grim specter,
I cannot quiet keep
And cry in shrieking tones
O boy, cease your anger,
I am going to sleep
You will not need your weapons."

Here we find the common symbol of arrow for member, of
death for the sexual act.* The anxiety corresponds to the
pent-up life-desire. The dreamer flees from the dream into
reality as the swoon, the dream, the neurotic symptom are to
be understood as flight into the unreal automatism.

Freud has shown how intensively the acumen of psychologists from Aristotle and his monograph on dreams and dream
interpretation down to Havelock Ellis, Sante des Sanctis and
Vold has been employed on our subject.

* Representation by contrast, simultaneously suggesting disappearance of the sense. The love-death is typical: E. T. A. Hoffman has his
hero say: "You believe too that the highest beatitude of love, the fulfillment of the mystery, is consummated in death." (Elixiere des Teufels, Berlin-Leipzig 1908, p. 157); Novalis says: "In death, love is the
sweetest; for the loving one, death is a bridal night, a secret of sweet
mysteries" Heilborn, Novalis, p. 160). He speaks of a "mystical marriage of pleasure and death" (p. 116). Heilborn rightly adds that the
pairing of ideas of death and sensuality is the way of all mystics (p.
104). Compare Isolde's Liebestod by Wagner (see above p. 320),
Kleist's death, etc.

(B) THE DREAM WORK

The plain meaning of many dreams lies right at hand. When, in Ibsen's "Klein Eyolf," the hero sees his lame child who was drowned, healthy and jumping around in the dream, this is comprehensible to us. Why, however, are other dreams senseless or trifling?

For answer to this question, we turn to the psychoanalytic investigation. Let us take a few simple examples:

A teacher aged thirty-five, sees himself going through bad weather to a school-house from which many young people are coming. Beside the house stand two furniture vans of which one is already loaded and ready to depart. Through the door, one sees a carefully equipped drawing-board. The other wagon is not yet entirely loaded. On account of the rain, many objects were placed under the wagon. The cover of the vehicle was pushed far up in perpendicular slots. A friend stands alongside.

[Bad weather.] "We have had it for some days. I wanted to start on a mountain trip but felt indisposed and feared to be held back by rain."

[School-house.] "On the trip, a pupil from this one and a teacher from another school-house were to participate, namely, my friend F."

[Furniture van.] "On the day before the dream, my mother spoke of moving."

[The loaded wagon.] "My pupil has already gone to the mountain, my friend is waiting for me and I am not yet ready."

[Drawing-board.] "I wrote first 'Reisbrett' (for Reissbrett) = guideboard."

[The other wagon.] "The cover shoved up says: 'delayed is not prevented.' This applies to my trip."

[The objects under the wagon.] "They were protected from the rain. Waiting hurts nothing."

Now the superficial interpretation of the dream is plain. The sleeper is to be consoled for his ill humor. Behind the dream ideas, the so-called manifest content, lurk the hidden motives, the latent dream thoughts. The complete work of transposing the latter into the former is known to us, the so-called dream work. We find the condensation (mountain trip, moving of the mother, in the figure of the furniture vans), the symbolical representation, here accomplished by a word-bridge (Reissbrett—Reisbrett, lifted cover [aufgeschoben]—delayed is not prevented (aufgehoben). One motive for the dream always belongs to an experience of the previous day or next preceding day. Here it is a very insignificant one: a conversation. But it affords material for effective symbolization. The dream is without affect (lack of emotion). Not all the ways of manifestation found by us were utilized. The regression into the infantile may still be added: The dreamer as a child experienced many movings which went off well in spite of bad weather. Further, a deeper meaning may be suspected: F. is married to a youthful girl friend of the dreamer, now grown handsome and strong and was envied by the latter, since his wife is thin. On the other hand, F. has no children to expect while the dreamer, to his gratification, sees himself in this position (objects under the wagon). Finally, the peculiar furniture wagon is a functional symbol: The dreamer consoles himself that his unsatisfied longing for love will still be gratified. But so he has waited for years and does nothing to reach a better situation with his love, to attain a nobler relation to his wife. The over-interpretation was revealed only after the first interpretation, from associations collected.

A pastor friend of mine dreamed that he was amid a howling mob of negroes by whom Europeans were killed. A huge fat negro seized him and lifted him on high in order to dash him to the ground. N., however, grasped a branch of a tree and felt secure. Some men dragged a piano into the dining-room. Suddenly their leader braced himself in a certain corner with the assertion that if the floor should fall down now, the floor in this corner would hold securely.

Both dreams are to their creators, senseless and without connection to their conscious mental lives.

[Mob of negroes.] "Three days before the dream, I held a

lecture on the mission in Africa and rejoiced that Christian culture had overcome cannibalism."

[The negro giant.] "Black, Pastor Black, Pastor Z., Pastor C. The latter is large, dark skinned and very robust." (I might have named these persons for associations but proceeded) :

[The branch.] "On a sheet of pictures, an ape was pursued by a lion, but at the last moment, jumped on a branch, mocked and maltreated the lion. In the dream, I swung myself triumphantly on high."

[The piano.] "My seemingly heavy, black piano was really transported into the dining-room before the dream. The leader in the dream is the father of the real baggage-man. I spoke with both men on the day before the dream."

[The corner of the room.] "The favorite plan of my wife who assists the mission very cleverly.

"And now I understand the occasion of the dream. Pastor C., my neighbor, preached a sermon which was rather cool and detrimental to the mission. He is a large man, according to his own statement, inclined to corpulency, clothed in black and having a dark beard. Plainly, he is the negro. I felt myself attacked by his sermon since I was openly identified with the mission. A friend of the mission said to me: 'Now I shall give Pastor C. nothing more for the works conducted by him.' I thought: 'Pastor C. was a duffer to injure himself so.' Or no, I did not think so, I wished him only the result of his imprudent conduct but in the dream I made a duffer out of the pastor. Out of me whom he treated slightingly in the sermon, I made an ape who first feared the lion but then despised him, overcame him and raised myself high above him."

The second dream seems to have nothing to do with the first but confirms the unbreakable rule that all dreams of a night (even when they are interrupted by awakening) form one homogeneous whole.*

The piano is heavy and black like the negro and threatens the dreamer like Pastor C. in the preceding dream. The

* Freud, Traumdeutung, p. 261.

dreamer saves himself in the favorite plan of his wife who performs such excellent service for the mission. He identifies himself with the man who managed the moving of the piano and thus climbs to leader of his colleague. Thereby, he makes himself father of the real baggage-man because he will be something better, the spiritual father. Thus the first dream says: Pastor C. cannot hurt the mission and me, he injures only himself and I triumph. The second dream adds: My wife also helps me to gain this victory.

Both dreams depict also a transposition of inclination: The dreamer was previously very cordial to his colleague, to his wife, less so. Now the relationships are reversed, at least an attempt is made in this direction.

It has been said that dreams are unimportant, mere repetitions of daily happenings. Both statements are incorrect. There are no mere reproduction-dreams. The unconscious is much too autistic to devote itself to minutiae. Where it seems different, the dream has deeper meaning. As proof for this, we may offer two examples from a number of observations:

A gentleman of about thirty-eight years disputed the observation that a repressed wish is fulfilled in every dream and referred to a dream which merely repeated quite closely an experience of that day: ''I was going with my band of pupils to the station but the train had just gone. Later I turned back and mounted the train.''

[I know absolutely nothing of the affairs of your life except that you are married. Were you something of an elderly ''young sport'' when you had the dream?] ''That is so.'' [And were you afraid that you might already have lost the power for connection?] ''I remember perfectly that this thought often troubled me at that time. How do you know this?''

I will disclose to the reader that ''station'' is an exceedingly frequent sexual symbol. At the station are the trains which run in and out. The literature shows a mass of proof for this, in itself, surprising symbolism, which I myself have found substantiated times without number. Thus the dreamer consoled himself by still coming to marriage.

The reproduction-dream of a student ran as follows: "I was sitting on the stage of an auditorium. This has really happened in the afternoon. Only in the dream, I saw some gentlemen sitting on the benches."

[Plainly it is your dearest wish to become a university professor.] "That is a fact; it is the goal toward which I strive with all my power."

As with these two dreams, so countless others may be interpreted by the experienced analyst without more facts. Therefore, no one should tell his dreams in society. Inexperienced people disclose their innermost and most delicate secrets. Still in the beginning, one should not devote one's self to guessing but seek carefully, according to the fundamental rules of analysis, the material for interpretation.

Finally, a last example which may show how in the dream, without exception, an important affair of the dreamer's is treated even where not the slightest trace of it is to be detected in the content. The dream is, as a matter of fact, always egocentric.*

A theological student in love dreamed: "The Duchess of Angoulême is expected." Who this lady is, he cannot tell. [Angoulême.] "Angleterre" (England). "There, my beloved is staying. 'Angoul' reminds me of angelus, angel. Such, I consider the beloved. Angoul agrees also with angulus, angle. Yesterday, I sang the whole day: 'She is my thought by day and night and dwells by the corner of the gate.' This student song fits in, for my beloved lives beside a gate arch."

[Duchess.] "The duchess from Ekkehard who loved a theologian without winning him. In the legend which I read when a child, there were duchesses whom I naturally would

---

* Freud (Traumdeutung, p. 254) calls it, as we have heard, egoistic. Often, however, real moral performances which demand sacrifice, are the content of the dream. Probably Freud understands egoistic as we conceive of egocentric.

have liked to possess. I was long afraid of not winning my lady friend.''

[Angoulême.] '' 'Lême is short for: 'Elle aime.' She really loves me too.''

[Is expected.] ''I may hope that of the girl. Before the dream, she invited me to make a visit.''

[The Duchess of Angoulême.] ''I have no idea whether such a person ever lived.'' (The conversation lexicon gave the information that she was a daughter of Louis XVI, saw the beheading of her parents, and later, thanks to her preference for the side of a capable man, became happy.) ''Now I remember that as a child, I read of the history of the unfortunate girl and that I thought I would certainly have married her. For the rest, the parents of my friend are somewhat estranged from their daughter because they do not understand her mental peculiarities. I have hoped to be able to provide a substitute for her parents.''

Here we see the regression to the infantile, the hypermnestic performance of the dream. The dream here realizes a real childhood wish which Freud asserts of all dreams * when he says: ''The dream is the representative of the infantile scene changed by transference to recent material.''

It will be easy for the reader, by analysis of his own dreams or those of others, to find the other mechanisms of the manifestation in the dream work. That which distinguishes the dream is the dramatization, the arrangement of the material in a pictorial connection which is only interrupted when nothing more can be done with the material at hand because the latent idea would be betrayed or because the thing is too painful and a solution of the conflict is not found in the dream. In such cases, there occurs in normal individuals, a flight into reality, an awakening, which is then often accompanied by the thought: ''Thank God it was only a dream!'' This consciousness can also appear in the dream itself in order to quiet the dreamer.†

Since the dream condenses, symbolizes, represents by oppo-

---

* Freud, Traumdeutung, p. 365 f.
† Stekel, Beiträge zur Traumdeutung. Jahrb. I, pp. 459–466.

site and sublimates, the meaning of the latent content is not exhausted by a single interpretation. One can never say that one has found the deepest meaning.* Many dreams cannot in general be interpreted.† "The complete interpretation of such a dream coincides with the analysis." ‡ "In the interpretation of every dream element," according to Freud, "it is doubtful whether

(a) it is to be understood in positive or negative sense (contrast relation)

(b) it is to be interpreted historically (as reminiscence),

(c) symbolically, or

(d) its estimation should proceed from the wording." ‖

For reassurance, the author adds: "In spite of this possibility of many interpretations, one may say that the representation of the dream-work, which is indeed intended not to be understood, offers no greater difficulties to the translator than the writers of the old hieroglyphics gave their readers."

Stekel asserts on the contrary that as a result of the "bipolarity of all psychic phenomena," each of the two possible interpretations which every dream fragment may claim, may be correct.¶ "Everything in the dream is bipolar. To the masculine impulses there correspond feminine, to the proud, humble, to the good, bad, etc." Certainly the ambivalence extends very far but that it covers everything, I do not see.

We must still say something regarding the origin and later fate of the dream. Great importance has been atrributed to bodily stimuli by the non-analytic side. Analysis, however, shows that every physical irritation passes over into the manifest dream content only when it affords the unconscious opportunity for elaboration.

A girl dreams of a band which she is following on X Street. A moment later, she awakens to the sound of a passing bugle corps.

---

* Freud, Traumdeutung, pp. 108, 223, 350.
† Same, p. 350.
‡ Freud, Die Handhabung d. Traumdeutung i. d. Psa. Zbl. II, p. II.
‖ Freud, Traumdeutung, p. 267.
¶ Stekel, Die Sprache des Traumes, p. 535.

[X Street.] ''There, many elegant but bad girls parade. I am glad that I am not like one of them. When a child, I liked to follow bands.''

The girl is in moral distress. She is fond of dress and passionately erotic in high degree. She envies elegant prostitutes but represses the unallowed desire. In the dream, she sees herself on X. Street wherewith the wish to be a prostitute comes to account. But she sees herself as innocent child running behind a band so that her conscience is satisfied. The dream thus reveals itself, as always, as a compromise between two mutually contending repressing, instinctive impulses.

A gentleman dreams at the moment of awakening that his wife is borne into the room dead, whereupon he feels great anxiety.

The door was opened just at this minute. Already the crash caused by this had often frightened him but never in such degree. His wife entered. He was considering dissolving his marriage to the unloved one. Hence the death-wish which came to expression in the dream.

A normal individual dreamed very clearly in the summer resort on awakening that someone said in front of his window: ''It is not quite six o'clock.'' He convinced himself, however, that some Italians were speaking outside who could not speak a word of German. He had gone to sleep with the resolution to get up at six o'clock in order to go mountain climbing and had been afraid of oversleeping. One might ask whether this was a hypnotic-like dream or a hypnoid illusion.

Such utilization of unexpected external irritations as also cryptography and cryptolalia, convinced me that these manifestations are formed with great rapidity.

To the sources of the dream, suggestion is also to be reckoned. Silberer's hypnagogic dream investigation (page 241) and Schrötter's artificial dreams in hypnotized persons (Zentralblatt II, page 638 ff) afforded evidence that ordinary dreams are also dependent on suggestive influences. As a matter of fact, the variety of dreams which appear during the analysis with different analysts betrays very plainly the effect of suggestion. One does well, therefore, to support the theory of interpretation mostly on first dreams or manifestations previous to the analysis.

Surprising and to me inexplicable is the fact that direct speech in the dream, as Freud found, goes back to such in reality.* I have very often found this statement confirmed.

It was urged against dream analysis that the dream was spun out and distorted after awakening so that an interpretation of the real dream would be impossible. In answer to this, it may be remarked that this subsequent dream elaboration as well as the forgetting of bits of dreams, is caused by the same forces which occasioned the dream. One keeps the dream so long as the complexes underlying it can invest themselves in this material. It does not matter at all if the dreamer phantasies in addition or lies somewhat about it. One may quietly admit such phantasies. If anyone dreams of someone present in the dream without seeing a single characteristic of him, then one simply says: "Imagine what this dream figure was like." These subsequent associations are as important for the explanation as the matter really dreamed. As a rule, they afford the key to the whole situation: they help to find the thoughts about which the disparate, diverging dream fragments group themselves and which they illustrate. (Herein lies the criterion for the correctness of the interpretation.) They lead to the unconscious which manifests itself in the dream.

Of great importance is Freud's observation on the aftereffect of the dream: "When, after a dream, the belief in the reality of the dream pictures persists uncommonly long, so that the dreamer cannot free himself from the dream, this is not an error of judgment occasioned by the vividness of the dream pictures but is a psychic act in itself, an assurance which relates to the dream content, that something therein is really as it was dreamed and one is right in believing this assurance." †

* Freud, Traumdeutung, pp. 134, 241, 247, 278.
† Freud, Gradiva, p. 48.

I gave an example of this in my first psychoanalytic publication, "Wahnvorstellung und Schülerselbstmord" * (Delusion and Suicide in Pupils). A fifteen year old boy dreamed that he had committed incest with his sister. No matter how vigorously he denied the accusation as impossible, he could not free himself from the feeling that the reality agreed with the dream. He fell into anxiety and doubt until, almost ready for suicide, he asked his sister on conscience whether he had committed incest with her. The indignant girl asserted that not the slightest immorality had occurred, whereupon tranquillity, even though not complete, appeared. Yet, three years after the dream, the memory of it brings tears.

Asked to fix his attention on the dream, the youth immediately remembered that his sister had enlightened him regarding sexual matters and spoke of incest between brothers and sisters which excited the brother sexually. The girl spoke repeatedly of similar things which every time occasioned voluptuous sensations in the boy. His phantasies were overemphasized. So far, a real occurrence corresponded to the dream, which may have been preceded by others in the early years of childhood.

(c) THE LOGIC OF THE DREAM

Since the dream dispenses with conscious apperception, strict logical thinking is in great part denied it. It possesses guiding tendencies, otherwise the artistic dream structure would not come into existence, but these are not conscious, however.

What we perceive as logical functions in the dream, fall into the following groups:

1. Quite simple pertinent performances, judgments, sequences, comparisons, computations, etc.

2. False logical activities. The simplest conclusions are drawn incorrectly. Computations which a child could do, have a wrong answer. Often a preceding correct judgment is up-

---

* Schweiz. Blätter f. Schulgesundheitspflege 1909, No. 1.

set by a subsequent false one and the latter finds firm belief in the dream.

3. From the waking life, logical performances are taken over in direct speech or without such. Conclusions in the dream have always arisen in the waking life.*

4. Logical judgment concerning the dream, for instance, criticism: This is nonsense, or: this is impossible, or: this is merely a dream. These reflections, which often appear upon awakening and conduce to new sleep, signify a flight into the form of the waking life and accomplish the purpose of protecting the sleeper.

Highly logical intellectual performances, as calculations, essays, poems, which were executed in sleep are not genuine dreams.

In order to manifest the finer logical relations of the latent dream thoughts, the dreamer makes use of special means which often serve their purpose with astonishing cleverness in witty or shrewd allusions. We have become familiar already with condensation, transposition of emotion, symbolic representation, representation by opposite and other mechanisms.

We may now describe how the logical relations come to expression. As pictography, for example the Indian pictorial writing, places the members of the logical chain side by side without visible connection, so does the dream. It can represent causality only by spacial or temporal juxtaposition. Temporally, by one dream fragment's containing the foundation of another.† Spacially, by placing cause and effect side by side or uniting them in a composite figure or by the representation of the cause passing over into that of the effect.‡ An element of the composite figure contains the cause of the hallucination of the devil on page 38. We met a good example also on page 194 in the dream of the courtyard of the barracks and the polyclinic.

* Freud, Traumdeutung, p. 301.
† Same, p. 248.
‡ Same, p. 249.

Two dream fragments may have various relations to each other. Perhaps they are joined in the latent content by: either—or, perhaps by: partly—partly, perhaps by: as—so. Throughout, it is to be remembered that the dream serves autistic interests, not real ones. But regard for phantastic gain of pleasure or the wish to carry out a repressed impulse in the dream can also take into account causal relationships when such exist in the repressed motives.

Hallucinations, we have already recognized in sufficient numbers. They constantly presuppose mental conflicts since they persist in getting their own reality.

The waking phantasies are of high value in judging the mental condition. During a single dream, only a momentary situation is represented, and in the morning an entirely new disposition of libido may appear; the day dreams are marked by strong tendency to persist. A single phantasy may be elaborated for months or years with immense expenditure of affect, until finally a whole romance is spun out, while the stereotyped dream occurs less frequently and does not undergo any such extended elaboration. Such day dreams, which regularly point to lack of gratification in life and should be held innocent of the deficiency in reality, are constantly invested with much affect. As the performance of waking life, the day-dream is less distant from the domain of possibility than the sleeping dream, so is it less bizarre and absurd. Hence it is often more difficult to interpret.

A girl of sixteen years was haunted for years by the following phantasy: She is the head of an oppressed Huguenot family. She is imprisoned and must renounce her faith. She stands heroically for her faith and dies a martyr.

It is striking that she dreams of herself as spiritual leader. The termination betrays the melancholia which rules her waking life also. To imprisonment, she associated father, a higher official who had been imprisoned for fraud and had shot himself when the child was nine years old. The spiritual rôle meant an identification with the grandfather who was a pastor but had gone over to a life insurance company, thus in the eyes of the child, had been unfaithful to his office. Further, the little one found a passionately adored father-substitute in her pastor. Thus in the waking phantasy, the daughter elaborated her great childish grief by expiating in her heroic deed the misdeeds of her father and grandfather. The obsessing phantasy ceased from the moment of the analysis.

The youth described on page 265, who was pathologically shy of girls, frequently produced the following phantasy which I found in his letter: "The Swiss are in a bloody war with a neighboring State. I immediately enlist as volunteer while my comrades stay at home. I overcome fatigue and become ensign by brilliant execution of orders. In the final great decisive battle, I bear the colors in the foremost ranks and strike down every one with my right arm. We are victorious. In the parade in Zurich, I march ahead with the tattered, blood-stained colors. Nora gives me flowers; no one sees them, I conceal them under my shirt on my breast. Someone comes upon me. I strike off this person's head with my sabre. It resembled yours. In the name of the soldiers, I make a speech to the colonel, we give him three cheers. I come home. No one there. Nora invites me in. I tell her family of my experiences. Later, I go walking with Nora and give her a gold cross which I received as decoration. We have remained mutually true to each other. We are married and live happily. I never go to the tavern. We always go together. We have a daughter who resembles Nora in looks but me in character."

The resistances were great. The youth wished to become a professional officer. The sabre with which he can strike a man down impresses him tremendously (counter-reaction against repression of masturbation). [Nora gives flowers.] "In C Street. There I saw beautiful girls. One wore a beautiful dress which was torn below, however."

[Someone comes upon me.] "This I phantasied in addition only while writing it down. The man came from behind."

[The man.] "It is you. The parents are mistrustful of you

and assert that you only wish to pump me.* They were likewise beheaded on C Street near the former place."
[The place.] "My teacher H. Sometimes I can endure him, sometimes, not. Once we were coming from the railway. In the crowd, mother and I lost father. At the Place of Execution, father came upon us. Mother was weeping about him and cried that she would go the next day to a lawyer for a divorce. The people looked after us. I was also very angry at father. This happened many years ago." [The gold cross.] "Tannera tells of the iron cross; the golden is still more beautiful."

The wishes are plain enough. The bashful youth becomes conquering hero and lover, exemplary husband and father. He identifies me in his negative transference with his father and kills me as his perfidious enemy. The beloved, avoided in reality, becomes his own when he has killed the father-complex within him. In this, the dream is entirely right; it came to fulfillment later to the letter.

7. Cryptolalia and Cryptography

When I investigated the previously undeciphered productions of religious secret speech and automatic writing, I found that every one, though he made senseless syllables, flourishes and other signs, every time gave masked expression to the complexes ruling within him. Where dreams were denied, I often made use with the best results of this simple measure, to consider this refusal every time as the association in order to continue the analysis. The fact that in this way a forgotten dream was often again brought to mind, betrays the fact that the same forces were acting in both manifestations.

(A) Cryptolalia

An acquaintance, forty years of age, upon my request, wrote meaningless words, namely: "Parastintunga nodaratschiwu."

* This was so. Especially did the severely hysterical mother speak badly of me, since I had recommended her to a lady physician skilled in psychoanalysis, whom she did not visit. The hostility of the parents

[Parast.] Palace in Togo. I heard it related this after-noon of a Togo chief who built huts for his two wives north and south from his village. I also saw the picture of these women. One was not bad. [Parast.] Parasite. When a boy, I read Schiller's drama which bears this title. Here is found this verse: "There is room in the tiniest hut for a pair who are happy in love." Thus again a hut like that of the pleasing negress. When I read Schiller's verse, I already knew it, for a young admirer of my early widowed mother had recited it. When I was one to four years old and seven to eight, I dwelt with my mother in a tiny house (infantile root).

[tunga.] Tonkin. Here too dwell pretty black women of small stature but good looks, attractive. To-day I met a simi-lar looking girl who gave me the impression of a graceful, dark little witch, but of loose morals. She went into a questionable house. And now I recall a young lady who in my emotional life took precedence of my wife who unfortunately is unlovable. I could never make up my mind, however, to be untrue to my wife, no matter how much I was attracted to the kindly, dark little friend who was entirely respectable. The latter is highly attractive and passionate, her ethical compulsion still not re-moved. Now it occurs to me that "Parastin" exactly agrees with Greek "πάρεστιν," "he, she or it is there" except that e is replaced by a (on account of "Palast" and "Parasit"). The situation is really this, that I wish a little hut for a loving pair. I imagine this hut as real.

[tunga.] Dschungeln. I wished to give my wife the "Jun-glebook" by Kipling. [Junglebook.] A funny episode—hold! Now I notice that my wife behaves like the amusing group of whom I thought. Thus, by the present, I would ex-press my derision without knowing it. [tunga.] Hungary. Saint Elizabeth came from there as I found asserted in one of your books. She was an unfortunate masochist whom they should have left alone in Hungary. She died very young be-cause of the maltreatment she received. My wife also bears

made the treatment difficult. We have heard that the recovery finally resulted nevertheless.

with all piousness and nobility of mind self-tormenting traits which disturb our marriage. She too might have better stayed in her parents' home. She has little life and my efforts to unburden her spirit are fruitless. (The reader will fill out the repressed wish: "That she might also die early like the Hungarian."

[Nodaratschiwu] "no" = non, not, "daratschiwu": Derwisch, "iwu" = ich will (I will). "I will be no Dervish." Dervishes are foolish people who renounce marriage in favor of their vows. Nodara reminds me of Biblical Gadara, the place where the possessed dwelt, melancholy men who lived among the tombs. I too often suffer from attacks of sadness since my marriage has lost its value from the repellent behavior of my wife. I seem meanwhile like one who has no wife at all and from exaggerated conscientiousness only recoils from divorce because he promised her lifelong fidelity. Thus, I too am a Dervish who has pledged himself to celibacy. Now it occurs to me that the first syllables sound much like a place where I had a little adventure. On a mountain trip to Piz Morteratsch, I went with a sympathetic young lady whom I esteemed very highly, into an empty sheep-shed in order to see the interior. We were entirely alone. Then a peculiar feeling came over me. Here we had again a hut for a happy loving couple! Nevertheless, I was not really in love with the girl although I liked to tarry in her company.

How would it be if one inverted the word?

[uwischtaradon.] Adon is a name of a god. Adon = Adonis is the chief god of the Phœnicians, the husband of the love-goddess, Astarte, Babylonian Ishtar. Wonderful! Also the name "Ischtar" is in the secret word directly before Adon (ischtar-adon)! Now I understand also the syllables "schiwu"; they mean "Schiwa" the cruel husband of the fruitful love-goddess, Kali Durga, who in spite of her children, is still a virgin. My wife also has children but will have no more sexual intercourse and acts like a prude; her character is old-maidish. A sadistic trait in her is unmistakable. In view of her refusal, I am not gratified by sexual intercourse with her.

Sometimes I said to myself, now in the feeling of my superiority I will exercise my conjugal rights with a certain malicious joy, thus play the cruel Schiwa. Yet this afforded me little gratification. Ishtar is a right sympathetic figure to me. Her descent into hell, on which, she left behind her clothes piecemeal, is of great beauty. My wife is overprudish. Likewise my mother, with whom I shared the sleeping-room as a child and boy. I considered it a sin to see her when undressing and therefore fought against curiosity.

[Uw] the poem "Nis Randers" by Otto Ernst. "Mother, it is Uwe!" I too have a brother on the stormy sea. The newspapers announce to-day the destruction of ships. I hope my brother is saved. (Identification: "And I too!")

The cryptolalia can thus be interpreted in the statement: I will neither renounce love like a Dervish as a sacrifice to my marriage vow nor like a Schiwa, live beside my masochistic wife but will either live in a little hut with a beloved or like an Adonis, revel by the side of a goddess of love in order to be saved. In the second word, the contrast is very beautifully expressed: Normally read, there is the need from the complex, by inversion, the gratification of the complex. The thought that the word must be read backwards suddenly appeared with force. Probably few readers would have thought of this method. Philology recognizes it and names it by the word, reversal of sounds or metathesis. Karl Abel introduces in his investigation of the contrasting meanings of primitive words, a number of excellent examples (page 320). Freud, from whose work, I derive my knowledge of this phenomenon, calls to mind how often inversion occurs in the dream and in childish speech (we add: also in hysterical attack).*

(B) CRYPTOGRAPHY

The process of ecstatic speaking with tongues returns, as we saw, in the arbitrary meaningless speech of normal individuals. I decided therefore, to trace the automatic cryptography, the senseless writing in healthy mental life. My expectations were

---

* Freud, ü. den Gegensinn d. Urworte, Jahrb. II, p. 184.

completely fulfilled. I will give some tests in the following examples. The reader will recognize that the method of exploration is exactly the same as that which we apply to neurotic phenomena and the dream. That the analysis is repeatedly incomplete and the infantile material in particular is neglected, I regret. The resistance of my subjects of investigation, who were attached only by scientific interest, unfortunately could not be fully eliminated. We know indeed that for the overcoming of the resistances, a whole psychoanalysis is often necessary. I may consider it a gift of fate that the inquiry into some graphic symptoms should afford at least a clear insight into the genesis of cryptography.

A French artist who utilized his travels to become acquainted with psychoanalysis from his own observation, was kind enough to allow me to analyze a sketch drawn by him in my presence. I asked for some kind of a senseless drawing; thereupon, he sketched the following figure with his face averted:

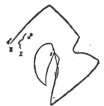

(I in the original is so lightly drawn that the line was at first overlooked.)

[Think hard of your drawing and tell your associations.] The line (II) shows head, throat and coiffure of a young girl who was drawn this morning in a painting-school for ladies. While I was drawing the line, I did not think of it at all. The girl sketched, possesses a fairly plump figure and bare throat. Throat and bust also give, however, the outline of a fairly plump shoe.

[The throat.] One of my friends, Mr. X. painted a singer of similar figure, Miss T.

[The plump shoe.] It reminds me faintly of a comic statuette which represented a vagabond with fat feet and legs, bent
backwards. One shoulder was up and forwards, the eyes were
staring and protruding as in Basedow's disease. Similar dis-
tressing eyes, I saw in a cow some years ago on a trip to the
country which I took with my that-time fiancée. My feet were
at that time in bad shape, I suffered from skin trouble and
could hardly leave the place. I had to bind up my feet and
limped pitifully. To my vexation, my fiancée paid no attention
to my condition and behaved heartlessly. (About one and one-
half years later: when small, I had great joy in pretty, shiny
boots. I received such once from my mother whom I surprised on the evening before a Christmas celebration when she
was arranging the present. From elation, I danced first on one
foot, then on the other, so that I was long laughed at by mother
and sister on this account.)

That is a brush-head or a plum. [Brush-head.] A little
Parisian who paints nicely. He is a neat little fellow, industrious, earnest, kind, tactful. Ah, now some traits occur to me
which he has in common with the statuette!
[Plum.] Or damson. It reminds me that this year I saw
on the tree below my studio only a single damson where ordinarily the tree is full of fruit.
[Glance at the whole again.] I can also imagine a face which
looks to the right. It is turned away, the angle at the right
under the top denotes the chin. [I do not see it as such.]
But I do. It is an unsympathetic head which reminds me of a
servant maid. My wife blamed me unjustly for an improper
relation with her. The maid had slandered me since she desired me. This leads me to a brunette model concerning whom
my wife likewise suspected me falsely.

Impression of a thumb. A teacher whom I know brought

me a similar figure which he had had one of his pupils draw. It
was an almost more than life-size index finger right well worked
out. To me, it looked like a male organ. The same boy, K. J.
by name, drew the back part quite like the one I made on my
sketch just now.

[Let us turn back to Miss T.] My friend X had painted her
and supported her with money. Then she left him in the lurch
over which he was quite cut up. Miss T. reminds me of how
my brother wished to get a divorce on account of another married lady. I sought to prevent the divorce by a visit and in
so doing got home too late for dinner. My wife accused me of
trying to take my brother's place and became violent toward
me. Then I held her hands, whereupon she bit me in the
finger.

[The profile first drawn.] The brow is that of my wife, from
whom I would be divorced. Otherwise nothing. Yes. An
old man with a little cap. I can think of no one under this.
Here is the face which I imagined. Hold! I think of Voltaire.
Our academy professor showed us his profile which was crowned
with a little cap. At that time, there stood beside me an attractive lady, a fellow pupil, who greatly favored me and gave
me to understand that she loved me. Further, the profile of
Leo XIII, who likewise wore a cap. In the studio of my friend
X, hangs the photograph of this pope; beside it was his money
box. Now Miss T. appears again, whom I once met there before the relation was broken off.

So far with the young Frenchman. Now we will attempt to
arrange the associations.

The subject begins with a day's experience, the sight of a
sensual girl who is portrayed. As I remind him of this one, it
suddenly occurs to him that he had also repeatedly wished to
paint his fiancée but never got beyond three studies. Unfortunately, she lacked complete distinctness, so that the girl represented to-day is killed in favor of the one-time wife.

The outlines of the head, neck and bust remind the artist
of the beloved of a friend who like himself had lost that fervently loved being and thereby squandered much money. The

profile of the woman (line I) is combined with that of Voltaire because thereby the pleasant recollection of a pretty seducer is awakened and with Leo XIII because thereby the consoling admonition on the analogous fate of the friend X is again emphasized.

The plump shoe will likewise help to mitigate the sorrow over the loss of the wife. The vagabond with the plump shoe and the staring eyes is naturally a caricature of the artist himself: when he was limping around with bandaged feet, the fiancée showed herself heartless. The identification of the staring eyes of the tramp caricaturing the subject, with those of a cow in the neighborhood, betrays a not very flattering compliment: you were a regular cow at that time because you did not appreciate the heartlessness of your fiancée and separate from her. The identification with the vagabond is that far consolatory as the subject now enjoys a sure income and is well clothed which was not the case earlier.

The brush-top refers to an elegant Parisian. This neat fellow who has traits agreeing with the vagabond, consoles for the tramp and cow: you are also a neat, earnest, industrious man.

The one damson refers in its sexual symbolism to his present eroticism in comparison with the earlier.

The face turned to the right which is hard for neutral people to imagine (in the drawing) simultaneously calls up painful scenes of jealousy with the former wife and awakens thoughts of the girl who desired him.

The finger hanging beside the damson realizes in connection with the associations the idea of a healthy, extraordinarily potent sexuality. There is also a by-play here referring to the wife biting the finger of the artist: now the finger is healed.

The cryptogram finally brings the following to expression: you are suffering from your divorce and the sexual deficiency caused thereby; but you were separated from a heartless, jealous and biting wife, whom you really should not have married; you are in the condition of your friend, are more potent sexually, a neater, superior man who won the favor of a worthy maiden and may therefore hope to win a much prettier and better wife.

My artist was at once convinced of the correctness of this explanation which disclosed his deepest, little understood feelings.

8. MANIFESTATION-ACTS

(A) SYMPTOMATIC ACTS

Many apparently senseless and accidental acts, which appear once or habitually, are disclosed by analysis as psychologically imperative manifestations. Freud gives such acts the name, "symptomatic acts" and defines them as those "performances which the person executes, as one says, automatically, unconsciously, without paying attention, as if playing, to which he would deny all significance and which he explains as of no account and accidental when he is questioned concerning them." *

Where we are dealing with habits of this kind—in Swiss speech, they are called "Mödeli," little mannerisms—they often have an obsessional character without their possessor's knowing it. He first becomes cognizant of this fact when he wishes to give them up but in spite of all his efforts, cannot do it.

A student who had fallen into a dissolute life had the habit, whenever he was in a restaurant in the company of ladies, of taking matches and bending them in three places so that the stick was at first a little curved. Then he brought the two ends together and formed an oval. This play he kept up until all the matches were used up. The analysis brought him to the recognition that he was deriving a male and female symbol.

A woman with obsessional neurosis wishes to show me a heart-shaped medallion. Unintentionally, she tears it from its chain and lets it roll at my feet. The confession concerned me and still as the discussion of the "transference" will show, not me.

Karl Hase relates in his autobiography that on the day that

* Freud, Bruchstück einer Hysterie-Analyse. Kl. Schriften II, p. 67.

the child of his beloved was baptized, the ring given him by her was smashed in the fencing room.*

Most people cultivate at a certain age a ceremonial of gait which I intend to treat in a special study. Sometimes, they count their steps in walking, up to a certain number, or they accentuate every second, third or fourth step or they devote special attention to the line of junction of two flag-stones in the side-walk, either avoiding it or stepping on it. In all cases analyzed by me, this refers to a process of diversion, the fund of energy of which springs from a complex and this has already occasioned an obsessional neurosis even though it may be a slight one.

One pupil always had to count his steps when he passed a trolley-car barn where cars go in and out (compare the station dream, page 358).

Another student remembers that he had the habit only on a certain street curve. With his attention concentrated on the place, he recalls that there were obscene pictures on the wall opposite which he wished to avoid.

We have already spoken of the neurotic patient who drew his finger under the nose (page 78). A teacher told me that one of his pupils, in spite of all admonitions, constantly· pushed his thumb through his button-hole. The motive is obvious. Nail polishing, picking of the nose and tearing of the skin from the finger (214) are comprehensible in this connection.

Many symptomatic acts are already obsessions before they are recognized as such. The educator can easily observe this by taking the field against certain striking habits in writing, for example flourishes, writing above or below the line, shading the loops, etc. That handwriting is full of symbolisms, no one denies; that it is closely connected with the complex, we saw in the variations of writer's cramp, as well as in the form of writing.

Since the literature, so far as I know, affords no analysis of handwriting, I will give a little example:

* K. Hase, Ideale u. Irrtümer. Leipzig, 1872, p. 47.

First, the previous history: A youth of twenty-one years suffered from downright anger at God because his father died, further, from anxiety when he found his dwelling closed. Then he hastened in violent excitement into the studio of his elder sister who quieted him.

[You stand before the closed door.] "My sister. She is engaged to a foreigner. I cannot endure him." [You stand before the door.] "The mother might be dead, therefore the door is closed. I would then go to the sister. I would like best to have her accompany me home. I always wait before our house until I see a light." [You stand before the door.] "The Sunday-School. I go there with mother. Now I detest orthodoxy. Mother is angry because I no longer go to church. She became excited and I said many things which hurt her. She said: I might wait until she was dead." [You stand before the door.] "My sister and her fiancé wish to take a dwelling of their own. I am anxious lest she be unhappy. Someone has come between my sister and me, she is no longer the same toward me as formerly. I loved her very much. Formerly I loved a girl who was unfaithful to me. Since then I have loved only my sister and hence her all the more intensely."

The anxiety over the closed door is related to the wish for the death of the religion-compelling mother. The sister is phantasied into the closed dwelling because she too forms the object of improper wishes. Her threatened misfortune is naturally only rationalization. In the studio, she is harmless: the brother flees from the image to reality. This young man has the following bad habit:

The loops of many large letters, especially of the D, but also of the B, P and G, and further the inner angle of the W, he is in the habit of shading although it delays him and offends his esthetic sense.

[Shaded letters.] "I do not fill my place, I might do more. Life has often seemed desolate since father died."

[D.] "Cover (Deckel). The cover of a coffin. It is lifted

from the coffin and stands at the side. I have repeatedly phantasied this. This view, I had upon the death of my grandmother. I fill out the empty place of the coffin. Now I see my grandmother in the coffin because I do not dare to see the mother there.''

More could not be obtained in this hour concerning the ''D.''

[Shaded B.] ''Biel. When my parents were there once, I remained behind with the strict, bad, hated grandmother.''

[B.] ''Bible. Father liked to read aloud from it. Mother held me in her arms. This pleased me. Sister did not care much for the Bible readings. She was therefore scolded by father. Then I was sorry for her. Thus the Bible lost value for me. I feel that I still constantly undervalue it. I suffer constantly from a feeling of guilt. For a long time after father's death, I wanted to shoot myself. Mother restrained me. I often got on badly because I deserted her.''

Next session:

[D.] ''Roof or ceiling (Decke). I imagine the ceiling of a room. Until the last (likewise the first) consultation with you, I had feared from my fifth or sixth year, the ceiling would fall down on me. All ceilings, even at school. When I was quite a small child, I saw the devil in the folds of clothes hanging there. I was in grandmother's room. It was her apron, from the upper opening of which, a devil's head looked out. (The drawing sketched at my request, showed the apron of cylindrical form held by its upper points.) The devil was thin with goat's beard and horns. In grandmother's room, there was a picture with rectangular slips of paper before it: looked at from in front, it showed Luther, from one side, Zwingli, from the other side, Calvin, who with his beard quite resembled the devil.'' [Reformers.] ''Nothing.'' [Ceiling.] ''It is white. Once, before the vision of the devil, a beetle or a mouse fell down from the ceiling upon me in bed. From that time, I was greatly afraid of fire and thunder storms, the latter up to the time of military service. Otherwise, nothing more.''

[Devil.] ''I knew that he tormented and scourged others.

The grandmother also whipped me much. In a Punch and Judy show, I saw how the devil took a woman across his knee, raised her skirts and spanked her."

Otherwise there was nothing else to be gained except a childhood dream: "When I was six years old, I dreamed during a fever that I was screwed to a carpenter's bench and worked with plane and hatchet. That probably means improvement." (The child still slept at that time in his parents' room).

The resistances were still apparently very strong. I ventured to give the youth the interpretation which he at once recognized as correct since he had already formed the thoughts expressed but had immediately rejected them.

The shading of the D went back to the same motives of hate and defence as the anxiety before the dwelling. Otherwise, the phantasy of the mother in her coffin could not occur immediately. Why the cover standing right beside the coffin made so strong an impression I do not know. Perhaps among other things, it was affected by the clang relationship with "Decke" (ceiling), which word has repeatedly been a critical one. The animal falling from the ceiling could naturally only set free a condition of anxiety already present, like the beetle on page 103. That the devil seen in the clothes and the dream of being planed and hewn are immediately associated with this, points the way for the student of anxiety-hysteria: The devil rising from the interior assumes on one hand the rôle of embodied "Schaulust" (pleasure in looking) (compare the obscene posture of the woman who was spanked), on the other hand, that of the hate-wish which the boy with a passion for whipping would repay in like coin. The scene on the joiner's bench naturally corresponds to a cohabitation-phantasy: The frightened child does not know the meaning of the process seen in the parents, his instincts are powerfully excited, as unfortunately not a few children show who even force themselves on the mother with physical signs of desire. I know of a youngster not yet of school age who held himself against his indignant mother: "Father does that too." The parents would probably have taken oath that the child had observed nothing.

The apparently insignificant writing hobby had therefore a very real background. Unfortunately, the anxiety vanished at once, the son assumed a correct attitude toward his mother, since he had recognized his hate and desire, and would not submit to more searching investigation as he now felt "entirely cured." I can therefore offer only a not uninteresting fragment.

Passion for travel is also very often a manifestation. A girl pupil of thirteen years longs passionately for the north, while she shows no interest for the south, no matter how alluringly one may picture it. She studies northern mythology assiduously which she has learned from a number of books. The analysis shows that she has easily brought her family into the saga of the gods. To Wotan, she associates: "He is a seemingly young man, kept young artificially by Freya's love apple, with one eye, in long mantle, with long pendant hat. I consider it improper that he took his daughter as wife. My grandfather was also old but he looked strikingly young, his cheeks were rosy."

[The mantle.] "As district judge, he wore a robe." [The hat.] "He also wore a lawyer's cap that hung down somewhat." [One-eyed.] "He was small and near-sighted and wore a monocle." [Half eyesight, at the same time, representation by opposite, hence Wotan the one-eyed is your grandfather.] To Loki, she reported: "He robbed Freya of the feather dress, the badge of her virginity, and turned himself into a fly; my brother took improper liberties with me. He was as persistent as a stinging-fly. Loki had the 'Fenrir-Wolf.': My brother liked to frighten me with our wolf-skin rug." To Thor, she associated: "When Loki had stolen the feather dress, he had to make the damage good. In so doing, he overcame dangers: A giant's daughter sent all streams against him, another concealed herself under his chair and raised him up to squeeze him against the ceiling but he pushed up with a pole and pressed the giant's daughter together."

[What comes into your mind to all this?] My father must make good what my brother, Loki, is guilty of. Mother and I often wept whole streams, he remained untouched."

[The giant's daughter under the chair.] "When small, I once crept under an upholstered chair to spy out what the parents did. My father sat down on the chair." The evil wish against the consciously hated father here comes to plain expression. A number of other relations came to light and explained the pathological preference for the north and the travel-fever. Thus, I find confirmed in this analytic subject, as in others, what A. von Winterstein says concerning the unconscious motives for travel.*

Keen students of humanity have long known the facts disclosed by Freud with scientific means. Very prettily says Rousseau :

"We probably never make a mechanical movement, the cause of which we could not find within us if we only knew how to find it. Yesterday, I went along the new street on the banks of the Bièrre to botanize. As I approached the Barrière d'Enfer, I suddenly turned to the right into the fields and went to the range of hills which border the little stream. In and for itself, this is nothing surprising; but when I remembered that I had already taken this by-way mechanically many times, I sought the cause within myself and had to laugh when I discovered it.

"Behind the Barrière, there was daily in her place a woman who sold refreshments. The woman had a poor little child who went on crutches." Rousseau liked for a while to converse with him, then this became irksome. "From then on, I did not like to go by and finally took the by-way quite mechanically. I brought this to light when I thought over the circumstances; for nothing of all this had been conscious to me up to this time." †

The poets also assign great value to the symptomatic act and we thereby feel esthetic pleasure, a sign that our own unconscious understands that of the master.

---

* Compare A. v. Winterstein, Zur Psychoanalyse des Reisens, Imago I, pp. 489–506.

† Rousseau, Rêveries du Promeneur solitaire. Zbl. III, p. 52, reported by E. Jung.

Jakobsen describes in his "Niels Lyhne," how a heroine who fell in love with the friend of her husband went carefully balancing along the straight line of the pattern in the carpet. Plainly, her action expresses the wish to remain in the right, straight path (reaction against the adulterous desire). This habit is familiar to the psychiatrist as obsessional act.*

Rudolf Hans Bartsch tells in his "Elisabeth Kött" of a lover, who, not able to gain his beloved, separates her fingers and presses his kissing lips between them and has to sneeze in her presence. That the latter means the ejaculation, I know from some of my analyses and those of a colleague.

Here belong the many aversions against certain acts and foods, as well as mysterious appetites, etc. We have already given occasional instances of these (215).

(B) ERRONEOUSLY-EXECUTED ACTS

Symptomatic acts in which an intention is inadvertently and strikingly disturbed, without visible external cause, are called erroneously-executed acts (Fehlhandlungen), thus for example, errors in speech and writing, losing things, coming too late. We have already spoken of forgetting. But the other erroneous acts as well, go back to intrigues of the unconscious.

An adherent and an opponent of psychoanalysis met each other in an inn and at once got into a lively discussion. The opponent exclaimed excitedly: "How can you assert that behind an accidental movement there is an unconscious intention? That is unscientific, entirely unscientific." At this moment the emotionally gesticulating man knocked his glass over the clothes of his vis à vis, the analyst. The day after that the same gentleman made a mistake which betrayed him, by proclaiming: "In the year 1893, Breuer and I—ah—Breuer and Freud published the discovery . . ." I am indebted for both these pretty examples to a reliable eye- and ear-witness. Now the reader may ask himself whether it is sensible to debate scientifically with any one who betrays his true motives so plainly.

* Maeder, Psycholog. Unters. an Dem.-præc.-Kranken. Jahrb. II, p. 197.

Brill gives an interesting case: He was questioned by another psychiatrist: "I would like to know what you would do in the following case: I know a nurse who was involved as co-respondent in a divorce proceeding. The wife sued her husband for divorce and named the nurse as co-respondent and he received the divorce." Brill interrupted: "You mean: she received the divorce," which was affirmed. He now expressed his surmise that his questioner was the hero of the story if he had not previously said that he was unmarried, for then the error in speech would be explained by the wish that his wife, and not he, had lost the case. The suspected person denied his connection with the case described, did it, however, with exaggerated affect reaction so that Brill and a third physician who was present, Dr. Fink, were strengthened in their suspicions. Later they learned on reliable authority that they had interpreted entirely correctly. The new witness was convinced by this experience of the correctness of the Freudian mechanisms.*

Freud calls attention to the fact that Schiller recognized the deeper meaning of the error in speech. In his "Piccolomini" (I, 5) he describes the excitement of Octavio over his son who is on Wallenstein's side, since he accompanied the latter's daughter into camp. To the Emperor's emissary, he says:

> "Come, I must
> At once follow the miserable track
> With my eyes see—come—
> Questenberg: What for, whither?
> Octavio (hurriedly): To her!
> Questenberg: To—
> Octavio (correcting himself): To the duke! Let us go!"

The error in speech shows us that the father saw through the erotic motive of his son.†

Rank found a similar estimation of erroneous act in Shakespeare. The latter in the "Merchant of Venice," has Portia, hindered by an oath from an open avowal of her love, say:

* A. Brill, Zwei interessante Fälle von Versprechen. Zbl. II, p. 33 f.
† Freud, Z. Psychop. d. Alltagslebens, p. 48.

"One half of me is yours, the other half yours—
Mine, I would say." *

In addition to Freud, one finds in the Zentralblatt für Psychoanalyse a great number of further examples. An unbelievably
large number of secrets can be read by the analyst in his fellowmen and by the analytically trained educator in his pupils without their knowing it. But one is glad not to have to pry into
complexes without necessity and judges the symptoms of his
neighbors with the charity which one wishes for his own im-
perfections.

(c) THE MANIFESTATION IN THE CONDUCT OF LIFE

Even the most important and best considered decisions often
prove to be the effects of subliminal instinctive impulses, the
carefully formulated reasons being rationalizations.

A fourteen year old youth who wishes to become a chemist,
showed in his earliest years an extremely strong interest for
feces. Countless times, the two year old child said that the
"disgusting ravens" had eaten horse manure. Later he
showed abnormally strong disgust for fecal odors. When about
eight years old he visited a chemical laboratory and wished immediately to become a chemist. As reason, he gave only that it
smelled so good in its vicinity.

We saw in many examples (197, 268) how the choice of husband or wife is influenced by the unconscious and indeed by
infantile fixation which precedes the educator.

I will add a few other illustrations: A just jailer, about
twenty-five years of age, fell in love with one of the female
prisoners, seven years his senior and not very pretty, who had
been brought in on account of prostitution and cheating and
who, as a result of spinal disease, was anesthetic to the knees
(251). He procured his discharge at once and married the
prisoner soon after her release. The man had a fixation upon
his mother and had nursed her in her long illness until her
death. The wife, too, whom he chose as substitute, he treated

* Rank, Ein Beispiel v. poet. Verwertg. d. Versprechens. Zbl. I, p.
109 f.

with touching solicitude. An analysis in this case would naturally have been inexpedient since the good man was well.

The best representation of a brother-sister complex is given by Ibsen in his drama, "Klein Eyolf." My observations confirm the psychological view of the great student of humanity in every point. The editor and former teacher, Allmers, has fathered his crippled Eyolf while he tormented him with instruction. He could not complete a book on human responsibility since the higher duty impelled him to devote himself wholly and exclusively to his little son to mitigate this one's bitter loss. From his wife, he withdrew his love except a remnant which could not satisfy her. After the death of the crippled child, the doubting father sought consolation in the sister whom he called his dear true Eyolf and the love for his wife died entirely. Why the abnormally strong concentration on the child? Plainly, Allmers seeks to silence his feeling of guilt as he had already undertaken by his book on responsibility. But the true reason, consciousness does not admit. He had allowed himself to be enticed aside for a moment by his wife as the child lay peacefully sleeping on the table. While he yielded himself to love, it fell. The sin of the father is consequently not so great as the mother's. A cruel fate has utilized a little carelessness on the part of the parents.

The motive for the guilt lies deeper: Allmers gives his child the name which his sister would once have borne if she had been a boy. He loves her, as the sister feels, not as a sister ought to be loved. The living with her he calls a particularly rare holiday. His wife, too, he took only to care for his sister. No doubt he has remained in his infantile attitude toward the sister, therefore he can transfer no real love to his excellent wife. The brief love frenzy, in reality, applied to the sister. The child who bore her name, he had wished from her. Therefore, Mrs. Allmers cannot love it. She herself explains that the aunt stands between her and the little son. The motivation that the sister-in-law had fascinated the child naturally does not correctly express the state of affairs. This attempt at rationalization has failed. Rather, the unhappy wife suspects that her rival is bound to her beloved husband in repressed incestuous love. As a matter of fact, Allmers' feeling of guilt goes back to this incestuous desire. He cannot finish his book on responsibility, as the sensitive wife rightly says, because of distrust of himself. The brother-sister complex which also hinders the sister in her transference upon another, goes back in Allmers to the mother- and father-complex: He wishes to atone for the harshness of the father toward the mother and sister. In the endeavor to make good the father's fault he identifies himself only too well with him, in that he treats his own wife badly.

This is all, most true to life. The pastor who analyzes, sees many marital misfortunes proceed from unconscious interchange of persons dictated by complexes of relationship. Jung gives splendid examples of the father-complex in his fine paper: "Die Bedeutung des Vaters für das Schicksal des Einzelnen" * (The Significance of the Father for the Fate of the Individual).

These things, too, were long familiar to poetic intuition. I mention only the masterly novel, "Die Tochter vom Oberbühl" by the Swiss poet, Jakob Frei.

That which we assert of the great decisions of life, applies also for all the highest productions of the mind, even for philosophy. We cannot take up this problem in this book. One example of Platonism and Kantianism conditioned by complexes I have already given on page 312. Similarly, Fichte's theory of the absolute ego, solipsism, pessimism, etc., may be shown to be manifestations. "Materialism, which denies the ego and has its rise wholly in the 'outer world,' one can consider as the most complete projection imaginable; the solipsism which denies the whole world, i.e., receives it into the ego, is the highest stage of introjection." † The most sharp-sighted of all profound psychologists, Nietzsche, even ventures

* Jahrb. I, pp. 155–173, also separate imprint.

† Ferenczi, Philosophie u. Psychoanalyse. Imago I, p. 521. (In the projection, one feels subjective processes producing discomfort as influences of the outer world, in the introjection, inversely, processes of the outer world as one's own (p. 520). Unfortunately, Ferenczi understands the concept of philosophy in a very low sense, for he separates

the declaration: "One must reckon the greatest part of conscious thinking under the activities of instinct, even in the case of philosophical thinking; . . . the most conscious thought of a philosopher is secretly guided by his instincts and forced into certain channels. Further, behind all logic and its apparent independence of movement, stand estimations, plainly spoken physiological demands for the preservation of a certain kind of life."* Freud's,† Ferenczi's, ‡ Putnam's ‖ and Schrecker's ¶ articles on a psychoanalytic comprehension of philosophy should at least be mentioned.

9. Art

With unsurpassable succinctness and clarity, Freud summarizes the results of analytic investigation of the psychology of art in these words: "The artist is originally a man who turns away from reality because he cannot directly make peace with the renunciation of gratification of instinct demanded by reality and preserves his erotic and ambitious wishes in phantasy life.

it sharply from science, indeed asserts that the two belong to different principles, philosophy (as at least is hinted) to the pleasure-principle. (Ferenczi, Phil. u. Psa. Imago, p. 521.) Is the concept of the atom, of law, of causality, invented from the substance of the pleasure-principle and is there an exact science which does not have to work step by step with philosophical concepts? So far as one assigns to philosophy the task of withdrawing from the contradictions existing in the (always naïve) concepts of experience and deriving a conceivable system of concepts, no penetrating scholar can get along without it. That natural science has been able to exclude autism entirely, even Ferenczi will not assert. Putnam has defended the just claims of philosophy against him in excellent manner. (Putnam, Antwort auf d. Entwiderung des Hrn. Dr. Ferenczi. Imago I, p. 527 ff.) Silberer has also warned against the error of wishing to solve the metaphysical problems of truth by psychoanalytic interpretation. (Silberer, E. prinzip. Anregung. Jahrb. IV, p. 802.)

* Nietzsche, Jenseits von Gut und Böse. (First Part, 3.)
† Freud, Traumdeutung, p. 375 f.
‡ Ferenczi, Introjektion und Übertragung. Jahrb. I, p. 430.
‖ Putnam, A plea for the study of philosophic methods in preparation for psychoanalytical work. Journal of Abnormal Psychology 1911, Oct.-Nov., pp. 249–264.
¶ Paul Schrecker, Henry Bergsons Philosophie der Persönlichkeit, Munich, 1912.

He finds, however, the way back from this phantasy world to reality, in that, thanks to special talents, he molds his phantasies to new kinds of realities, which are allowed to pass current by people as valuable likenesses of reality. Thus he becomes, in a way, hero, king, creator, favorite, whom he would, without taking the tedious route of real changes in the outer world." * I limit myself to a few cases.

Franz J. is an intelligent youth of eighteen years with whom I have repeatedly conversed on religious, philosophical and ethical topics. Sprung from pietistic circles, he had attained to freer views. Since the beginning of our two years' acquaintanceship he had met me with confiding frankness so that I concluded that there was a favorable transference relation. Some months ago his behavior toward me changed. His criticism, which I had previously heard gladly, assumed a grumbling tone and expressed fundamental negativism in scornful opposition. When the youth finally explained all ethical values as nonsense and almost in the same breath, complained of the lack of moral earnestness in his comrades, I recommended analytic treatment to him, which, after brief resistance, he accepted. It is, of course, preferable that the subject for analysis should come of his own volition; but many times a direct summons is not to be avoided.

At his first appearance, Franz confessed that life was most distasteful to him. He had fallen out entirely with his parents, and of his comrades, with one exception, he would know nothing. He often meditated on suicide. If he had not hoped to visit an academy of art in three quarters of a year, he would long since have taken his life. The visit to the institute to which he belonged, had become almost impossible to him; only this week, from inner compulsion, he had shirked two days. His condition was a fearful one, he could not possibly endure it for three more quarters. Hence, it were best that he make an end of his life. Nietzsche had completely destroyed the hold of religion on him, all life values had since disappeared.

* Freud, d. zwei Prinzipien d. psych. Geschehens. Jahrb. III, p. 6.

The youth presented a number of oil paintings and drawings which I, in accordance with good analytic procedure, had him at once exhibit and explain to me. The material which I give in the first part of the following section is a part of the results of the first three consultations; in the fourth session, new pictures indicated the metamorphosis of the complexes.

1. Self-Portrait

First we analyzed the self-portrait which had been painted in two or three hours on the day of the first consultation.

The drawing, in the original 50½ cm. x 64 cm. in size, is well painted, except that the dark, threatening facial expression which has characterized our budding artist for some time, is replaced by calm resignation.*

Our attention soon turned to the group of heads hanging on the chain at the right. Franz asserted that they designated no distinct personalities known to him. Urged to give only his associations, he at once named the face on the front, his father, the one on the left, his mother, the one on the right, his younger sister. All three, as he frankly admitted, are hated by him.

Later, he said: Only the upper part of the face resembles the father somewhat. Looked at closely, only the shape of the forehead and the root of the nose correspond exactly to the same features in the father's face. (Not distinct in the picture.)

The nose is that of his elder brother, who, walking in the steps of the severely religious mother, leads a quiet, pious life, shut off from the joys of the world.

The wrinkles from the wings of the nose to the corners of the mouth belong to an uncle on the father's side who died when Franz was five years old. And yet, our subject still remembers vividly how his uncle raged in his epileptic attacks. The eyebrows also reminded him of this brother of his father.

The curved extremities of the mouth revivify a brother of our artist, likewise epileptic, who died six years ago.

The furrow under the nose, as well as the two points of the

---

* In the reproduction, the face was changed so far as was practicable without disturbing the comprehension.

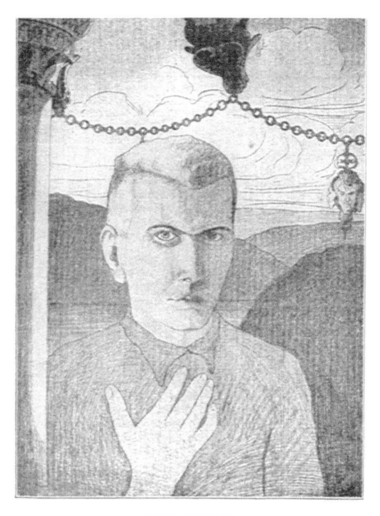

SELF-PORTRAIT

upper lip (indistinct in the reproduction), Franz explained as derived from the hated younger sister, who also had the corner of the mouth portrayed here. The downy beard was traced back to some disliked teachers. The facial expression as a whole showed a cynical smile which our artist attached to himself.

The face on the left reminds Franz of his mother, though strikingly enough, he finds none of her characteristics on our pendant. Only the hair which covers the vertex and encircles the face on the front, might correspond to that of the mother. Somewhat later, the lips of the mother are also added. Our peculiar portrait artist remembers how the mother constantly reasoned with him when he began to read Nietzsche, as well as how some aunts reproached him at that time. Now it turns out that the younger sister is also indicated by the same lips.

The nose bears a similarity to that of a gossiping neighbor. Once she mocked a boy who had a speech defect; immediately after, a similar disturbance appeared in her own child.

The whole face is deathly pale. The head on the right is associated with the hated sister. The hair over the frontal area comes to a point. The lower locks belong to a contentious, untidy maid, who, in spite of her church going, lived immorally and because of an illegitimate child, had to marry. The mouth also came from her.

The hated younger sister resembles this maid in so far that she is likewise distinguished by sensuality, likes to quarrel and gossip although she affects piety.

The neck of the figure bears an ornament which is recognized as a boy's lace collar. The boy struck Franz on the head with a hatchet while framing a bench. Further, the neck indicates the goitres of several elderly relatives.

So far, we have collected only the associations of our artist and have allowed none of our surmises to come to expression. The interpretation of our group is now easy for every one who has tested empirically the theory of psychoanalysis: Franz has cleverly put to death a number of hated persons, first of all, his father, mother and a sister, by (1) beheading, (2) hanging, (3) spitting (a spit runs through all the heads) and (4) crucifying them (the cross over the heads is interpreted expressly as reference to the piety or hypocritical piousness of the relatives). Two brothers, an uncle, a bad neighbor and a comrade fall victims to the massacre or at least the father shall find the end of the two epileptics.

Besides this sadistic procedure, all kinds of little meannesses come to expression.

We turn now to the ornament which hangs down from the center of the upper border. Again we hold the object before Franz, though he may find it tedious, and collect his associations.

In front, we see a heart which the artist describes as hard, ironlike, wounded. It is indented and looks as if it would tilt forward so that one might see what is behind it. It must belong to the father.

At the right, a second heart leans against the figure. "One can consider it as a withered breast devoid of love." The mother is indicated thereby.

Between the two parts of the ornament, a strange creation is inserted which Franz cannot interpret. It seems to him, nevertheless, that a wonderfully beautiful girl dwells opposite it. The association is inexplicable to him. The bow toward the left, he suddenly interprets as knee; then only does he discover that he drew the girl inverted, standing on her head. The reader sees also at once that the ordinary and the gravid womb is plainly shown, at least they come into Franz's mind.

The whole thing would represent a dragon.

The explanation runs thus: On the hard-hearted father, leans the mother, deficient in love. Both have a secret in common that is just unfolding. Into view comes the naked mother as girl and gravid woman. The Œdipus complex which is seldom absent in a psychoneurosis, may be clearly recognized: Franz is fiercely jealous of his father. In the love for the mother, so plainly colored with incest, lies the foundation of his neurosis. This reprehensible inclination is the dragon which threatens to devour him.

Finally, the self-portrait came to discussion. The costume is that of a monk. Franz long cherished the wish to become a Buddhist monk. He imagined it as something "immense" to enter a cloister or to be merged into nothing. The monastic garb in which the artist disguises himself, is also that of the parricide in Schiller's "Tell." What that name signifies, Franz is unwilling to know for some time, which seems to him "curious." Suddenly he remembers that parricide is called "father-murder."

The hand is that of one imploring mercy. The model is the publican who beat his breast, praying: "God be merciful to me a sinner." (Luke, xvi.)

The little finger is drawn incorrectly. It occurs to Franz that the mistake aids in giving the hand the form of a male genital organ which is about to relax after masturbation.

The bit of iron dependent from the chain penetrates the head of the artist and puts him in the same position as the members of the family killed in four ways.

The meaning of the portrait may be given in the following sentence: I confess repentantly the guilt which I have brought upon myself as murderer of my father and relatives, as well as masturbator, implore mercy and will expiate my sins by my execution or as Buddhist monk sink into nothing.

Thus the three chief points in the drawing contain: 1. Guilt (murder of relatives, strengthened by masturbation); 2. Cause (incestuous love for the mother, hate for the father and onanism); 3. Expiation.

If one would summarize the essential content of our picture in a sentence, after the manner of a dream, one might say: Since I am consumed in a criminal, threatening love for the mother and wish a violent end for my nearest relatives, I repentantly confess myself worthy of death and will expiate my crimes by flight into the nothingness of the cloister.

A month later, we analyzed the recent instigators of the portrait. Five days before the drawing, Franz visited an art-exhibition with his father and the hated sister. Before the pictures of Böcklin and Segantini, he became angry since he was thinking of his bad relation to his parents. Bitter and with the intention of inflicting injury, he said before the father that it was a shame that they first let an artist be almost ruined and then admired his paintings.

As he looked at himself in the glass next morning at eight o'clock, as he was making his toilette, the furrows running from the root of the nose straight over the forehead struck him. Even earlier, when he was still a boy, it occurred to him that his father drew these lines when he was filled with trouble and sorrow over his son. Now he asked himself what would the father say if he knew that his child of sorrows played truant. Two hours later, the inspiration suddenly came over our artist. He hastened immediately to buy a pad of paper and set to work. One sees how the lines of care on the father's face are strongly emphasized. The sympathy striving for expression is discharged by the negative father-complex by means of a sadistic elaboration. The wrinkles on his own brow may represent a justification of the cruel deed: "You have already caused me much more sorrow than I you!"

Thus, this artistic conception displays, exactly like the dream, a recent root, while the complex plainly goes back to earliest childhood when the strictness of the otherwise excellent father influenced the Œdipus attitude for the worse.

2. *Requiem*

This gloomy oil painting (45 cm. x 37 cm.) was done some seven to eight months before. The sketch on the ground of artistic intuition was dashed off in an hour, the whole uncommonly effective picture took only eight hours. Franz remembered that while painting it, he often wished to disappear in the river which rushed past his home town * as at the time when domestic strife tormented him. Further, he was angered because they made so much of Christianity while his prayers remained unheard. He wished himself buried with Christianity. Then, however, he heard beautiful organ tones floating from the chapel he had just painted.

* It occurs also in picture number 1.

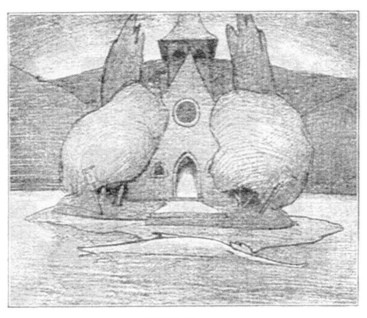

REQUIEM

The chapel makes Franz think that the father might be present. Where, he does not know how to say. Still, the round window brings to his mind the eye of God surrounded by a triangle on Albrecht Dürer's etching "The Holy Family in Egypt." Further, it reminds him of one-eyed Wotan, as well as of Polyphemus who swallowed the companions of Odysseus in his cavern and sought to kill with rocks Odysseus fleeing from the cave into water. This eye is also that of his own father who looks down gloomily upon his son.

The two cypress trees recall his two brothers, the two round trees, his sisters, of whom, one, the one whom we met in the preceding picture, was boasting how good a daughter she was, how she made herself useful to the parents, while she sought to get as many benefits as possible from them; the elder, nobler sister, however, corresponding to the tree on the right, does not behave so strikingly. The officiousness of the hated sister is expressed in the position of the left tree.

The chapel next turns out to be the chapel of an institution for the incurable insane. The institution building had previously been a cloister. There, a gifted artist lived, who, like Franz, painted and wrote poetry, until he was brought to this institution. And now, our subject confesses his burning desire to visit this man and be himself interned for life as insane. For hours at a time, the youth sat before the little church and dreamed of the happiness of being freed from all care in the adjacent asylum and continuing his splendid phantasies. Repeatedly, after some hours of day-dreaming, he went to distant places. The pointed church of the insane asylum is not on an island. The latter reminds of the castle Wasserstelz in Gottfried Keller's "Hadlaub." The young troubadour was concealed in the castle so that he would not be discovered by the recruiting Count of Rapperswyl. His beloved came to Hadlaub, brought him an infant and became his wife. This story led Franz to a beautiful girl of his home town who lived in an "exceedingly quiet" house off the street and pleased the father very well. Thus, Franz hoped as in Keller's novel, to get the better of his father.

The interior of the chapel is brightly illuminated. Wonderful music peals forth. Again, strangely enough, the pretty neighbor comes into Franz's mind, who had hidden himself behind the hearts (in previous picture) of the parents, as representation of the mother. Then our subject jumps to the Christmas festivals which he celebrated at home as a child. All the interest which he has in the picture, is concentrated on the light which streams from the church upon the dead. In connection with this, Franz imagines that his elder brother must still hide in the church. Finally, it occurs to him that he has always thought the same about the mother. At present, he has no love for the mother.

The two crucifixes are the brothers; the posts stick slantingly in the earth. Soon they will fall. The poplars (brothers) do not touch the church (mother) although they incline toward it (inartistically symmetrical).

The corpse, naturally Franz himself, lies in front of the island with outstretched arms like the true Christ, much too large for the perspective.

The three stars (circles) recall to mind again father, mother and hated sister (they are indistinct in the reproduction).

By way of explanation, it should be said that the father is trustee of the church (president of the church association) and that Franz is quite familiar with the expression, "Mother Church."

The oil-painting expresses the death-wish and its origin in the boy's attitude toward his family. Franz wishes to die and as corpse to draw to himself the mother love denied him in life. The other masochistic, likewise pleasurably toned, wish, points to his living henceforth entirely in the church (= mother). The parallel longing for the insane asylum seems thus to be a desire for the mother-womb. In both places, he is hidden, escaped from reality, in a certain sense, dead.

This phantasy corresponds on one hand to active cruelty, on the other hand, to self-aggrandisement. In the first respect, we notice the death-wish against the father, mother and younger sister (the three stars), the identification of the father with

Polyphemus, in whom, Odysseus (Franz), before swimming away, bored out his one eye, the representation of the brother destined for downfall, the ridicule of the officious sister. A tendency to grandiosity is suggested in the desire to be like the gifted insane patient, to supplant his father in the esteem of the village and especially to be discovered and mourned by the mother as the great, true, crucified savior beside the false messiahs, the brothers.

As in the self-portrait, the artist compares himself to the father by wrinkled brow, so here, there is brought to attention a wish-comparison which is not painted. During the drawing, Franz hears wonderful music proceeding from the church. The (hysterical or catatonic) mother hallucinated similar music, formerly often, now occasionally.

One notices the religious sublimation of the death-wish and the phantasies directed toward the relatives of the family.

Some weeks after the ''Requiem,'' Franz did a very pretty drawing, to which he gave the significant title, ''Let the Dead bury their Dead.'' A drowned youth is floating near the bank of a stream lined by poplars. A veiled woman is holding her hands over the dead body as if blessing it. The artist has no difficulty in recognizing himself and mother in the two figures; the mother is characterized in the title as spiritually dead. Later, the anger advances even to wishing the death of the erotic object passionately loved in secret. In the Aare which flows by his home village, Franz has long wished to go to sleep. Every swimming bath becomes a death orgy. The river becomes a mother symbol and assumes the rôle which is played in the other paintings by mother-womb, cave, insane asylum and cloister (compare Ibsen: ''Die Frau vom Meere'' [The Woman of the Sea]).

3. Madness

Pen and ink drawing, 36½ cm. x 26 cm., drawn five months before the analysis.

The picture as a whole reminds Franz of the magnitude, the violence of madness, of his visit to the insane asylum, in which he revelled in the sight of the patients, especially their eyes. Opposed to the powerful wish to be insane, is the clear insight into the absurdity and inferiority of the desire.

The eyes of the figure first arrest the attention. They betray the insanity, but also remind the patient of his own eyes as they look in moments of enthusiasm.

The mouth shows his own under lip. The reason for this substitution, I cannot give. The creases at the corners of the mouth are those of an uncle, with whose cane, the patient was whipped because he would not eat the oat soup. On that occasion, he called out to his father: "Strike me dead!"

The finger under the chin is at once named as sexual member which is trying to get to the lips. Franz is thinking of an act of masturbation. To the same gain of pleasure, lead the serpents which at the same time express something devilish.

To the weeping woman, Franz associates first himself who is complaining, then the cemetery which is near his parents' house, then the sister and the "wonderfully beautiful chapel of the insane asylum, thus the mother."

The hand is abnormally large. It holds and controls all the threads which run over the curtain (the world). It can press all together. It belongs to Franz.

The whirling lines represent "downward flowing dirt from which strength proceeds so that all is illuminated." Franz sees himself and his mother in the midst of the same pleasant filth of improper sexual activity.

The perpendicular, snake-like figures, drawn from below upward, are rising from unknown dark filth, attracted by the light. (I cannot interpret them with certainty. They are caused by the folds of the curtain. Perhaps they refer to the sexual instincts which, set free by open sexual pleasure (see below) ascend from their hiding place).

The inscription, "I know," relates to the insight into the secret of his own condition.

History of the picture.

The picture was drawn at the residence of an elderly gentleman who overwhelmed Franz with attentions, invited him on

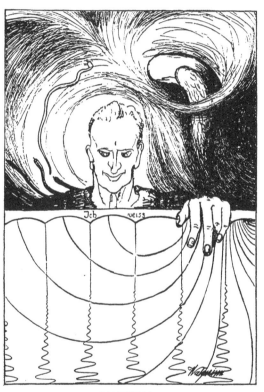

MADNESS

long journeys and promised to pay the expense of his academic education. Shortly before the sketch was made, our subject made the discovery that the man was homosexual and had bad intentions. Upon leaving the room, as the youth was going in advance, the man seized him and pressed himself against him. This repelled the surprised youth who decided to separate from the old sinner. At the table of the homosexual, he began to draw the picture without knowing what would come of it; usually his inspirations appeared to him like a shot, clearly defined.

Interpretation.

Disgusted by the homosexual attack, Franz experienced the most intense introversion. Dementia præcox is excellently symbolized by his drawing: The patient withdraws from the outer world behind his curtain, revels in the wildest auto-eroticism (masturbation and masochistic pleasure in the suffering of the mother) and incest, as the all-wise one who (paranoiacally) controls the destiny of the world with masterful hand. Franz states that such trains of thought have repeatedly filled his mind, though not during the composition of the sketch.

Space forbids reproducing here the whole analysis which dealt almost exclusively with drawings and poems, as well as (quite incidentally) with the life condition of the youth who was plainly gravely threatened with insanity.* Also the gain for the psychology of art cannot be presented here. It may only be pointed out in this regard that the introverted one, informed of the seat of his trouble, immediately sought with astounding energy to free himself from it. The subsequent pictures showed with great clearness the different steps in the struggle. The previous motives were again taken up according to the law of the remolding of complexes to be discussed later (Chapter 17, II) and elaborated in an opposite, life-giving sense until finally the rebirth of the rescued hero celebrated the triumph with splendid decision. The very inde-

* It is published in the second year of the journal, "Imago" (1913) under the title: "Die Entstehung der künstler. Inspiration."

pendent youth felt healthy and happy but from that time on, would hear nothing of further analysis. When, some months later, external relations of life shaped themselves unfavorably, his mood suffered a clouding, which, however, occasioned no relapse into the earlier introversion. With great energy, the young artist solved his life problem, got himself into the long desired position and has since worked industriously and well in the best of health and in good relations to his parents. His whole attitude toward life underwent an entire change. Whether the cure of the sorely threatened individual is a definite one, the future will show. After many experiences, there has been to date no occasion for fear. The analysis of drawings which were made unintentionally, as for example, during a lesson or consultation, is interesting.

10. POETRY

This section also will interest the educator. The pedagogue experienced in psychoanalysis can draw many valuable conclusions concerning the mental status of his pupils from their essays. Even in play there is a bit of poetry which betrays the repressed instinct.*

That the greatest poetry comes forth from hidden depths of the mind, has already been mentioned in Schiller's words (page 8). Its automatic character is, at least in regard to the great conception, even though not in its later elaboration, indisputable. Goethe confesses: "Every productivity of the highest kind, every great thought which brings fruits and has results, is in no one's power and is elevated above all power ... it is related to the demoniacal power which, endowed with superior force, does with a man what it wills, and to which he yields *unconsciously*,† while he thinks he is acting on his own initiative." ‡ Goethe relates that he wrote down most of his poems at night as in a dream; he sprang out of bed to his desk

---

* Freud, Der Dichter u. d. Phantasieren. Kl. Schr. II, p. 197 ff.
† Italicised by me.
‡ Cited by S. Kovacs, Introjektion, Projektion und Einfühlung. Zbl. II, 263. Rank, Inzest-Motiv; p. 475.

and without pushing the sheet of paper straight, wrote the poem from beginning to end, diagonally, for which purpose he used a pencil in order not to be awakened by the pen.* It is certain that Schiller was found lying on the floor twitching convulsively as he was busy with the scene between Eboli and the prince.† Similar half-pathological symptoms are reported of Goethe, Kleist, Turgenieff and A. de Musset.‡

The content of the poetic production also proves to be a manifestation. In the hero, we recognize, often without difficulty, the poet himself: Goethe is the original of Tasso and Antonio, Clavigo and Carlos; he lurks in Faust and Mephistopheles, both are personified libido characteristics. Schiller treats in the majority of his great dramas, in the Räubern, in Fiesko, in Don Carlos, in Kabale und Liebe, in Wallenstein, in Tell, of the struggle with the father, usually in the form of a father-substitute, because he himself suffered under a father-complex.‖ Grillparzer describes in many works the man divided between two women, Richard Wagner, the woman divided between two men passing over to the new-comer, because both authors thereby expressed their own erotic situations: Grillparzer remained for a lifetime devoted to the Fröhlich sisters, of whom he was engaged to Kathi to the end of his life; he could marry neither from inner reasons.¶ Wagner has Senta go over to the Dutchman, Elizabeth to Tannhäuser, Sieglinde to Sigmund, Isolde to Tristan, Eva to Stolzing, Brünhilde to Siegfried, because he himself desired the love which prejudiced a third person (Mathilde Wesendonk, Kosima von Bülow). This tendency, on the other hand, may be derived, as Max Graf § probably did, from the fact that Wagner, who lost his father when six months old and was passionately fond of the stepfather whom he soon gained, the comedian Geyer, thought of the wished-for possibility that he

---

* Stekel, Dichtung und Neurose, p. 3.
† Rank, Inzest-Motiv, p. 476.
‡ Same, p. 477.
‖ Same, p. 87 ff.
¶ Like Goethe he remained attached to his mother (see above p. 120).
§ Graf, Rich. Wagner im "fliegenden Holländer," p. 28 ff.

might be a child of Geyer. Ibsen's constant handling of the
marriage problem may be elucidated from the history of the
poet's marital conditions.* Konrad Ferdinand Meyer writes:
"I use the form of historical novel simply and solely in order
to embody in it my personal experiences and emotions, . . .
because it gives me a better disguise. In all persons of Pes-
cara, even in the common Morone, there is something of K. F.
Meyer." †

The analysis has also attacked the psychological riddle of
poetic art. I mention the problem of Hamlet because of its
high pedagogical importance. Freud says in one place that
Hamlet in no way represents the type of the dreamer made ill
by the specters of his thought for we see the prince act vigorously twice (killing of Polonius and the two courtiers).
Rather, Hamlet who is capable of doing everything else, cannot accomplish his revenge on the murderer and successor of his
father because he committed the same crimes in his phantasies
and so covered himself with guilt.‡ The English psychiatrist,
Prof. Jones, has elaborated ‖ this argument in a monograph
which excites the delight of the historians of literature by its
profoundness and lucidity; Otto Rank illuminates the problem
in its connection with other creations of Shakespeare.¶ The
judgment of these works will only be given for certain by the
analysis of living Hamlets, of whom the educator, unfortunately, knows not a few.

The reader will find an enormously extensive and most interesting material in the monumental work of Otto Rank: "Das
Inzest-Motiv in Dichtung und Sage," (Elements of a Psychology of Poetic Creation; 1912).

With the many problems of the psychology of art, the solving of which is rendered possible by psychoanalysis, we do not
have to concern ourselves. Yet on the other hand, it may be
pointed out in this connection that poetry, like every manifesta-

* Same, p. 27.
† A. Frey, K. F. Meyer, Stuttgart, 1900, p. 284.
‡ Freud, Traumdeutung, p. 192 f.
‖ Jones, D. Problem d. Hamlet u. d. Ödipus-Komplex.
¶ Rank, Inzest-Motiv, pp. 45 ff, 204–233.

tion, represents an attempt on the part of the artist (painter, author, poet, etc.) to free himself from the demands of his complexes. Goethe kills himself as Werther and thereby guards himself against suicide. Complete happiness, absolute salvation for a free life is seldom really attained by the poet. He remains a tragic hero. Schiller testifies: "How feeble still is the highest grandeur of a poet against the thought to live happy." Richard Wagner makes the shocking confession: "Dear friend! Some thoughts regarding art often come over me now and I cannot usually avoid finding that if we had life, we would have needed no art. Art begins just at the point where life ceases; where nothing more is present, there we call in the art: I wished. I do not understand at all how a truly happy person can come to the thought: only in life can one create art,—is our art not for the rest merely a confession of our impotence?" * Another time, he says: "Yes, to be always in strife, never to attain to complete calmness of soul, to be always baited, enticed and repulsed, that is really the ever bubbling life process, out of which the artist's inspiration bursts forth like a flower of despair." †

Although the poetic creation is a manifestation, the artist is not, as Stekel asserts, a neurotic. Rank rightly says "that the artist's achievement, which acts both as a relief for him and at the same time contributes something of great value to society, is always so sharply differentiated from the incapacity for achievement of the neurotic that even the most intimate relationship in the prerequisite conditions cannot obliterate these plainly visible distinctions." ‡

I conclude with two quotations from Hebbel who here again shows himself to be a thorough student of humanity: In the passage quoted at length on page 116, where the contribution of the unconscious to artistic creation, the infantilism, the regression, and the repression are so well pictured, the poet laments the fact that "even intelligent men do not cease from

* Rank, p. 482.
† Same, p. 482.
‡ Same, p. 479.

quarreling with the poet over his choice of material, as they call it, and thereby show that they always conceive of the artistic creation, the first stage of which, the conception, lies deep below consciousness and at times recedes to the dimmest distance of childhood (regression), as a making, even though it be a noble one."* The other quotation is: "My idea that dream and poetry are identical finds ever new confirmation." †

11. THE MORAL MANIFESTATIONS

The psychoanalytic investigations concerning the moral consciousness and its scientific regulation are unfortunately not yet far enough advanced to allow us to devote a long section to them. Only two investigations are at hand: my analyses of hate and reconciliation which appeared in 1910, furnished the proof that hate, by one-sided direction and fixation of interest, impoverishes the personality, destroys the mental power by growing dependence upon dark compulsion, cripples the will, weakens the moral energy by volatilization into autistic dreams, strengthens sadism and masochism and isolates the individual. Reconciliation, on the other hand, removes all these injurious influences and creates sublimation.‡ Evil proves thereby to be biologically useless, good to be the healthy condition. Naturally, this individualistic mode of consideration is not the only one which is ethically demanded. Into consideration there comes that which is hygienically approved for the community, to which the individual life has, under certain circumstances, to be sacrificed.

In the year 1912, there appeared an important investigation by Karl Fortmüller, entitled "Psychoanalyse und Ethik." ‖ Starting from Adler's fundamental hypothesis, he seeks to explain the ethical imperative as a defence process erected

* Hebbel, Preface to "Maria Magdalena," cited by Rank, Inzestm p. 125.
† Hebbel, Tagebücher, June 3, 1847, cited by Stekel, Dichtung und Neurose, p. 2.
‡ Pfister, Hass und Versöhnung, p. 46 f.
‖ K. Fortmüller, Psa. u. Ethik. Eine vorläufige Untersuchung, Munich, 1912.

against the feeling of inferiority (Minderwertigkeitgefühl). The demands made upon the child for order and subordination strengthen in him the feeling of inferiority which is now reacted not only in defiance and passive submission but also by the acceptance of that external command into his own will. The feeling of inferiority is thereby overcompensated, however, in that this inner imperative is expected of everyone as a moral command. A tendency toward assurance is also manifested by the moral consciousness to the extent that the imposed prohibitions form a defence against the covetous instincts and their dangers.

It seems to me that Fortmüller has developed his ideas, which are interesting and may be correct for certain cases, in a one-sided manner. When the father gives an eight months-old child a little command, it may perhaps playfully acknowledge his greatness, yet the reaction is certainly not primarily a heightened feeling of inferiority but one of joy. And thus are many, even if not all, moral emotions, both admonishing and warning, aroused on the path of pleasure and indeed so that the feeling of greatness, the pride, is strengthened. Still, Fortmüller indicates in very commendable manner dangers in the moral education.

Psychoanalysis has led to a number of moral facts without intending to deal with ethical considerations, by the duty of healing the sick. We spoke of lying, stealing, love and hate, Don Juanism caused by complexes. We are not dealing merely with pathological processes.

I want to point out here only one phenomenon especially important for pedagogy, by which, the whole direction of life, the greatest part of the happiness of life or of the tragedy of life is determined. I mean the plan of life conditioned upon complexes regarding its moral character. We have already discussed the life tendency in general on page 385. We have often seen the whole life devoted to the service of a completely unconscious tendency. We heard of the place-seeker who elaborated for a lifetime an infantile inferiority complex and wished to compel from humanity the recognition which his father had denied him (110); of the Don Juan who sought unknowingly to gratify his high emotional needs in his erring love and thereby exposed his own life and the lives of others to the greatest dangers and hardships (329). We called attention to the avaricious, over-exact, analerotic individual, totally incapable of conjugal love (200), to the homosexual individual and his peculiar life development (202), to the choice of vocation determined by complexes (326), to the unlucky fellow (110), to the quarrelsome individual (246), to the fundamental themes of the poets (parricide in Schiller, the woman between two men in Wagner, the man between two women in Grillparzer, etc.), to the predetermination in religion occasioned by repressions of childhood (Zinzendorf, etc.). One might refer further to the reformer who will quit scores with his feeling of guilt by a zealous combat against immorality (385), to the army of reaction builders (321), etc.

Still a number of other unconscious plans of life may be named. The knowledge of such connections imposes mighty tasks upon the pedagogue. The whimsical eccentricity in the choice of a vocation, often so mysterious, now becomes comprehensible and instead of belaboring the youth by pressure and compulsion with tiresome lectures which do not annul the inner need, he will banish the illusion analytically in such a way that the pupil may breathe again in freedom. For the boy who is absorbed in a burning passion for the problem of flying, he will, if the wish cannot be sublimated to valuable achievements at the proper moment, analyze a flying-dream; for the aspirant for the stage who has little talent, he will analyze an exhibition dream. For the youth who is excellently suited for the profession of medicine and shows great inclination toward this profession, but is restrained by aversion for wounds and corpses, he dissolves the inhibition by analysis. The man imprisoned in a "life-lie," to use the expression of Bertschinger * adopted by Ibsen, who wishes to make believe that he is an angel of purity,

---

* C. Bertschinger, Ü. Gelegenheitsursachen gewisser Neurosen u. Psychosen. Allg. Zschr. f. Psychiatrie u. psychisch-gerichtl. Medizin, Vol. 69 (1912), pp. 588–617.

gallantry, magnanimity, and in this feigned rôle, receives severe injury, he enables to fight an honest battle against his internal enemy.

For the first investigation of a plan of life, we are indebted to Sigmund Freud, who, under the unpretentious title, "Eine Kindheitserinnerung des Leonardo da Vinci" (A Childhood Memory of Leonardo da Vinci) traced the peculiar life development of the great artist and thinker back to infantile sexual influences. Alfred Adler institutes far-reaching investigations of the theory of the plan of life in his book, "Über den nervösen Charakter" (Concerning the Nervous Character). According to Adler, every neurotic and psychotic individual is under the rule of a uniform life plan which proceeds towards the mastering of the feeling of insufficiency. "The character traits, especially the neurotic ones, serve as psychic means and forms of expression for bringing about the guidance of the life opinions, acquiring a place, gaining a fixed point in the fluctuations of existence, in order to attain the final goal, the feeling of superiority."* Thus the neurotic creates assurances for himself. "To these assurances belong also the fixation and strengthening of character traits which, in the chaos of life, form working guides and thus lessen the uncertainty." † "Feeling of guilt and conscience are fictitious guiding lines of caution, like the religious emotions, and serve the tendency toward assurance." ‡ "Still more firmly does the nervous individual keep his god, his idol, his ideal personality in view and cling to his guiding line, thereby losing sight of reality, while the healthy individual is constantly prepared to give up this assistance, these crutches, and reckon unprejudiced with reality. The healthy individual also, can and will create his divinity, feel himself drawn upward, will however, never lose sight of reality, and calculates with it as soon as the moment of action and effort arrives. Hence the nervous individual is under the rule of a fictitious plan of life." ‖

Aside from the previously mentioned one-sidedness with

* Adler, Nerv. Charakter, p. 8.   ‡ Same, p. 25.
† Same, p. 14.   ‖ Same, p. 36.

which Adler makes the limitation of the ego-instinct conditioned on organic changes, the foundation of the plan of life, and purposely denies the erotic influences, aside also from the insufficient religious psychological construction, Adler's theory of the fictitious guiding line is highly fruitful and valuable. But it must be qualified by a consideration which allows the instincts for self-preservation and for perpetuation of the race to have their rights.

12. RELIGIOUS MANIFESTATIONS

Psychoanalysis performs two services for religion: one in the domain of religious psychology and one in that of biology. It helps to understand religion and to estimate its significance. On the other hand, psychoanalysis gives no explanation of the content of truth in religion, although it eliminates neurotic forms of religion which do not hold their own against the reality-thinking, much quicker and more surely than all historical and systematic theology.

We have repeatedly had occasion to disclose the origin of religious experiences. Page 36 crown of thorns, 37 vision of angel, 38 vision of devil, 66 anxiety-hysteria as the effect of improper religious instruction, 71 obsessional praying, 76 prayer with negative result, 83 laughing during religious services, 83, 92, 135 correspondence between profane and religious love, 93 disturbance of prayer, 92 piousness, loss of the adoration of Jesus, stoicism, 129 pantheism, 136 madonna fanaticism, 145 religious scruples, 194 disappearance of love as result of religious influences, 203 oscillation between religious and homosexual emotion, 213 anger against God, 247 phantasies concerning the face and figure of God, 252 religious explanation of a sexual wish in a dream, 326 longing to change churches, 275f the symbol in religion, 327 dogmatism, 255 disjection in religion, 331 clothes fetichism in connection with religious conversion, estrangement from God, turning to Jesus, 379 juvenile hallucination of a devil. I will add a somewhat complicated but highly instructive example:

I was asked by a gentleman of excellent character, aged

thirty-nine, member of a Christian communion, who was on the point of joining a new sect, to explain a number of passages in Daniel and the Apocalypse. Naturally the attempt failed at the first citation. Apparently diverting, I learned that the man, some weeks before, after attending a religious lecture, had felt a kind of sticking pain in his stomach at the moment he asked himself if he were not sinning by denying the devil. At the same time, a violent anxiety appeared which compelled Bible reading for hours at a time for the purpose of overcoming the anxiety. The words of the demoniacs at Gadara occupied much of his attention: "Why do you come to punish us before the time?"—a speech which had caused him much thought since his sixteenth year but now had become an obsessional idea. The so-called prophetic (apocalyptic) part of the Bible, as well as the observation of the Sabbath and the refraining from pork, exerted on him an irresistible magic. Withdrawing from analysis, he actually transferred to the sect. Only after months did I obtain a continuation of the analysis. Then it came to light that the man, in addition to the obsession over the demon question named above, was obsessed by the saying: "The night cometh when no man can work." The prophetic part of the Bible was the most important to him so that he published a very definite plan of God which culminated in the second advent of Christ. The observance of the Sabbath was sacred to him as exact observance of divine command. He was especially impressed by the statement that the dead should sleep until the second coming of Christ. The belief in the devil, previously denied, became very important to him. One while, he feared to have committed the sin against the Holy Ghost but could not decide in what this consisted. Now, he felt, after long distress, happy and healthy. The analysis had therefore, a priori, little prospect of changing the manner of thought.

Whence came these phenomena? When twelve years old, the boy practiced masturbation, which, three years later, after he had read a warning article, weighed heavily on his conscience. The pains in his stomach appeared at this time, never to disappear again for good. For a half year, he successfully fastened his hands at night with a cord. In his sixteenth year, three sayings frequently occupied his thoughts, among them the absurd song:

> "To combat the Kingdom of Lust
> Be my wisdom, O Highest!
> It is a poison for our life
> And turns our joys to pain."

Further the maxim:

> "Everything in its place
> Saves much time and many an evil word."

Finally the saying of the demoniacs of Gadara already mentioned. In the analysis, it proved that all these sayings had attained such great emphasis because of their relation to the sexual complex. The two last named, attained their obsessional character because they expressed allegorically the unpleasant sexual function and its results.

As a young fellow, he had been disgusted with the brothels into which he had allowed himself to be enticed. In his marriage, his wife compelled him to practice coitus interruptus. The result was, as described on page 208, extreme partiality for nature-cure methods so long as the improper marital inter- course lasted (over-compensation for the unnatural sexual practice) but only so long.

Passing over the interesting dilemmas of the period immediately following, I will mention the circumstances under which the transfer into a new communion occurred. As a result of his religious sublimation, the patient had been free from his old hysterical pains in the stomach for two years but showed during this period a nervous tic. Some months after the death of his wife, the demons' question: "Why do you come to punish us before the time?" again gained control over him, an expression of the sexuality violently raging within him and the damming up of his sublimated compensation. He became dissatisfied with the sect which he had previously loved, because he thought he discovered in it anxiety over death. Hence, figuratively expressed, his eroticism flowed back into infantile channels, the old complex-functions awakened and sought new gratification. Such a gratification, the new sect afforded. Its teaching gratified him for many reasons which corresponded to his complexes. I will name only a few: 1. The Apocalyptic plan of salvation in God includes death, after that, the sleep of the dead in the night when no one can work, thus where the "premature punishment" is ended, and finally the second advent of Christ. We have recognized the sexual necessity, the unsatisfied libido, as foundation of the obsessions, hence the ideas of death-sleep and of the parusia as recipients of the complex-gratification become comprehensible to us as expectations of sexual peace and later of gratification. The second advent was thus a sublimation of the wish for a second marriage.

2. The reality of the devil corresponded to the experience of the tormenting eroticism as the second advent of Christ satisfied the longing for a second happy marriage.

3. The Biblical orthodoxy was a symptom of the anxiety-neurosis (compare Freud, "Zwangshandlungen und Religionsübung." Sammlung kleiner Schriften zur Neurosenlehre, 2d Part) as the patient himself admits. For the estimation of orthodoxy in history, such cases are very important.

4. The observance of the Sabbath, of the tithes, of the refraining from pork, form, like the fanaticism in the practice of the nature-cure method, in its time, an overcompensation which would make up for the ethical deficiency in the marriage. For the rest, the patient was (like another of my patients) as result of sexual repression, a vegetarian; so much the more willingly did he now submit to the religious demands of abstinence. The prohibition of meat commonly corresponds to sexual denial.

The mentally weak, though studious, man agreed with me point by point. But he felt happy in his piety. He left his lucrative post for the sake of the Sabbath. A few years later, the official who had previously been well off financially, was ruined. Concerning his inner state, I know nothing.

. We see how well that the sublimated form of religion was adapted to the primary fixation of the libido. Very often, the repressed unmoral material returns in the center of the religion, for example, in the disgusting masochism of many ascetics and the sadism of many judges of witches and heretics (above page 311). Novalis justly remarks: "It is remarkable that the association of sensual pleasure, religion and cruelty and the common tendency of these has not been noticed long ago." * E. T. A. Hoffmann puts these words in the mouth of his "Medardus": "Thus I spake of the wonderful mysteries of religion in glowing pictures, the deep significance of which was the voluptuous frenzy of the most ardent, longing love." †

One must, however, guard against wishing to consider religion as altogether only higher directed libido. Kant based it on the ethical demand, understanding God as the real basis of the moral postulate. The metaphysics of practically all great philosophers from Plato and Aristotle down to Leibnitz, Hebbel and Herbart, indeed even to Wundt, Theodor Lipps and Riehl arrived at a concept of God by way of reality-thinking, which concept agrees in essential outlines with the Christian one.

Psychoanalysis in no way violates the claims of truth of the Christian religion as such. Of course, as already noticed, it destroys many spurious religious experiences by showing the illusory complex-function at the bottom of these. It must do this in order to banish misfortune. It would be all too small for Christianity to think that harm is to be feared for its future from analysis. The new method teaches us rather to understand many a form of current piety rejected as monstrous or ridiculed as laughable, to consider them causally in their necessity and estimate their deeper meaning. It comes to the assistance of religious psychology which is in its infancy. Even to-day, it has given us the solutions for a mass of myths, religious hallucinations, inspirations,‡ prohibitions, bizarre new formations, ceremonials, ancient enigmas like automatic glossolalia, etc. And it will accomplish still much more.

---

* E. Heilborn, Novalis, p. 160.
† E. T. A. Hoffmann, Elixiere des Teufels, p. 73.
‡ Pfister. Glossolalie. Jahrb. III, p. 440.

Psychoanalysis also teaches us to estimate the value of religion anew. I confess that the beauty and the blessing of a healthy, ethically pure piety have only become overwhelmingly clear to me from the investigations here described. Religion, in favorable cases, guards the libido repelled by the rude, avaricious reality, against conversion into hysterical physical symptoms and against introversion into anxiety, melancholia, obsessional phenomena, etc. Freud speaks of the "extraordinary increase in neuroses since the decline of religions." * I would much rather have unfortunate people whom I cannot really cure by analysis, in an extreme sect or a cloister than in a psychoneurosis. Of course there is also much neurotic misery in cloisters and religious communities.

Stekel also attributes to religion a high ethical mission: "Religion serves to bind these (original) impulses of hate in the form of anxiety (tendencies toward assurance of Adler). The inhibitions increase to consciousness of guilt when the individual does not succeed in utilizing his hate; thereby he rationalizes it, converts it into love or sublimates it." †

We have already discussed how Jung assigned to religion the task of making fruitful for ethical achievements, the forces bound up in "incestuous" constellations (299). Of Christianity, he says: "In a time, when a great part of humanity is beginning to deny Christianity, it is well worth while to perceive clearly why it has really been accepted. It has been accepted to escape eventually the grossness of antiquity. If we lay it aside, then the unbridled license is already at hand, of which life in modern large cities gives us an impressive foretaste. The step thither is no progress but a retrogression. . . . To-day, the individual feels himself inhibited by the hypocritical public opinion and hence prefers to lead a secret life apart, publicly however, to represent the moral code; things might be quite different however, if people in general should find the moral mask too foolish and should become conscious of how dangerously their beasts lay in wait for one another; then a

---

* Freud, D. zukünftigen Chancen d. Psa, Zbl. I, p. 5.
† Stekel, Sprache d. Traumes, p. 53.

debauch of depravity might readily sweep over humanity—
that is the dream, the wish-dream of the morally restricted person of the present: he forgets the distress which robs the human
being of breath and which with harsh hand would interrupt
every pleasure.'' * The religious myth, Jung calls ''one of
the greatest and most important institutions of humanity,
which with deceptive symbols gives man security and strength
against being overwhelmed by the vastness of the universe.'' †
He wishes therefore to carefully retain the religious symbol
''after unavoidable elimination of certain antiquated parts, as
postulate or as Transcendental theory and also as object of instruction but fill it with new content in such measure as the
status of the cultural life of the time demands.'' ‡ This is a
position which has also been assumed by Wundt ‖ and Eucken ¶
and especially by Paulsen. The latter says, for example:
''The great symbols which already interpret the meaning of
the world to the child, again become vivid. The systems of
the philosophers, the theories of the scholars, the systems of
the theologians pass away, as between evening and morning
the clouds come and go, while the great symbols remain like
the stars of heaven when they, too, are momentarily hidden
from view by the passing clouds.'' § Many theologians are of
similar opinion, for example, A. E. Biedermann, Lipsius,**
Rauwenhoff,†† Trotltsch.‡‡

While psychoanalysis may disclose the emptiness of religious
errors, it is helpful to a healthy piety which increases moral
strength. It has compelled more than one physician, who, in
the bonds of materialistic thinking had discarded religion as a
bygone superstition, to adopt a more just estimation, yes, even

* Jung, Wandlungen. Jahrb. IV, p. 273.
† Same, p. 275.
‡ Same, p. 276.
‖ Wundt, Syst. d. Philos. pp. 668 f, 674.
¶ Eucken, Wahrheitsgehalt d. Relig. p. 405 ff.
§ Paulsen, Einleitung in d. Philos. p. 340.
** Lipsius, Lehrb. der er-prot. Dogmatik, Paragraph, § 72 ff.
†† Rauwenhoff, Rel.-phil. p. 468 f.
‡‡ E. Troeltsch, D. Absoluth. d. Chr. u. d. Rel.-gesch., Tübingen, 1912,
p. 149.

admiration, for the mental phenomenon. Where, outside of psychoanalytic circles, would you find a society of physicians, teachers and theologians which would discuss the religious problem in a series of evenings devoted to earnest conferences? To me, it is a mystery how anxious souls can fear damage to religion and morality from psychoanalysis. How closely the results of the latter stand to the commands of the Gospel, we will show later.

CHAPTER XIII

THE MEANING OF THE MANIFESTATIONS

In manifestations as a whole, we may differentiate a psychological and a biological significance.

1. THE PSYCHOLOGICAL MEANING

(A) IN GENERAL

1. The Manifestation as Wishfulfillment

In every manifestation, we recognized as compelling force an instinct which acted along indirect ways instead of mastering reality or adapting itself to reality. So far as every instinct proceeds to gratification, we may unhesitatingly call every manifest symptom, the pathological as well as the normal, for example the dream, a gratification of the complex. In so doing, it would naturally not be declared that an actual gratification should occur but it is at least striven for.

So far as the instinct is directed toward an object unattainable at the moment, it becomes a wish. Since with every gratification of instinct, pleasure is released, even though this is not the direct goal, it yields a gain of pleasure.

According to the first aspect, every manifestation must be a wishfulfillment, since gratification of instinct occurs only when the longed-for thing becomes at least relatively reality.

That which we would expect from our insight into the laws of complex-reaction, Freud found substantiated by direct analysis of neurotic phenomena. His statement that every dream represents a wish as fulfilled, has been treated very slightingly. And as a matter of fact, everyone who thinks of the painful situations experienced in the dream, may at first find Freud's assertion absurd under the one condition that he does not

416

trouble about that which Freud wishes to say and does say plainly enough. With Freud, the accent lies on the points that (1) it need in no way be a conscious wish which is fulfilled in the dream, but often an unconscious one; (2) the wishfulfillment does not occur in that which is really dreamed but the latent wish comes to expression only symbolically in veiled form, metaphorically, like a charade. He who leaves these two fundamental considerations out of account, does an injustice to psychoanalysis with his jest. In the sense indicated, which is clearly and plainly defined by Freud, the significance of a wishfulfillment appears not only for every dream but for all neurotic symptoms,* no matter how tormenting they may be.

In some dreams, which Freud describes as infantile, although they apparently occur also in adults,† the dream content corresponds to a manifest wish, for example, the father sees his unfortunate lame child jumping around. Usually however this is not the case.

He who only looked at the dream of the two furniture vans (355), or that of the negro and piano (356), or that of coming too late and arriving at proper time at the station (358), or that of the awaited Duchess of Angoulême (359), might find it difficult to see a wish realized in them. But if one takes into consideration the associations, the whole mental situation, then he can scarcely miss the autistic gratification of a strong desire, unless he is greatly prejudiced beforehand.

Or if one had said at the beginning to the hysterical girl whose psychogenic deafness we described (96): ''Your suffering corresponds to your wish''—she would have justly rejected this silly assertion. For under ''your wish'' she would have had to understand a conscious wish, while the wishes:

---

* An exception may be formed by anxiety which Freud seeks to elucidate physiologically in a manner clever, but for me, not convincing. (Freud, "Angstneurose," Kl. Schriften I, p. 76 f.) Jones derives the anxiety not directly from repressed sexuality but from an "inborn instinct of fear which is excited to excessive activity (as defence mechanism) as answer to the danger from repressed sexual wishes." (Die Beziehungen zwischen Angstneurose und Angsthysterie. Internat. Zschr. f. ärztl. Psa. I, p. 13.)

† Here they are in need of an overinterpretation, however.

"would that I might no more hear the raging father, the groaning mother, the dissolute brother, the base gossip and especially the unloved fiancé who makes sexual demands" in their connection with the suffering were unconscious. Further, the actual deafness was not wished for, but only a relative deafness, even though the hysterical girl certainly often used the expression: "Would that I might hear nothing of the whole thing!" Just as little did the dreamers wish a real furniture van or the historical Duchess of Angoulême.*

Let us take another example characterized by extreme simplicity. A refined lady, married for some months, is suddenly seized with great anxiety lest burglars be found in the garden. Who would wish anything of that sort? The explanation is that the husband is impotent and that she can therefore love him no more although she lays no blame on him. The lady suffers also from severe pains in the pelvis (imaginary defloration- and birth-pains) and is operated on for vaginismus, since the hymen is still present, without the pains being helped in the least. I cured the husband, a woman physician with the aid of psychoanalysis, the wife, who naturally wished for burglary in her organs and the couple which had been married about a year, at once experienced the joy of normal marriage and parental happiness (124).

I have always found confirmed without exception where analysis was possible, that the manifestation, as a whole, represented as real something which was secretly wished for, often without the subject's knowing it. Many times, one will not consider it possible that the impulses displaying themselves in the dream can really be present, until one is convinced by acts in the waking state or a series of other arguments. It is shocking to many subjects of analysis to have demonstrated by infallible proof what vulgar impulses were now and then present and repressed in their minds. The analyst must often console

* A very beautiful example, in which a physician sees his index finger as syphilitic, is given by August Stärke in his communication: "Ein Traum, der das Gegenteil einer Wunscherfüllung zu verwirklichen scheint, zugleich ein Beispiel eines Traumes, der von einem andern Traum gedeutet wird." Zbl. II, pp. 86–88.

with the assurance that one is not responsible for the repressed material and that everyone, without exception, carries within himself his demons.

Often there comes to fulfillment in the dream, a wish which is still entirely unconscious but which later becomes conscious. Freud calls such dreams, prophetic dreams, of which we also heard Hebbel speak, page 352, "annunciatory dreams." Maeder gives some good examples of these.*

The indicative instead of the optative is also used in ordinary life. "You do that" is emphasizing the imperative: "do that." When a skittle ball misses its goal, the unfortunate marksman who is accustomed to act out his impulses is the personified optative in the indicative.

A more frequent special case is that when a repressed thought, a fear, is expressed by some harmless phenomenon of related nature. From a certain date, a gentleman suffers from the annoying and vigorously combated habit of leaving the door open on leaving the house, when he intended to shut it, so that he would have to turn around and draw it to; or he has forgotten something and must turn back, for example, to get a pencil or to brush his hat or to close a cabinet which he thought was open, etc. Often he was vexed at himself for turning back for such a bagatelle but originally the intention seemed important. The analysis shows: His marriage is unhappy, further he takes little pleasure in his children. He would like to free himself from these relations but does not dare to make the plans, chiefly because the external difficulties seem insuperable. Further, he shoves aside this thought: "I cannot escape from these relationships." The symptomatic act says: "Quite right but it is only the house from which you will not so easily get free." Perhaps it also means: "Guard against tearing yourself from your family."

A peasant, aged fifty-three, suffered from violent pains in his arm. The physician made the mistaken diagnosis of beginning muscular atrophy. I found: his son whom he called his "right arm" gave him much pain.

* Maeder, über die Funktion des Traumes. Jahrb. IV, p. 694 ff.

The same man showed an uncommonly frequent hysterical symptom: pains in the loins (Kreuz). They are only an expression of the phantasy: "you must bear a heavy cross (Kreuz), yes but only in your body." According to this construction: "yes, but only," many neuroses are formed and thus fulfill a relative wish.

Especially in the beginning of the analysis when the deeper mental motives, the most intimate needs, are not yet recognized, the dream contains fairly plain wishfulfillments. The more the attachment in infantile phantasies is released by analysis and the instincts turn to a future corresponding to the inner imperative, just so much the more does the dream-content assume the character of a proposal which one might designate as prophecy, if the possibility of new, preferable life-plans did not exist. Thus, the wishfulfilling in the manifestation may then be called a kind of *ballon d'essai*.

2. *The Manifestation as Acquiring of Pleasure and Avoiding of Pain*

This title, too, may cause those who saw the enormous physical and particularly mental suffering of profound neurotic and psychotic patients, to shake their heads. And yet the superscription expresses a truth. In the depths of grievous tortures, there often lurks a high degree of pleasure which we have to understand as masochism. Goethe was far too keen a student of humanity to have missed the universality of this desire for the sweet torment. He remarks that man has a kind of lust for evil and a dim longing for the pleasure of pain.*

Often, the morbid symptom itself is obviously pleasant and unpleasant at the same time. We heard above of the girl who scratched herself to the hair-roots, tearing out whole pieces of skin and tufts of hair, thereby obtaining a high degree of pleasure, however (34).

The hysterical man who admired the hallucinated nixies' veils so greatly and was indifferent to the nixies themselves

---

* Goethe, Wilhelm Meisters theatralische Sendung. Reports by Gustav Billeter. Zurich, 1910, p. 93.

(331), often goes into the forest in the evening. Then the trees change into ghosts who pursue him through the thickets and frighten him terribly. But in the depths of his soul, there plainly lurked pleasure. He invited a lady to a ball, retracted the invitátion at the last moment and wept miserably over his misfortune but revelled in his phantasy that he tasted richly of "sweet torment."

A normal young girl who wanted to gain moral strength according to the advice of a teacher of Catholic morality, cauterized a burn with the prescribed substance in quadruple strength. The pain was frightful but the pleasure gained, outweighed it.

A physician whom I know tells me that a waitress appeared at night in great excitement with the beseeching entreaty to open her stomach for she had swallowed a fragment of glass. After four days, her request was complied with and no foreign body was found. The mishap was purely imaginary. Six weeks later, the hysterical person appeared to the physician again with the same demand.

How a hysterical person can torture herself for decades with indescribable torments and yet secretly enjoy ecstasies "with immeasurable sweetness" in her adoration of the heavenly bridegroom, I showed in Margaretha Ebner (1291–1351).*

Frequently, this gain of pleasure is hard to find but it is seldom lacking. A conscious intention to gain pleasure and avoid pain may not, as a rule, be ascribed to the subject of the manifestation. When an analytic patient perceives that getting well demands much sacrifice, namely, the renunciation of the autistic release from the duties of life which should be performed with moral strength in actuality, the hate is rationalized upon the analyst. But such neurotics who make the most of their assertions of misfortune, are not as a rule, conscious swindlers, for intentional automatism would be a contradiction and neuroses are, from the standpoint of consciousness, automatisms. Still, there are also moral imbeciles among neurotics.

Not in all psychoneuroses, does one find as plain motive, the

* Zbl. I, pp. 468–485,

flight from reality and its demands with the aim of a phantastic and dramatic solution of the conflict. But very often, one meets such unconscious pleasure-seekers.

Bed-wetting, for instance, when there is neither bladder weakness nor epilepsy, is usually a nocturnal exaction of attention, as I have been able to demonstrate many times. If the child is given over to a nurse who affords him no erotic gratification, the wetting often ceases at once. The habit may, however, according to an infantile theory of reproduction, represent a sexual act and is then curable by analysis. An eighteen year old girl with neurotic anxiety, who had suffered from eneuresis since a small child, of late years had had her symptom every time a boy had called to her a greeting or jest during the day. I carefully allowed the girl, who was not especially intelligent, to discover the state of affairs for herself and was surprised to see how little assistance was necessary. The recovery resulted at once.

The sparing of discomfort is often striven for by physical sufferings which save an ethical struggle; if the conflict is worked out consciously, the suffering is far greater and terminates in melancholia or neurosis of higher order. I once met two sisters who, as strangers, embraced the opportunity to pour out their hearts to the pastor. Both labored under exactly the same mental needs. The younger suffered from violent migraine but came off satisfied with the difficulties of life, since, as she said, she banished the disappointments from her mind and laughed. Thus she was, according to the testimony of her sister and her own assertion, always cheerful and in spite of the migraine, a happy person. The other sister, on the other hand, was free from hysteria but in its place, moody and melancholic. She fought out the life conflict in great part consciously and became unhappy. Naturally, her mental suffering was also enormously strengthened by subliminal contributions. For the rest, the example shows the protective character of hysteria.

A young husband was mean to his wife before asthma broke out but then became proportionately kind toward her. When the physical trouble receded, the previous irritability returned. This interchange happened repeatedly.

Many times, it is not an ethical longing but resistance against some kind of duty, hard to perform, which drives the person into the infantilism of the neurosis. That such a result is very bad, is obvious enough. He who wishes to get through life cheaply and seeks to escape the moral command of his inmost soul, must constantly pay heavy damages. One puts off from week to week the composition of an unpleasant letter, has to repress many unpleasant feelings and finally writes it when the situation is just so much the worse. Freud indicates the significance of the repression-process shown in this section when he speaks of an attraction from the unconscious.*

(B) THE SPECIAL MEANING

"According to a rule which I had always found substantiated but had not the courage to set up as a general one, a symptom signifies the representation—realization—of a phantasy with sexual content, thus a sexual situation. I might better say, at least one of the meanings of a symptom corresponds to the representation of a sexual phantasy, while for the other meanings, there is no such limitation of content." † "The morbid phenomena are, to put it bluntly, the sexual activities of the patients." ‡

My experiences support the contention that these statements very often prove correct, still, in view of the insufficient number of my observations, I venture neither to explain Freud's rule as universally applicable nor to consider the sexual significance of the cases seen by me as the deepest ones. Let us recall at this point the broadness of the definition of the sexual given by Freud. That very strong sexual and erotic energies may be invested in manifestations, as well as in sport, art and religion, is obvious. Only in this way, can we explain the tremendous intensity of the compulsion to senseless acts or

* Freud, Z. Übertrag. Zbl. II, p. 170.
† Freud, Bruchstück. Kl. Schriften II, p. 39.
‡ Same, p. 102.

phantasies, to hysterical pains and other complex-reactions. Further, the pent-up instinct for assertion and execution often manifests itself in symptoms.

A fifteen year old girl became ill with severe dysmenorrhea which the physician wanted to relieve by operation. A woman physician who practiced analysis fortunately advised analysis however, which soon revealed the purely hysterical character of the disturbance. The girl plainly acted out a birth-phantasy as her accompanying dreams proved. She repeatedly had a red spot, about one centimeter in diameter, on her throat, very often during the analysis. She once surprised her parents together. At that time, the embarrassed mother said: "Father has lost his collar-button and is looking for it." Soon afterwards, the trouble began.

Many similar examples might be introduced.

2. THE BIOLOGICAL MEANING OF THE MANIFESTATION

The biological purpose of the instincts consist in the preservation of the individual and of the race. We observe this also in the effects of instinctive activity which proceeds from the unconscious.

(A) THE MANIFESTATION AS MEANS OF ASSURANCE

Freud considers every manifestation as a final, even though not always suitable, measure to avoid discomfort, to protect the individual against pain. He speaks of defence-neuroses and considers the neurosis as an attempt at healing which has miscarried. Adler pursued these thoughts farther in a one-sided manner. According to him, every neurotic manifestation seeks, as we know (407), to secure the individual against the organic inferiority which is present.* One might also speak, to select a thought of Freud's, of an assurance against the demands of life, against the impelling force of conscience (Jung). The combat against the enormous dissipation of moral energy practiced by healthy and sick, belongs to the most important tasks of education.

* Adler, Nerv. Charakter, p. 11.

(B) THE MANIFESTATION AS AN ATTEMPT AT HEALING

We have just pointed out that the complex-formation may represent a defect in the moral sense. The ethical impulse can, however, be executed so vigorously in the compromise which every manifestation signifies that its tendency predominates.

We have already given examples. I recall the Don Juan who endowed himself with pains in arms and legs, the former probably the latter certainly, to escape base love affairs and to guard against new ones (126).

According to Maeder, the dreams contain in great part such unavowed ethical attempts, unconscious imperatives, in order to solve the life conflict and represent the moral demand corresponding to the law of the personal nature. (Jahrbuch IV, 692 ff., V, 647 ff.). My own experience has not found so great a universality of the moral problem named. Only by applying force and rejecting the associations given, can I bring every dream into this scheme. For the therapeutic aim, this method may be harmless, but not always, since it renders difficult the analysis of the attachments lying in the past and leaves them to good luck. Scientifically, that Procrustean method is always dangerous.

Freud showed in his "Gradiva" the process of spontaneous cure of a neurosis. We pedagogues are very interested in this important conception but do not feel ourselves called to settle it.

Our examples showed that the instinctive connection desiring expression in every manifestation is to be traced back not merely to the purpose of sparing consciousness painful thoughts, thus discomfort. Besides this repression, we observed a positive factor, an attraction: that of subconscious pleasure. Further, we found—and in accord with Freud—that the manifestation has not merely (as regression) a backward-looking significance but also a forward-looking one, in other words, not only a causal character but also a final meaning. Also, we now recognize the intimate connection between morality and health, disease and moral delinquency. Far removed from the position that this insight, gained by pure empiricism, may cause ethics to degenerate into naturalism, it shows us rather the power and worth of the fulfillment of duty in surprisingly sublime light. Has not Jesus also called himself a Savior?

PART II
THE TECHNIQUE OF PSYCHOANALYSIS

SECTION I. THE METHODS

CHAPTER XIV

THE FUNDAMENTAL RULE OF PSYCHOANALYSIS AND ITS APPLICATION

THE content of the fundamental rule of psychoanalysis has already been given in the introduction (6f). We will now discuss it somewhat further and examine its application.

When one has reached the point with the patient where the analysis can begin, he says to him something like the following: "You are to direct your attention to that which I shall say to you and simply name the first thing which comes into your mind; do not ponder over what is said to you but merely say without critique that which first comes into your mind, regardless of whether it is nice or ugly, clever or stupid, relevant or irrelevant, important or unimportant." It is advisable to give this instruction more than once and to emphasize that we are dealing with the very first associations or when several appear simultaneously, with the very first group of associations, entirely without the exercise of any criticism of the content of the associated idea or the rejection of anything as inferior.

One carefully avoids, therefore, all suggestive influences which might cause the patient to be guided in his associations by the tone, attitude or facial expression of the analyst instead of by the idea proposed. As we shall show, suggestion cannot generally be entirely eliminated. But it should be restricted as much as possible. Hence the analyst maintains as uniform an attitude as possible and does not betray his emotional impulses, especially not by voice and facial expression. In obtaining associations from the patient, one makes use of fixed formulæ, as "What does X bring to mind?" Or simply, "X, further."

One can either analyze a definite manifestation systematically or allow such an analysis to be produced; for example, taking associations from any word, a chain of associations, a cryptogram or something similar may be formed. As a rule, the patient is full of his symptoms. Freud has the patient tell,* first of all, of the origin of the symptoms and beginning here, collects the conscious causes. "When we proceed from the last material which the patient remembers, to seek a repressed complex, we have every prospect of guessing this, if the patient puts at our disposal a sufficient number of his free associations. Thus, we allow the patient to tell what he wishes and we hold fast to the presupposition that he will have no associations except such as depend directly upon the complex sought for." † There is never an absence of associations.‡ But the patient often keeps silent or represses his associations as they appear, the former under neurotic compulsion. Of this, we shall speak later. To each association, one has one or more others given, according to need, which can be considered singly or in groups (constellations) until one has sufficient material to be able to approach the interpretation.

The procedure in dream-analysis is similar. Preferably, one has the dream repeated a second time and notes the deviations because they indicate the points of strongest repression, the seats of the critical secrets, that is, when we are not dealing with a mere matter of style. Now we can proceed in various ways. The sequence does not matter. Stekel first asks the dreamer what the dream brings to mind. If the beginner answers, "Nothing at all," Stekel asks further, of what actual experience the dream may recall, whereupon, most patients tell of an event which appears in the dream changed and falsified. Or he ascertains what significance this or that person acting in the dream may have for the life of the dreamer.||

* Freud, Studien, p. 234.   ‡ Same, p. 31.
† Freud, Über Psa. p. 30. || Stekel, Sprache d. T. p. 513 f.

Often, one names the part of the dream which is most striking and proceeds farther from that. Or one has the dream considered bit by bit and uses these parts as instigators for other associations. If one gets little or nothing from an idea, he can come back to it later. Many a dream fragment reveals its secret only when one has dissected it into separate characteristics. Hence one has the manifestation described very clearly and in detail.

Soon, it will be seen that a number of associations to the dream fragment point to one latent dream thought. If further associations follow, one holds back with his assumption for awhile and also does not betray his surmise by any gesture and allows further material to accumulate until a view of the whole dream or of an essential part of the dream-content can be gained. Much which is still obscure, becomes elucidated by the discovered meaning. New associations are gathered and thus one gains first an interpretation which exhausts one dream stratum. We know now, however, that overdetermina- tions are always possible. One tries to determine by obtaining further reactions whether a deeper meaning may not be conceivable, for example, an erotic meaning behind a religious one. Every interpretation allows the entrance into consciousness of other unconscious ideas in case the conductibility has not been previously exhausted. If one wishes from theoretical reasons to penetrate deeper, then in the next session, he turns back to the object. Still, it is more to the interest of the patient to decipher the new dream, so far as it reveals its secret, since the unexplored remnant returns with infallible certainty in this or that disguise when one needs it.

During the analysis, whether it proceeds by free rapport or by stepwise treatment of individual contents of the manifestation, one pays attention to the complex-indicators which we described in discussing the association experiment (page 335). The whole analysis is indeed only an extended association experiment. One pays particular attention to physical reactions, for example, blushing, twitching, twisting around, and also to mental ones, as omissions, misunderstandings, transferring attention to some object in the surroundings or to a distant idea which is at once analyzed again. This jumping to an object which apparently does not belong to the subject at hand, in particular affords the analysis excellent stopping points. Further, lingering long over the same object (perseveration) is a valuable indication.

If the conversation lags, we can have the patient make up phantasies, fictions, sequences, general impressions, etc.

One should allow the patient to discover the interpretation as much as possible by himself. He thus obtains earlier the feeling of security and rejoices in his discovery. One thus prepares him better for subsequent autoanalysis and self-education.

Falsifications of memory, for example, chronological errors, should be noted carefully and analyzed.* Conscious untruths should not be censured, otherwise the resistance is aroused. One simply gives the patient to understand that one sees through them readily and considers them as a resistance-symptom which injures the patient. Many persons who are liars at the beginning of the analysis, prove later to be highly honorable and agreeable patients, while many others who are frank at first, suddenly erect a barrier and wish to fortify themselves behind it. Those who are liars because of moral deficiency, cannot in general, be deeply analyzed.

In certain systems of manifest contents, it is often impossible to decide which interpretation is correct and most important (see page 361).

On page 181, I described the hysteria of a girl who suffered from severe fatigue, convulsions of laughing and weeping, as well as pathological dislike for touching wool and silk. I beg the reader to imagine that episode, the death of the little brother who snatched an object from our hysterical patient and in so doing, fell into a tub of hot water, so that the reader may share in the interpretation of the following fragment of analysis:

[Wool.] "Wool bites. I could never put on woolen stock-

* Freud, Kl. Schriften I, p. 220.

ir.gs. I wept when I had to put them on. This peculiarity I had from a little child, like many children."

[Wool.] "Disagreeable, thick. When one's nails are freshly cut, it clings to them." (End of the session. Next time:)

[Wool.] "It is always so hot in it, in stockings and dresses." (The father entered and gave information. Next session:)

[Wool.] "I cannot wear it, not touch it. It is rather because of the dress." (Ambiguous.) [Little dress.] "Small. I mean rather a child's dress such as quite small children wear."

[Imagine one.] "Yes. It is white. I do not know whether it belongs to a boy or a girl." [White, small child's dress.*] "I see one before me on a body. I see no head, however. I see the dress lying down. On the same body are gray stockings."

[The body.] "Yes, it would be horribly unpleasant if it were wet. If it were so tightly wrapped in swaddling clothes and woolen things. It would be hot."

[Thus you phantasy the body of a little child lying with small white dress, the head invisible, and you imagine: if it were wet, hot and tightly wrapped; now?] ˙ (Long pause.) "Nothing. Perhaps I was once so." [May there not be another bit of reality, this wet, tightly dressed, hot little body?] "You certainly mean my little brother but I do not think so. The little body which I see, is much smaller and younger."

[Have you had this phantasy long?] "No, only to-day. No, also at the last hour when you said wool."

[Where is the child?] "On a table. I was told once that when quite a small child, I rolled from a table but was not hurt. At that time, I probably had on a little dress and swaddling clothes like the child that I imagine. Perhaps I rolled off by myself because I was thick, perhaps someone gave me a push. Perhaps father had to lay me down to dry me and did not attend to me properly in so doing."

---

* If a manifest object is described more precisely, one has the newly given characteristics apperceived.

The mother confirmed later that they had to dress the scalded little brother wet and wrap him up thickly. The daughter thinks she recalls this sight. On the day of the accident, the little boy did not wear woolen stockings.

It seems to me that without further experiences, according to our logical arrangement, all possible interpretations of this material are admissible.

With the "cathartic" forestage of psychoanalysis (Breuer), one might say, the tragic accident acted like a foreign body. The phantasy proved then something like this: it happened to the little brother only as to yourself. You too were allowed to fall. That is only fate.

Janet might assume under such circumstances, so far as he considers a counter-suggestion as healing, "Your little brother was not dead, he only lay there like yourself."

In accordance with a later expression of Freud's, one may speak of a withholding of affect, but our little patient showed no sorrow over the fatal accident, while the somnambulistic repetition of the scene in the laundry, like the convulsions, betrays the powerful impression.

One might, if one knew no other facts, think with Stekel of repression of primary hate. If one notes that the girl is jealous of her celebrated sister and her favored brother, then the most superficial interpretation runs something like this: "May it go with me as punishment for my hate and my impious joy as with the unfortunate brother! I was indeed once near to it!" With this interpretation agrees the fatigue which always symbolizes, where it is psychogenic, being tired of love, thus being tired of life. Freud confirms the finding that in apathy, love and hate often inhibit each other.*

Adler too would be in a position to see his theory of the neurosis as a result of a complex of inferiority organically conditioned, confirmed in this case. The girl actually felt helpless against her brother and let him have everything without the slightest resistance. Later, she considered herself dis-

* Freud, Bemerkungen ü. e. Fall v. Zwangsneurose. Jahrb. I, p. 415.
Pfister, Analyt. Unters. ü. Hass u. Versöhnung, p. 46.

agreeable and in so doing, did herself an injustice. By the fear of contact, she secured herself against the violent torment of the memory of the creature who made the most of his weakness, regardless of everything and compelled tenderness, since that little brother on account of nervous (epileptic?) phenomena, enjoyed special attention.

Freud could find his "nuclear complex," the "family romance" corroborated. For the little brother did actually block the way to the parents' love. Therewith, the "incestuous root" would be unearthed.

Jung would be in a position to consider the phantasy figure as libido-symbol: The patient wishes to assert herself in reality by sacrificing herself as a little child, i. e. her infantilism.

At the time of the analysis of this case, I was just making the acquaintance of Freud and expected the cure from "abreaction," from the affect-laden conversation. Nevertheless, I did not neglect to emphasize strongly the error of the feeling of inferiority conditioned on infantilism, the possession of abundant love on the side of excellent parents and the right, as well as the possibility, of making herself properly efficient. Thus I made good in part as consoling and counseling pastor what I lacked as analyst. At all events, the phobia disappeared from that hour and the other symptoms were soon overcome.

I would call attention here to the fact that cure does not guarantee the correctness of the analysis, as the results of various interpreters and places of pilgrimage and charlatans testify. This fact has been emphasized from remotest times.

The reader will see from our example how difficult it is, under certain circumstances, to obtain absolutely reliable interpretations or to take a position in the successive theses of the leaders of analysis.

In consolation, one may point out that not everything depends on the particular interpretation. The unsolved conflict manifests itself again and again and gives occasion for correction. It often happens that an uninterpreted symbol keeps reappearing with obstinate persistency until the right explanation succeeds and a better outlet for the life-force is found.

CHAPTER XV

SUPPLEMENTARY METHODS

1. EXTERNAL AIDS

In the beginning, Freud made use of a little artifice when the flow of associations stopped, which he later abandoned: he assured the patient that the memory which would come at the moment he laid his hand on his brow would be the right one.* He gave up this tedious method, however. I attempted to coax out an association by promising that it would come immediately after I had counted three, since actual touching the patient, because of the transference to be discussed later, seemed to me from the beginning to work unfavorably. This forcing also is superfluous. There are better means of overcoming the resistance.

Even to-day, Freud and other analysts, chiefly for reasons of quietness, have the patient lie on a couch and seat themselves at the patient's head in order not to be seen. Freud asserts in recommending this method: it has historic meaning as a remnant of the hypnotic treatment, from which, psychoanalysis developed, it spares the analyst the tiresome condition of being stared at, it guards the patient against the danger of interpreting the mien of his analyst.† Stekel and many others have given up this practice and offer the visitor a chair or armchair. I have even analyzed pupils with great success while walking with them, since facts sprang up which would have been sought in vain in a room. For the pedagogues, having the pupil seated is decidedly the method of choice.‡ The recum-

* Freud, Ü. Psa., p. 19.
† Freud, Weitere Ratschläge zur Technik der Psychoanalyse. Internat. Zschr. f. ärztl. Psa. I, p. 10.
‡ In connection with Freud's arguments, it should be noted: A mere historical memento of the hypnotic period has no great value. For a

bent position produces anxiousness and phantasies in many patients which must first be overcome. Girls are embarrassed and are afraid to lie on the sofa before their teacher even when they do it unhesitatingly before their physician. Most of them feel themselves placed in a subservient, helpless position. Sexual phantasies are easily aroused. Very important for the decision is the rôle which one imputes to the analyst for the educational process. Hence, I am of the opinion: the natural conversational position, in which one sees every movement best, is probably the one most to be recommended to pedagogues.

2. HYPNOSIS

Forel, Frank* and other psychiatrists who agree with the analysis in the main, find fault because hypnosis has been given up. I cannot accept this view for the following reasons:

1. Hypnosis is not successful in all cases. Freud, himself a master of the technique, whose appreciation went so far that he translated into German † two works of his teacher, Bernheim, calls it "a capricious and as one might say, mystical aid." ‡

2. Hypnosis does not penetrate as deeply by far as a correct psychoanalytic treatment in the waking state. He who compares the analyses of Frank with those of Freud, Ferenczi, Rank, Jung, Riklin, Maeder and other real analysts, sees at once that the former is satisfied with an entirely superficial analysis. This may suffice for the lighter cases but is insufficient for severe ones.

3. Hypnosis penetrates only to the symptom while psycho-

great number of analysts, being-stared-at is not in the least disagreeable, as little as in daily conversation. The actual expression of the analyst who knows how to control himself, is less disturbing than the artificial ones. As it is not the real father but the father-image which injures, so with the analyst and the image of him created by the patient's wishes under certain circumstances.

* L. Frank, Die Psychoanalyse, Munich, 1909.

† H. Bernheim, Die Suggestion u. i. Heilwirkung. Further: Neue Studien ü. Hypnotismus, Suggestion u. Psychotherapie. Both from the press of Deuticke, Leipzig and Vienna.

‡ Freud, Ü. Psa., p. 18.

analysis aims at a thorough educational work which makes all restricted life-energy available for ethical purposes. For us pedagogues, the pathological symptom is often a matter of secondary importance. We recognize a hundredfold that it is great good fortune for a person when he is afflicted with a malady which compels him to search out the deeper-lying inner conflict which muddles his whole attitude toward life and duty and to relieve it in the sense of an ethical, often religious, solution. This noblest gain is largely lost in hypnosis which aims at an external result. The deep, inner dissension remains, nevertheless, and often creates new, perhaps worse, disturbances which may however, escape the attention of the physician but are therefore so much the more important for the educator and pastor. Especially for autoanalysis and self-education as a whole, the follower of the cathartic method with his hypnosis accomplishes far less than the psychoanalyst.

4.   The results of hypnosis are also less permanent than those of psychoanalysis.

5.   The analytic physicians also practice hypnosis, probably even to-day, and indeed often the light hypnosis recommended by Frank * as well as occasionally, the deeper. Thus, they have the best opportunity to make comparisons. On the basis of their numerous experiences, they apply hypnosis only to those individuals whose mental level, judged less in regard to knowledge than to insight, is not high enough for analysis, or where the time for proper analysis is lacking, but they do not conceal the fact that the result is far less thorough and permanent. If they could attain the goal by the shorter way of hypnosis, they would do so gladly, but as a matter of fact, they obtain by following Forel's and Frank's recommendations only such superficial analyses as these investigators themselves, and in the interest of their patients, cannot and will not be satisfied with these.

* Frank, Psa. p. 20. Since Frank emphasizes that this light grade of hypnotism distinguishes him from Breuer and Freud, it should be pointed out that these too expressly apply the "light hypnosis" (Studien 14).

Hence I consider the hypnotic position, which for the rest holds the "abreaction of affects" as the vital point, as out of date, although it can certainly do much good in practice, but in scientific investigation, much less. At all events, we teachers, out of consideration for our internal and external competence, (medical law) will not meddle with hypnosis.

3. SUGGESTION

(A) PAUL DUBOIS

It is well known that Paul Dubois, neurologist of the University of Berne, has produced the valuable proof that many organic maladies and most nervous attacks depend on mental stimuli.* According to him, therapy depends on the law: "The nervous patient is on the way to health as soon as he has the conviction that he can be cured; he is to be considered as cured on the day when he thinks himself cured.† The means for attaining this "fixed idea" are fairly indifferent: religious faith, suggestion by charlatans, suggestion by medicaments and physical agencies, scientific psychotherapy by the education of reason, all help if they bring about that fixed idea.‡ Religious faith would be the strongest prophylactic against the diseases mentioned if it occasioned a true Christlike Stoicism (202). Rational psychotherapy applies itself simply to the healthy human intelligence of the subject.|| One must know how to become master of the patient at a stroke and really inoculate him with the fixed idea that he will be healed.¶ Everything depends on the power of the conviction.§

A simpler method than this suggestive taking possession and persuasion is scarcely conceivable. The search for causes disappears: the physician works according to the same prin-

---

* P. Dubois, Die Psychoneurosen u. i. psych. Behandlg. Bern, 1905, p. 101.
† Same, p. 202.
‡ Same, p. 202.
|| Same, p. 214.
¶ Same, p. 223.
§ Same, p. 427.

ciple as the charlatan and Christian Science healer, the Zionist or Mormon sects, except that the former appeals more to healthy reason. In this concurrence, the poor physician plainly often shows up to disadvantage, since, "the healthy human reason" in the majority of people is by no means the strongest power. Those individuals of weaker intellectual gifts would do better, according to Dubois, in their nervous troubles to go direct to charlatans and religious therapeutists, many of whom are given to a miserable swindling, indeed it would prove the fraudulent advertising, on account of its suggestive effect, to be an actual benefit.

No one can deny the results of suggestion. Every Christian, Buddhist and Mahommedan place of pilgrimage, every priest of fetichism and quack afford proof in abundance. But behold the reverse side:

1. In the application of suggestion, one experiences many relapses. "Only too often are the symptoms banished for only a short time, the suffering likewise glossed over." * These experiences which soon bring so many wonder-workers and shrines into discredit when they are not kept silent, may also be read in Jesus' words: Mat. xii, 43–45, "When the unclean spirit is gone out of a man . . . and when he is come . . . then goeth he and taketh with himself seven other spirits more wicked than himself . . . and the last state of that man is worse than the first."

2. Many troubles which cannot be cured by the method of Dubois and religious therapy may be overcome with analytic aid. Not a single victim of obsessional neurosis could Dubois cure, only a decided improvement could he obtain (429), while I have observed a long list of cures by pedagogic analysis of this highly interesting and often frightful malady. Further, patients who have gone away uncured from recognized Christian healers in spite of strongest effort, I have seen healed by analysis.

3. The application of the Dubois method is very painful to

* J. J. Putnam, Ü. Aetiol. u. Behandlg. d. Psychoneurosen, Zbl. I, p. 140.

teacher and pupil during its duration. The monotonous assertion of the psychotherapeutist by authority becomes, in the face of maladies countless times persisting unchanged, farce and torture. The results are moderate. Beside the method of Dubois, always driving at the same "fixed idea," the analytic method is as a rule exceedingly mild.* My experiences after all kinds of disappointments (I practised Dubois' method as convinced adherent) have made me very reserved toward the practice.

4. Dubois proceeds to attack only the symptom and a single condition, which is usually not present in reality at all, namely, a false theory concerning the nature of nervous maladies, while analysis seeks the actual seat of the trouble.† I shall not enter upon the astoundingly one-sided rationalistic psychology of Dubois.

5. The assertion that the psychoneurotic malady is removed by the belief in the possibility of being cured, is absolutely incorrect. With the strongest faith, we often see the disease persist, while with psychoanalysis, we often see a cure result in doubting individuals.

6. The stoicism recommended by Dubois, with its tendency toward introversion, signifies usually a bad canalization of instinct. Above we saw stoicism as symptom and cause of disease (93).

The suggestive suppression of a symptom under threats and punishments is obviously dangerous in the highest degree. A mother told me triumphantly that she had driven out by sternness a nervous tic (twitching of the face) in her daughter. Forthwith, three new ones appeared.

---

* The assertion that psychoanalysis is painful, is not, according to my experience, true. Only clumsy boring and compelling acts painfully. Also the excitements come more at the beginning of the analysis. But he who will console, need not be disturbed by the fact that the telling of the causes of suffering causes excitement. Almost always, the analysis brings either immediately or after the first hours, relief.

† Dubois leaves the causal need of the normal psychologist entirely unsatisfied. He does not once hint what the meaning may be when a patient with obsessional neurosis will not venture to stick his hand into his portemonnaie (p. 427) etc.

(B) SUGGESTION IN PSYCHOANALYSIS

(*a*) Unintentional Suggestion.

Obviously, the psychoanalyst cannot exclude sugestion.* Profession, examination, preconceived opinion already suggest. It is known how powerfully the consultation-room of the dentist works in this direction.

(β) Intentional Suggestion.

1. In the preliminary stage of the actual analysis (the constellation). That the attitude belongs to the fundamental rules of analysis has been shown.

2. In the actual analytic procedure. Here the suggestion cannot be too carefully avoided by tone and gesture, particularly also the autosuggestion. One must also guard against the theoretical instruction which one must give, dictating the associations, since the consideration for these instructions, the expectation of their coming true or the hope of their proving false, influence the direction of the associations. The sharper the patient has his attention fixed on his manifestation or his free rapport, so much the more surely does this foreign suggestion recede.

3. In the synthetic part of the analytic procedure. Freud considers it proper for the educator to give suggestions intentionally and consciously to point out life-paths and invite to the following of these. He should not compel, however, but rather allow the love of the pupil (transference) to act.† How this suggestion has to work in the new canalization of the instinct will be shown later.

Nevertheless the analysis is differentiated from the suggestion technique by the avoidance of strong pressure. It merely coaxes and invites. Herein it is an exact contrast to Dubois. How often does one experience that a symptom disappears without the slightest persuasion, while before, it persisted against all pressure in spite of strong faith. This is particularly important for moral improvement. That which cannot

* Bleuler, Jahrb. II, p. 642.
† Freud, Z. Dynamik d. Übertragung. Zbl. II, p. 172.

be attained by rack and thumbscrew, since a neurotic obsession exists, psychoanalysis often attains without any violence and self-torture.

(C) DUBOIS AND FREUD

(α) In comparison with the Old and New Testaments (Law and Gospels).

Dubois endeavors to force a fixed idea. For many individuals, the forced belief means a heavy burden. The impulses forcibly given signify a new "Thou shalt." Inversely, Freud wishes to take away a burden already present. Dubois shovels coal into the furnace of the leaky steam-boat which is half filled with water; Freud plugs the hole and pumps the water out. Then it can be seen whether coal is still needed.

Dubois represents the pedagogy of the Old Testament, Freud, that of the New. There: "Thou shalt!" here: "Thou mayest!" There, new demand, here, salvation. There, command, here, love.

(β) In their Relation to Buddhism and Christianity.

Dubois lays great stress on renunciations: "The stoicism, if it would really lead to health, cannot rest on mere auto-suggestion . . . rather it must be founded on the enduring fundamental propositions of philosophy which can serve as plumb-line for the whole life." * Thus the renunciation of illusions is certainly necessary, hence stoicism certainly cannot be the final word. Jesus does not, like Buddha, recommend the cessation of thinking, feeling and volition but rather the maximal self-efficiency in the sense of sublimation, yet without the negation of the primary instinctive life. Now, Dubois is certainly far distant from Buddha's absolute introversion, but he stands decidedly nearer to it than psychoanalysis, to which, the most abundant instinctive activity in the sense of sublimation and an ethically valuable primary eroticism seem to be the right conceptions.

---

* Dubois, Psychon. p. 404. In his book, "Selbsterziehung," (Bern 1909), Dubois praises more the freeing from egoism (for example, pp. 107–120, 261, 267).

(γ) In their Positions toward Authority and Freedom.
While Dubois leads his medical authority into the field full tilt, Freud allows the patients to find the truth themselves as much as possible. The former holds his patients in the father-complex, the latter sets them free. The former wishes to free by a "fixed idea," the latter by re-education to have the patient find for himself the law of his own inner self and the best possible realization of his capabilities. So in this regard, the two men represent the difference between heteronomy and autonomy or between Catholicism and Protestantism. Thus, the beautiful word, self-education, has with Freud a much deeper significance than with Dubois: The man does not force and persuade himself to a larger life, he loves himself into it. Dubois points in the direction of resignation and asceticism, of autoeroticism, Freud in the direction of transference and sublimation, Jung quite similarly in that of the independent comprehension of the individual law of life, to the chief demands of which, love for others belongs.

4. THE DISLOCATION

In contrast to Dubois and most psychotherapeutists who provide for the patients in sanatoria, psychoanalysis leaves its pupils in their civic relations and at their work. Further, it places little emphasis on the diet. While many physicians wish to lead their patients to health by forced feeding and others by fasting and sometimes also succeed, Freud imposes only rational life-conduct. We know that even severe physical lassitude can arise from mental causes (181), as in other cases, it can arise from overwork or physical defects.

If bad relations exist at home, however, or an uncommonly strong father-, mother- or sister-complex prevails, then, removal from home facilitates the treatment, indeed it is often an actual prerequisite. I have repeatedly seen convalescence, rendered possible by the analysis, immediately appear after the patient's departure. Very often the meddling of foolish people forms an obstacle which must be met. Strong natures find the new adaptation to reality, the solution of the inner conflict, the actual utilization of the libido, even in very unfavorable relations.

The change of surroundings, often health-bringing for mentally ailing individuals, even without analysis, oftentimes assists the analytic work because it imposes a new attitude toward life. Still, it is usually superfluous.

In conclusion, it should be remarked again and emphasized that Freud does not at all mean to say that psychoanalysis is always and in all cases the only therapy possible or necessary.* On the contrary, he and probably everyone who has mastered this and the other methods, is of the opinion that "it acts most thoroughly, has the most far-reaching results and is the method by which one attains the most intensive changes in the patient.†

Obviously, psychoanalysis presupposes the previously known pedagogic methods and merely joins them in learning and teaching.

* E. Hitschmann, Freuds Neurosenlehre, Leipzig and Vienna 1911, p. 117 f.   Eng. translation in Monograph Series of the Journal of Nervous and Mental Disease, N. Y.   Freud, Ü. Psychotherapie, Kl. Schriften I, p. p. 211.

† Hitschmann, p. 118.

SECTION II

THE EFFECTS OF THE PSYCHOANALYTIC PROBING

CHAPTER XVI

THE ABREACTION

"WE found to our great surprise that the individual hysterical symptoms immediately disappeared, and that without return, when we had succeeded in awakening to full vividness the memory of the causative event, therewith also arousing the accompanying affect, and provided that the patient described the event in the most detailed manner possible and gave verbal expression to the affect." * With this sentence, Breuer and Freud describe in their first communication their method of treatment. In so doing, they proceeded on the assumption that the hysterical individuals suffer, in large part, from reminiscences which are pent-up in the unconscious like foreign bodies, because they are neither discharged by physical movements of expression nor in normal manner by associative elaboration. That which remains behind at that period, the analysis has to search out. It aids in this discharge, or as we say, in this "abreaction." †

The experiences of almost two decades have taught us, however, that this abreaction is not exactly correct, though the original assumption to-day still seems intelligible. In order to gain lucidity, we will proceed from our insight into the nature of the repression and fixation.

* Breuer und Freud, Studien, p. 4.
† Same, p. 13.

1. Necessity for the Abreaction

If an idea accompanied by strong emotion is repressed and fortified by its autistic gain of pleasure, the instinct to which this idea belongs, suffers, within a certain circle of activity, a damming up which often persists for a lifetime. One finds many elderly people who have possessed their hysteria, for example, vertigo, automatisms of the muscles of the jaw, astasia, etc., for decades. Freud makes a comparison from Jensen's "Gradiva" which illustrates this state of affairs beautifully: the repression, he says, resembles the burial of Pompeii.* That which was buried, remains unchanged under the thick covering. Upon excavation, it disintegrates. Thus the repressed material persists, the fixed instincts can develop no farther. The analysis first creates the possibility of freeing the imprisoned instinct. Frequently, however, neurotic symptoms disappear without analytic assistance. Of course this is far from saying that the attached force with its full contribution of energy has been conducted to a free life development. Rather, the repressed ideas persist or more correctly expressed, the instincts fixed at one place (the complex) by repression (negative) and automatism (positive) in their relative fixation, find new channels, under certain circumstances, highly valuable ones, in order to expend their energy.

Thus for example, a religious cure can eliminate the pathological phenomena. In this case, the demand of the instinct, which is in conflict with the internal and external forces, is sublimated. The retention of the repression is no longer necessary and possible because the demand of the instinct when sublimated, is satisfied.

Or the dammed-up instinct breaks a way into reality and knows how to enjoy itself there. Hysteria, resulting from burning desire without gratification, may be extinguished in marriage.

Or the repressing force may be released. The onanist finds that his spinal cord is not destroyed, the adulterer finds an

* Freud, Gradiva, p. 42.

easy peace of mind in the promise of good conduct. Since, according to our findings, the inner motives for repression and fixation are more important than the external ones, so the overcoming of the repressing force by pastoral instruction is to be named among the best methods making for mental health. Hence the indisputable results of the consoling Christian Science which combats anxiety, of the invoking of the saints and similar religious healing forces. Also the barrier which causes the forward-longing instinct to ever regress into infantilism may be surmounted by a moral venture, a strengthening of the ethical nature.

All these outcomes are possible, without the unconscious conditions having been previously transferred to consciousness. Proceeding from such experiences, many educators hope to get along without analysis and to eliminate the disturbance of morals, religion or health by simply opening new channels.

Whether this is possible cannot be decided by general theoretical construction but only by experience. I am constantly amazed anew at those numerous educators, neurologists and psychiatrists who, on the one hand, discuss with extreme modesty, indeed with evident resignation, the possibilities of their professional skill, but on the other hand, however, announce to the world with proud plerophoria that psychoanalysis may be dispensed with in all cases.

The facts decide. They afforded us the proof that a great number of patients whom previous methods, applied by recognized physicians and educators over long periods, had not helped, were cured by analysis.

Let us examine more closely the non-analytic release of pent-up life-instinct in patients and healthy individuals.

The religious cures have done good to countless individuals and made them happy, healthy, ethically valuable people. Where this end has been accomplished, no unprejudiced educator, pastor or physician will urge analysis. But do we not see among the personalities who have caused the needs of their complexes to flow into religious channels, besides great phenomena, an immense number of troubles and· moral defects?

Innumerable monks and nuns suffer from severe hysteria, obsessional neurosis or other tortures. Countless strictly religious men and women get into awful sadism and masochism so that the history of religion drips with blood. One needs think only of the burning of witches, persecutions of heretics, wars over faith, self-torture even to suicide (for example, Saint Elizabeth) in which the repressed material ever emerged in the center of piety, the ghastly deed was performed in the name of God! Countless persons come to foolish, immoral, bizarre ideas, to orthodox and ceremonial fanaticism, in which the life-instinct is wasted in immoral, unproductive manner in automatism. Countless more fall to a great narrowing of the mental horizon, other multitudes to a weak flight from the world, a cowardly, inefficient attitude toward the future life which leaves this one desolate. Religion, grand and wonderful as it stands before us in its pure form, often changes, according to the testimony of history, from a benefactress to a seducer and instigator of grievous injustice. The position of Jesus toward marriage, toward neighbors, toward self-love show that he denied the investing of all love in God. If you will do God the highest honor, love thy neighbor as thyself. This is His profound conception of the destiny of the life-instinct.

Much less still, can the direct discharge of the instinct in sensuous activity save people. Freud expressly proves that the psychosexual is the most important.* He affords the proof that the highest mental powers participate in sexuality and seek gratification in it. He has shown the eminently moral character of the sexual life and the relatively subordinate importance of the animalistic side of it in a manner to cause every unprejudiced ethicist to rejoice, even though other thoughts of Freud cannot find so much approbation.

In general, the change in the life-relationships can happen so favorably that the life-instinct ventures out of its subterranean hiding place into the life struggle. But who would wait for this dispensation coming from without? Is it not

* Freud, Ü. "wilde" Psa. Zbl. I, p. 92 ff.

wiser to put the person in a position to frame a useful life with the means at his disposal?

Finally, the wisest religious and moral pastoral training is not sufficient in severe cases. Indeed Jesus recognized this fact as mentioned on page 440, and he who knows the foundations of health perceives that it must be so. The skilled analyst is far superior to the best non-analytic pastoral instructor against many manifestations. If he is strongly religious and has an energetic religious person to deal with, a pure, healthy piety will probably be the end result of the treatment while much morbid religious fanaticism must fall by the way.

The ethical and religious demands, the admonition, punishment, reward, instruction concerning the results of the action, etc., are nevertheless entirely ineffective when an inner fixation exists, to release the instinct. If one speaks to certain victims of the obsessional neurosis, who suffer from a feeling of guilt, of God's grace and forgiveness, one acts like a child which would wish away the spots of light on the wall instead of removing the source of the light. The conscious guilt is not at all the real one (compare above, page 75 pathological lying, page 76 kleptomania). Or if one wishes to convert with Bible and reason a person who wants to transfer to a bizarre, immoral sect, one usually accomplishes little because the actual forces acting in that piousness lie below the threshold of consciousness. I have seen many persons who strained every nerve to free themselves from moral defects by means of ascetic practices, repentance and prayer, accomplish nothing except doubt, pathological crippling of the will (abulia) or strengthening of the vice. Analysis brought them salvation without compulsion and torture.

Therefore, for a great number of moral, religious and hygienic defects, psychoanalysis is not only the surest, shortest and relatively pleasantest method of treatment but indeed the only possible and hence imperative one (compare chapter 26).

2. THE PROCESS OF ABREACTION

(a) The abreaction as outlet by expressive movement and associative connection.

The results which the abreaction is meant to accomplish, the telling to other persons, has been warmly recommended from antiquity by people who understood human nature. Not only the New Testament and Catholic confessional but also certain great poets have so treated it. Shakespeare (Macbeth V-1) testifies as we heard:

> "Unnatural deeds
> Do breed unnatural troubles: infected minds
> To their deaf pillows will discharge their secrets:
> More needs she the divine than the physician."

Goethe says:

> "The disease of the mind
> Most easily resolves into complaints and confidences." *

To Frau von Stein, he writes on Sept. 25, 1811: "Yesterday evening I did a very clever feat. Herder was all the time strained to the most hypochondriacal state over everything unpleasant which had happened to her in Carlsbad. I had her tell and confess to me everything improper in others and herself with most minute details and results and finally I absolved her and made her cheerful, comprehensible under the formula that these things were now done with and thrown into the depths of the sea. She became very gay over it and is actually cured." †

In his religio-psychological romance, "Theobald oder die Schwärmer," ‡ which is highly interesting, Goethe's friend Jung, called Stilling, describes the cure of a melancholic hysterical person. The pastor Bosius converses with the patient in uncommonly sympathetic manner and guides her to the con-

---

* Goethe, Tasso, III, p. 2.
† From Stekel, Angstzustände, p. 7.
‡ Heinrich Stillung,. Theobald oder die Schwärmer. Frankf. and Leipzig, 1802, I, p. 259 ff.

ception that love is the supreme end of nature. "Everything loves in the order in which the Creator has placed it." "Are you not stirred by the fact that the Eternal Love pours love into all creation? What do you understand by the word, love?" The patient answers: "Impelling force (instinct) to union, to be one with the beloved." The pastor continues: "You feel, deep in your soul, the instinct for union with something which you love; obstacles which stand in the way of your love make you shut-off because you consider them insurmountable; hence you are melancholic."* He expresses fundamentally the whole situation, lets the girl open her heart, cleverly defends the rights of sensuality, as well as the sublime significance of marriage and helps her to obtain the beloved.†

We find similar confessional efforts in the writings of

* Same, p. 264.

† Jung-Stilling has the correct insight into the nature of hysteria. He has his pastor say: "Your (the patient's) weak body is not strong enough to bear the passion which burns in your soul, the imagination busies itself unceasingly with the beloved object, you may struggle against it as you will, thereby the feeling only increases. . . . When the feelings mount higher than the nervous system, already weakened apart from this by many pious ideas, can bear, then a fever must result. As soon, however, as there is a fever, the cause of which, as in this case, can be removed by no other medicine than the gratification of the love, then the symptoms of the fever ever continue, these again have their results and thus the malady becomes ever more complex. . . . A girl is held back by shame from speaking of that which principally engrosses her mind, namely of her beloved, the longing for him remains ever deeply hidden; he who does not know of this circumstance, and also does not recognize the cause, never guesses the cause, the physician says: the person is hysterical, that is about the same as saying, she is sick—something which everyone sees. Now the cause of this illness lies in the imagination, something which borders nearest to the nerves; because of shame, this cause never comes to light, on the other hand, the other ideas which in good and pious girls, ordinarily concern religion, reveal themselves so much the stronger; now the external senses are very weak because the nerves are weak, while on the other hand, the internal senses or the imagination are so much the stronger, so much the more lively—what is the result? Dreams—and indeed of a particular kind. . . ." (There follows a corresponding theory of hallucination and religious ecstasy.) "You see that the feelings of love are the whole cause of these supposedly heavenly revelations." I, 290–292).

Justinus Kerner * and of Pastor Blumhardt, father and son, in "Bad Boll." †

Bismarck writes: "It is laudable and praiseworthy to break one's self of useless or injurious outbreaks of feeling, or to give them another more acceptable form, but I call it self-compulsion which makes one ill within, when one stifles his feelings within himself."

Before Freud, however, attention was fixed almost wholly on the conscious painful material. Only gifted students of the mind like Jung-Stilling, penetrated deeper. The Catholic confessional is, moreover, one-sided in other respects: It fixes its attention on the guilt instead of also taking into consideration the suffering. It makes the confessional compulsory and leads to punishment by the Church; thereby, the resistance against the disclosure of the unconscious material is powerfully strengthened. It is satisfied with cursory examination instead of carefully seeking the circumstances which led to the origin of the evil. And yet it does untold good while the Protestant pastoral instruction, which is in a far more favorable position, stands hesitating in the midst of wickedness. When I have had unhappy people confide in me, their hearts overflowing with need, I have been reproached that this was a regression to Catholicism! For the evangelical pastor, the aim in question is not a cultistic servitude to the confessional as a means of supernatural grace, but an ethical, hence really God-pleasing, purification purpose and hygienic process which will gain a great amount of inhibited forces for the affairs of God and therewith for the affairs of men. In this sense, the teacher must also be religious instructor and who denies that there have always been spiritually-minded educators? ‡

The follower of the cathartic method and the psychoanalyst go a step farther still by exposing the unconscious to the light

---

* H. Silberer, U. d. Behandlung einer Psychose bei Justinus Kerner. Jahrb. III, p. 725 ff.

† A. Muthmann, Psychiatrisch-theologische Grenzfragen. Zschr. f. Rel-psych. I, p. 136 ff.

‡ In this direction, psychoanalysis is only a scientific refinement of a method practiced intuitively.

of consciousness. By so doing, they obtain a series of new results which would have been impossible before.

To-day, however, no experienced physician and educator doubts that merely with the full expression in words, even though accompanied by tears and affects, the healing of the trouble caused by fixation is not always accomplished. One symptom very deeply analyzed may persist unchanged, while another one disappears upon superficial exploration, even without analysis. Thus, there must be still other forces acting besides the associative outpouring.

(b) The abreaction as mental outcropping of the unconscious.

The analysis penetrates into the depths and discovers the mole which throws up its piles of earth on the surface. It shows not only the latent thoughts but also the repressing thoughts, the original instinctive tendency as well as the opposing tendency arising from within or without. Now we know that the symptom was a means for concealing the unconscious thoughts and at the same time for giving them some measure of expression. Thus, we shall expect that the unmasked symptom will disappear like a developed but unfixed photographic negative in the daylight. An associative connection is simultaneously joined to the mental outcropping. Thus with the becoming conscious and acceptance of the analytic interpretation, the manifestation will have to fade, somewhat like life according to Uhland's saying:

> "He who sees only truth, has lived to the end,
> Life is like the stage, there as here,
> When the illusion fades, the curtain must fall."

As a fact, we see a multitude of simple and gravely severe signs of disease disappear as soon as they have lost their incognito, as a thief disappears from the field of the camera as quickly as possible when he knows that he is recognized.

Why may other symptoms remain? One might assume that there were still deeper overdeterminants than those discovered. This view is irrefutable for one can never pursue a symptom to the absolute beginnings of all the threads in its enormously ramified network. Every analysis is incomplete. Thus one might conceive of an inner fixation from past causes. But as often as we carefully investigate a symptom, we also find present causes, according to Freud, the foremost are the striving for avoidance of discomfort and the resistance against the analyst who is unconsciously identified with the father, according to Adler, a tendency toward assurance, according to Jung, resistance against fulfillment of duty connected with the sacrifice of precious infantilism, according to all three men, fear of reality. The neurotic individual knows what he has in his automatism but he does not know what may happen from the abandonment of it. Fear of the unknown constantly drives him back into the regression. Hence he represses with astounding force the results gained by analysis, forgets them, throws suspicion on them with miserable rationalizations and incorporates new phantasies in the symptom. He acts like an invited guest who brings forward a thousand excuses in order to remain at home. Under some circumstances, he creates new symptoms, or, and this is the most fatal, he withdraws still deeper into his complexes. The latter can occur particularly in dementia præcox. Where the isolation from the outer world increases, the educator is under obligations to call the psychiatrist into consultation at once.

With the pure analysis, the end is not at once attained. Freud remarks: "It is a conception long ago exploded and dependent on most superficial appearances that the patient suffers from a kind of ignorance and that when one removes this ignorance by communication (concerning the causal connections of his malady with his suffering, concerning his childhood experiences, etc.) he must become well. This ignorance is not in itself the pathogenic agency but the foundation of ignorance in inner resistances which have first occasioned the ignorance and still maintain it." * Analysis shows where the instinct is attached and thereby renders possible its release. It resembles the sword of the prince which cuts through the

* Freud, Ü. "wilde" Psa. Zbl. I, p. 94.

hedge surrounding the castle of the Sleeping Beauty. But the liberating force is still lacking. The analysis shows whither the attack should be directed, it performs scouting service but it does not at once drive out the enemy. In what direction the life-instinct will apply itself, that is the great question, upon which the relief of the inhibition of the instinct depends. That this fact was not visible at first, is due to the circumstance of the fortunate, spontaneous new canalization of the life-instinct in the cases observed at that period.

Generally, one allows the patient to say as much as he wishes. The more he produces, the better. And if he speaks ever so meanly of his father, ever so vulgarly of God, women or of any subject, one quietly allows him to proceed. The dirty stuff should be abreacted, at all events, it should be told to the educator as much as possible. The physician has the most disgusting stomach-contents emptied out by vomiting. Jesus says: "Judge not that ye be not judged" (Mat. vii, 1). These words, the analyst should keep in mind, for he knows that the evil impulses of the unconscious are everywhere present in greater or less degree and that many high and noble powers make their appearance when these can be utilized.*

* He who believes that psychoanalysis reveals only the bête humaine in men, is greatly in error. Freud has shown in the capacity of men for sublimation, how far man transcends the lower animals. The dark background of the instinct is not the whole man. The countless illnesses from moral conflicts (fundamentally, all neuroses are the results of ethical complications) show that the ethical trend belongs to the fundamental tendencies of the human soul.

CHAPTER XVII

COMPENSATION, RECASTING OF THE COMPLEX AND TRANSFERENCE

WE háve perceived before that analysis opens the cell of the prisoner. That he leaves the cell, analysis does not vouch for. Some have become so accustomed to prison life that it would be too unpleasant to venture out into reality. Their will to health, the indispensable condition to the overcoming of the inhibition, is too small to exert a counter-pressure against the complex. They like to remain in infantilism. They submit to automatism according to the principle of the least expenditure of effort. They disclose the fact that even severe neurotic suffering affords a certain, even though unpleasant, protective measure against moral demands and mental needs and they would escape the hard struggle for the ethical life content. What the educator has to initiate in such pupils, for example, lazy or rebellious boys who vent their hatred of their fathers upon the teacher, the second chapter following (19) will show. For the time being, we have to deal only with the changes which the analytic probing brings about.

1. COMPENSATION

The life-instinct, frightened by external or internal changes (not merely by the analysis), seeks a substitute manifestation. If the repulsion which proceeds from the humdrum uniformity of life is too severe in denial or too unpleasant, if further, the attraction by pleasurable relations, partially or wholly unconscious, is too powerful, then a neurotic symptom arises, in which, perhaps, one can hardly perceive its near relationship to the antecedent conditions. We have already shown a number of such symptom-formations appearing during the analysis or independently of it.

(Clucking, itching of the scalp, skin eruption 33f, tearing the skin on the thumb, eating carrots, playing the violin 215).

A particularly fine example may be added: The youth mentioned on pages 90 and 331 showed in the first two analytic sessions the following changing forms in his writing cramp occuring immediately during the analysis:

1. Strong tension of the hand, fourth and fifth fingers anesthetic. Motive:, The hysterical youth, because of inner conflicts (negative father-complex, fetichism) cannot "fulfill" his external duties. The cramp creates an excuse. The writing teacher, a specialist for writer's cramp, advised him to correct the faulty position of the hand by India rubber bands which were placed about the last two fingers. Thereupon the fingers went to sleep. The wished-for emancipation from sexual desire is symbolically expressed.

2. Only the thumb suffers from tension. Pretended motive: "If the rubber rings are removed, I still remain inhibited."

3. Automatic drawing back of the fourth and fifth fingers. Motive: "I fall back into the old fetters and am retired."

4. Fatigue of both hands: Motive: Tired of life.

5. Weak tension, pronounced sweating of the two last fingers. Motive: "Though I sweat from endeavor, I do not escape the enfeeblement. I sweat as soon as I have to speak with a lady, I accomplish nothing."

6. Feeling that the bones of the hand, particularly those of the middle finger, are broken. Latent thought: "If I am a broken man, nothing can be expected of me."

7. The whole arm is drawn backwards, hand normal. Motive: "What help is it to become free in one place if the whole person is inhibited?"

8. Tension in only one joint of hand which is pressed towards the right. Latent cramp thought: "You were shoved aside."

9. The same tension with sweating. Association: "The position of my hand is faulty, that throws me into anxiety."

10. Contracture of the hand toward the left. Motive: "If I am not repudiated on one side, I am on the other."

11. Tension in the middle of the hand up to the elbow.

Motive: "The inner inhibition remains, even though I am shoved neither toward left nor right."

The subsequent test of the writing turned out exactly the same. One sees that the analysis of symptoms, in severe cases, accomplishes nothing so far as the complex is not hit in the center and the resistance lowered. We find plainly the phenomenon of compensation and recall that we also found above (90) spontaneous change of symptoms in writer's cramp resulting from changes in the unconscious wishes at the moment of symptom-formation.

The forms of the compensations are very manifold. Each manifestation can be considered as such. Ferenczi has collected a pretty group of rapidly interchanging substitute formations occasioned by analysis.*

Many of these formations are new additions of symptoms previously present, many, quite new. Many have come by paths of inner association, many by those of outer ones.

The law of compensation applies also to normal individuals. A drinker is to be considered as cured only when he has found a substitute of similar or superior value, for example, religion, friendship, music, authority, family life. Also for the onanist, a superior value must be made accessible. Without such an "inducement" (Freud), many a person does not decide on separating the life-instinct from the inferior function.

Highly valuable substitute formations, especially sublimations, to which a patient directs his life-instinct, should, therefore, not be disturbed. I made the acquaintance of a patient to whom the analyst had forbidden charitable work while she longed for it. In its place she was to live fully in the marriage relation. The effect was that her love turned passionately to the physician and regardless of how forcibly he explained to her the unreality and origin of this inclination, she clung to him; with this love and gratitude, of course, a truly raging wrath went hand in hand. Hence she felt immeasurably unhappy and incapable of living. She called psychoanalysis a

* Ferenczi, Ü. passagère Symptombildungen während der Analyse. Zbl. II, pp. 588–596.

pleasant but base method since it brought the patients into slavish, immoral dependence upon the physician and showed the person the vileness of his own nature only to consign him to his disgrace. Two hours sufficed to dissolve the fixation on the physician who had treated the very sick patient in vain four years according to Dubois and three years according to Freud, and to substitute a sublimated relation to me as well as to give her self-esteem by participation in philosophical works and religious reassurance. Further, an hysterical symptom of twenty-two years' duration disappeared. One year later, she confirmed her continuing health, happiness and proper attitude toward God, family, fellowmen and life in general. For psychoanalysis, she had only words of astonished admiration. She was entirely independent of me. She promised to inform me immediately of the slightest disturbance but never let me hear anything from her again.

The analyst should allow the compensations to be retained so far as they do not bring with them new dangers and inexpediencies and not try to see if he can guide the life-instinct into paths which suit himself personally best.

2. MOLDING AND REMOLDING OF THE COMPLEX

It has been shown in various places how the unconscious tries to adapt all possible experiences and ideas to its complex. In dreams, waking phantasies, morbid symptoms, reactions, cryptolalia and cryptography, etc., one finds an enormous amount of such contents which are estimated in the sense of gratification of the complex or of the wish. In my ''Analytic Investigations of the Psychology of Hate and Reconciliation,'' * I formulated the following law:

The repressed hate of certain individuals forms phantasies out of suitable contents of experience, either actual or imaginary, according to the laws of the dream-work, by which procedure, it creates for itself imaginary gratification. This gratification of complex comes about through the mechanism of a disguised wish, directed toward the injury of the hated per-

* Deuticke, Leipzig and Vienna, p. 25.

son, being represented in the content of the waking-dream as realized. The sexual component of the hate appears in the form of sadism and masochism. The "pleasure of hate" reveals its secret to the analysis.

To-day, I am ready to amplify that law and express the law of the molding by the complex in the following form:

Every complex forms phantasies from suitable contents experienced or merely imagined, according to the laws of the dream-work, by which mechanism it aims to create for itself imaginary gratification without understanding the true meaning of the phantasies.

The mechanism of the complex-molding, we describe as follows: These phantasies, sometimes wholly, sometimes partially, unconscious, are occasioned by an inhibition in the present and utilize the regression into the recent and ever more remote past (infantilism) in order to gain autistically favorable perspectives for the future.

We add the new formula as generalization of the assertion previously expressed: * "During longer duration or sharpening the complex ever makes use of new contents in order to deck out the previous phantasies or to create entirely new ones. These new formations express the variations of the complex with the finest nuances."

Good examples were afforded me by the artist whose cryptographic series I have described elsewhere †; further examples by the religious speaker with tongues mentioned in my monograph.‡

We recall also that the complex-molding, as autistic performance, represents (459) a compensation for actual gratification and thus far signifies a compensation.

Particularly noteworthy is the fact that with the change of the complex, not simply new phantasies are assumed but that

---

* Same, p. 40.

† Kryptolalie, Kryptographie u. unbew. Vexierbild b. Normalen. Jahrb. V. (1913), p. 130 ff.

‡ Die psychologische Enträtselung d. rel. Glossolalie u. autom. Kryptographie, pp. 19–92.

a regression to the earlier phantastic manifestations occurs, in order to extend the change to them. This happens before any analysis but comes to view in it. A new love relation, for example, is not conceivable without reversion in the dreams and phantasies to the earlier analogous situations and the characteristics of earlier objects being superimposed upon the later ones.

In my analyses of hate and reconciliation phantasies, I saw for the first time in what astonishingly clever manner the elaboration of the earlier pictures is executed when the complex changes suddenly to the opposite: All phantasies are, as one might say, provided with a negative sign and rendered innocuous. Therewith the earlier scene is either retained, accompanied by tears, or the criticism of it covered by a black wall: Previously, the complex-ruled poet saw his brother as dying diver (344), now he comes by the stimulus word, "Erde" (earth) to the secret, water, etc. Associated with water, he sees the dying diver hidden by a black wall.* It also happens that the picture seems dissolving, transient. Many times, the tragic figure is replaced by one similar to it but not tragic, perhaps even comic. Or the scene may be split into several harmless ones, or inversely, several horrible phantasies may be welded into one harmless one. Further, sublimation with condensation and disjection may occur.

A further interesting example is the sudden change of religious ideas in the case of conversion; up to a certain degree, this must be considered as manifestation. Considered purely psychologically, conversion is a reaction-formation. Hence it does not surprise us that after the conversion, the religious ideas suddenly change into the opposite, thus, are not entirely new where they are formed independently and are not mere products of suggestion. Rather, the one-time religious contents persist, but in the sublimation they are changed into their opposites. The Apostle Paul shows this very beautifully. As a Jew, he suffers from an anxiety-neurosis because he cannot fulfill the "law of the flesh" or the "law in the members" accord-

* Same, p. 27, compare also p. 337, 399.

ing to the law of the spirit (Romans vii). So much the more fanatically does he hold to the "Law of Moses" (obsessional neurotic displacement). He hates Christ because the latter replaces the law by the free demands of love and therewith disturbs the asylum of the complex-need, the ceremonialism and orthodoxy; Christ must be the accursed one because the law condemns everyone who hangs on the tree or changes a letter of the law. After his conversion, all these ideas return, recast: instead of the flesh, spiritual dominion and heavenly body, instead of the law, freedom, instead of Christ the Wicked One, Christ the Holy One, the Spirit, the Son of God, who had to be born of the flesh and was saved in the resurrection from the flesh—this too betrays the need for express revocation—instead of the ignominious elevation on the cross, elevation to divine majesty in pre- and post-existence,* instead of the cross, a pillar of shame, the cross, a power of God (I Cor. i, 18). The letter killeth, the spirit (previously powerless) maketh alive (II Cor. iii, 6).

It seems to me that we can sum up this very important law of complex-remolding in the following formula:

When a complex changes its direction or loses in intensity, the earlier complex-phantasies are in great part, perhaps altogether, not simply replaced by completely new ones, but first of all subjected to an elaboration which manifests the new complex-attitude.

Proceeding from the standpoint of ideas, we can formulate the proposition: Every new psychic content arranges itself with earlier analogous contents while it is conditioned by them in its conception and elaboration, or recasting them, seeks to bring them into harmony with itself.

This law, in which the organic unity of the mental life is expressed, I call the psychological law of reference.

Before a thought or endeavor has executed this active or passive arrangement, it does not belong to the fixed mental possessions.

* H. Holtzmann, Lehrb. d. neutest. Theologie, Freiburg and Leipzig, 1897, Vol. II, p. 81 ff.

The significance of punishment, of expiation, indeed of the analysis, consists chiefly in the circumstance that the contents of ideas and volitions to be denied are made clearly accessible, and thereby accessible to the conscious remodeling. From the necessity for relative confrontation is explained also the regression so far as it is not absolute. The regression is only a stage in the process of reference. From the same necessity, to establish the unity of the mental life, is explained also the important phenomenon which we have now to discuss, the transference.

3. The Transference

(a) Its Forms of Phenomena

A form of compensation proceeding from regression and indeed the most important for the progress and outcome of the analysis and the hardest to deal with, is the transference. Freud describes it in these words: "Transferences are new editions, copies of the impulses and phantasies which should be awakened and made conscious during the progress of the analysis, with a replacement, characteristic for the class, of an earlier person by the person of the physician. To put it differently, a whole series of earlier psychic experiences is revived, not as past but as actually pertaining to the person of the physician." * The transference occurs unconsciously in every close pastoral relation. Psychoanalysis merely discloses that which happens everywhere, but it must also awaken the hostile impulses and therewith feelings of denial which are projected upon the analyst † and easily change the affection (positive transference) into its opposite (negative transference).

In the transference, also, a manifest and a latent contribution is to be differentiated. It may happen that in consciousness there may be the strongest love for the analyst, while in the unconscious, grim hostility against him may hold sway. The transference is to be recognized most clearly when the charac-

---

* Freud, Bruchstüch. Kl. Schr. II, p. 104.
† Same, p. 105. Gradiva, p. 78.

teristics of other persons are openly attributed to the analyst, for example, the eyes of the seducer (246), or when he is even identified with another person, for example, with the physician who had performed an operation in the first year of life (123, 265). I will add a rather exaggerated example:

It concerned a youth of seventeen years, who, on account of severe melancholia, turning against all people, temporary excitements and all kinds of physical defects associated with these things, had come to me for special education. I limited myself to a very superficial analysis which revealed to him the causes of his condition and the necessity of a suitable utilization of instinct in the direction of religion, love for neighbors and fulfilment of duty. After the fourth session, he explained to me triumphantly that he felt entirely well and could henceforth help himself. Only later did I find out that he had at that time made the acquaintance of a fine girl and been kindly received in her family.

A year later, the depression returned, which did not surprise me in view of the previous superficial treatment. It proved that he had been thrown out of poise by a conflict with his beloved. When I sought information concerning further symptoms and asked especially after hallucinations, I discovered to my surprise that the patient had formerly for a space of three to four years, viewed himself in the mirror as dead, in the figure of a skeleton dressed in a white cloth. Previously, he had a strikingly strong fondness for a death's head. After the first conversations with me, the phenomena ceased. I remarked to my patient that we would speak next of his youth—a violence which was at once avenged, for the unconscious does not allow its tasks to be imposed by command.

My visitor told of his old hate for his parents, brothers and sisters. The father had handed him over to his grandfather for education up to his eleventh year and yet shamelessly drew for this, a kind of wage money, indeed from time to time, he had increased the amount demanded. The grandmother had died in the insane asylum.

Suddenly the patient's facial expression changed, his hair

stood up, terror spoke from his distorted features. He cried out anxiously: "Why do you look at me so sharply?" [I am not doing so at all.] "Yes! You are the skeleton, you wear a white cloth about your face and body, you are Death! I cannot look at you longer!" [Calm yourself; we will at once analyze this pretty hallucination. Imagine me as Death!] "My friend. The same thing happened to me with her recently. When I had a quarrel with her and she looked at me painfully disappointed, she seemed to me Death. I hallucinated the same thing when I awoke at night. I had to arise and leave the house. The friend is the only person I love. Even for you, I do not feel affection but esteem. With you, I never felt free but rather when I went away from you." [The facial expression of the girl.] "Reproachful, wish for reconciliation. I can never forgive her, however, for showing favor to another." [Your love is barred again, hence depression and excitement. You have previously wished for death, hence the hallucinations at that time. Your friend helped your life-desires to an outlet in reality. Since you thought to lose the loved one, you read death in her eyes and made the girl your murderer. Now consider the connection of your vision of to-day: You were telling first of the avaricious behavior of your father and of the death of your insane grandmother. Then you exclaimed: "Why do you look so sharply? Now?] "I explain it like this: I was raving at father. Then you occurred to me. I considered you as my father. To that, I come only this minute, I had thought the explanation in other regions. Now I can look at you quite well. Just as I found the solution, the white cloth went away, then the figure; the eyes of Death remained a moment longer but faded when I looked at you a second time."

We discussed at great length the position of the parents, their financial need, their worthy traits. After long inner combat, the youth begged me to speak with them and arrange a reconciliation. I would have preferred that the son had spoken his mind directly against them but could not expect too much. The reconciliation with the parents and girl friend came to pass but I lost my patient who was again feeling very happy.

Only ten weeks later, I received a second visit. I heard details of his pleasure in considering skulls and the wish to possess such an one.* The death-hallucination was not determined by Rethel's picture "Der Tod als Freund" (Death as Friend) for it occurred before the youth knew of the picture, the cloth also was differently arranged. Asked to associate to the latter, the youth mentioned first his beloved, whose facial expression nevertheless was different. The features reminded him of a prostitute whom he once saw on the street, and then of another. Only after I had him think of the cloth of the dead, did he exclaim: "Now I have it!" A girl relative had aroused his passions some four years before and claimed his consideration. This scene left behind a strong feeling of guilt. Scarcely had the cousin who wore just such a white cloth as the death's head in the dream, departed, than the hallucinations broke out for the first time.

Now, however, the analysis led to a surprising intermezzo. The youth found to his own astonishment, that he now phantasied me alternately in two different figures: at one time with a cloth, at another, without such. After some investigation, we found that I received the cloth as often as bending forward I sat before the evening sky but was free from the cloth when the white window post stood behind me. The face was imagined as a skull covered over with skin, with bulging eyes. The attitude in this hallucination produced the association that the father had looked sharply at his son after masturbation when both sat at table, whereupon the guilty one thought the father saw the practice in him; then every time, out of hate and expiation, he changed hallucinatorily the feared one into the death's head. Before the session, the boy had fallen back into his error and identified me with the father. The latter, too, he sees as death's head with and without a cloth, the latter at table, the former upon going to bed.

The white background reminded him of the second sexual trauma which followed soon after the first: Our patient sur-

* Compare Gottfreid Keller, Der grüne Heinrich, III, p. 104 ff: Der Schädel des Albertus Zwiehan.

prised his eight year-old sister as she was sitting on the sheet changing her shirt. The cousin on the other hand, who was accustomed to wear the cloth about her head, lay at that time on a dark sofa in the twilight. The hallucinations had often been called up voluntarily by wishing and had regularly appeared. The wish appeared, however, only after onanism.

Here, we plainly see the hallucination as identification of the analyst with the patient's father, wherewith the death's head served not only as expression of death but also as representation of the wish for highest life activity, for cohabitation, in relation to two objects who had excited him. The intermingling of the objects comes plainly to view here.*

The following example may show a positive transference: A sixteen year-old girl dreamed: I held out to the piano teacher a paper, notes or something which he needed, as if to say to him, "There you have it!" When he would take it, I always drew it away from him again."

[To the whole dream?] "We have such papers in the institute, programs, note paper. My brother says I am a piece of music: fine and long. He always vexes me. Therefore he cannot enter my room any more."

[The paper.] "Love letter. My teacher is officious and jealous of my friend." [The teacher.] "I formerly had one who had a little boy. Something concerning his marriage occurs to me. He idolized my mother as my father did formerly. My friend must also rave over me. Now my right eye smarts."

The piano teacher is myself since I too am admired by the girl like that teacher because of my performances on the piano, I have a son and agree with the dream figure in the detail given in regard to the marriage. I once called the mother of the refractory, hysterical girl a handsome woman when the daughter would unjustly refer to her as old woman. The comparison with the father also stands out plainly.

* We saw a fine example of negative transference in the phantasies of God, p. 247.

The paper which contains a love-letter or piece of music refers to the girl ("long and beautiful") and her love. She would like to provoke a counter-transference on my part and play with me. She will, however, also withhold her secret from me which really came to view at the next session. The friend must appear in the rôle of father and analyst in order to be fully accepted. The pains in the eye refer to defloration- and birth-wishes. The refusal of the transference resulted in the girl's attempting, when she thought herself unobserved for a moment, to push away my chair and she frankly admitted that she would be glad if I were boiled or ground up in a mill. Further elucidation eliminated the hate, whereupon the analysis advanced farther. The following dream brought the solution of a riddle which had been sought for weeks.

The analyst is accustomed to being now passionately loved, admired, deified, now hung, impaled or broken on the wheel with sadistic murder-lust. Ferenczi justly says: "A slightly less friendly remark, pointing to a duty or urging punctuality, or a little sharper tone on the part of the analyst, suffice to bring down upon him all the patient's unconscious hate directed against moralizing persons in authority (parents, husband)." *

Freud found that always when the free associations of a patient, not merely the reports of such, stop, the patient's attention is busy with the analyst. The stopping may be immediately eliminated if one pays attention to this state of affairs.†

(B) THE PSYCHOLOGICAL PROCESS OF THE TRANSFERENCE

The instinct ferreted out by analysis seeks, as we have heard, new manifestations. As compensation, the analyst comes into consideration as the nearest person. Every person bears within himself a portion of his life-force not realized, retarded in its development, which could find expression only autistically or remained in the unconscious. "He whose love-need is not completely gratified by reality, must attach himself

* Ferenczi, Introjektion u. Übertragung. Jahrb. I, p. 426.
† Freud, Z. Übertragung. Zbl. II, p. 168.

to every newly appearing person with expectant libidinous ideas and it is entirely probable that both portions of his libido, the conscious part as well as the unconscious, have a share in this attitude.'' (Freud.) *

It happens that the analyst, by virtue of his authority and his assisting attitude, appears in the place of the father and in the regression occasioned by the analysis furnishes an obvious carrier of emotion. He forms a composite figure with the father or if he bears mother characteristics (for example, tenderness or thoughtfulness) he is joined to the mother, is identified with the one or the other. The patient hopes also to be able to gain earlier autistic favors for the future. It may have been noticed already that the analyst should not play the father rôle with arrogant authority but treat the patient throughout as an equal, hereby affording the latter the consciousness of his self-determination, self-responsibility and value, unimpaired.

The emotions applied to the analyst (man or woman) are therefore not genuine. They belong to a totally different person. He who is no vain or love-hungry person will accordingly very soon become indifferent to the positive or negative transference as far as his own person is concerned. The love-hungry, vain beginner is violently affected when he sees himself ardently loved as he is vexed over the hate. In more sensible manner, one has to say, however, that one is not intended at all but the image which is projected into us.

(C) THE SIGNIFICANCE OF THE TRANSFERENCE

As little as we make for ourselves from the positive and negative transference an erotic application in so far as it has us as analyst for object, we esteem it of great importance for health and education. It belongs to the most important steps in the way of the psychoanalytic treatment.

Freud formulates the reason in the following way: ''In a residuum of love, the process of healing is carried out, if we

* Freud, Zur Dynamik d. Übertragung. Zbl. II, v. 168.

summarize all the manifold components * of the sexual instinct as love, and this residuum is indispensable, for the symptoms for which the treatment was undertaken, are nothing else than precipitates of earlier repression- or return-struggles and can only be dissolved and swept away by a new flood of the same passion. Every psychoanalytic treatment is an attempt to set free repressed love which had found a miserable compromise outlet in a symptom." † We remember to have heard that the life-desire, driven from the light of consciousness, can withdraw still deeper into infantilism and therewith be still more surely excluded from real elaboration. The analyst has now the opportunity of directing the life-desire, in statu nascendi, upon himself, thereby upon a bit of reality, and thus of building the bridge for a return to reality. He is thus at the decisive moment, since it is a question of still deeper introversion or return to real life, the knight who prevents the Sleeping Beauty from hiding in still more hidden castle chambers and who guides her back to the world.

One can therefore confidently say: That which is the most decisive factor in the analysis is not merely the thoroughness and correctness of the mental illumination of the unconscious, but just as much, indeed still more, the person of the analyst who temporarily accepts the life-desire of the patient in order to transmit it to reality, to healthy moral life activities. Where the personality, freed from complex-illusion, can win in high degree, it will tear the fixed life-desire free from its stagnation in weak fixation, even after slight analysis, indeed without analysis (by suggestion). Where the personality is weak, the patient can often by his own power take the good way. In severe cases, however, both the analysis for setting free the life-desire and the transference for the purpose of enticing and provisional adaptation of the life-desire to reality are necessary. Analysis without transference easily leads to introversion, transference without analysis to counter-reaction, to false, slavish sublimation, to deification of authority, mental bondage

---

* We would say: "active tendencies."
† Freud, Gradiva, p. 78.

and narrowing of the horizon, to incapacity for saving the soul in the highest meaning of the word and becoming a strong, free personality.

(D) THE TREATMENT OF THE TRANSFERENCE

The correct treatment of the transference must also be tested out in tedious investigations and complete agreement has not yet been attained.

We proceed from the consideration which we laid down regarding the transference: To guard the neurotic against regression and introversion and to further the actual utilization of his life-instinct. From these points, the following formulations result:

1. The negative transference is to be annulled

This is accomplished first of all by careful analysis. Warm affection often rules in consciousness while in the unconscious, bitter hostility holds sway. Hence all hostile impulses are to be discovered and stripped of their power. If they gain the upper hand, the resistance gains the victory. Perhaps the patient may break off the treatment under threadbare rationalizations or he may give himself up to regression. Under certain circumstances, he seeks to treat the educator badly if the latter is so foolish as to allow it. Hence it is the analyst's duty to make clear to the refractory subject, without the slightest show of affect, that he is only continuing the methods practised against the father or is erroneously ascribing to the analyst unkindnesses suspected of someone else.

The relation to the pupil should be cordial, guided by genuine human love. Still, one never attempts to compel love in order to combat hate—possibly the father may have already attempted that sort of thing so that the resistance, the mistrust, is only strengthened. One should never give more praise in momentary exaltation than one could give upon more calm consideration. One never allows one's self to be overawed or put in bad humor when the patient complains of pretended slights, capriciousness, etc. One appears as a strong man, conscious of his goal, with whom absolutely nothing is to be obtained by defiance, not even a little vexation.

2. *The positive transference is to be accepted in analytically purified and sublimated form*

Freud emphasizes that the unobjectionable and conscious components of the transference may be the "bearers of results" as in other methods of treatment.* If someone should ask why the analysis is still necessary then, it must be said that often the transference may not be strong enough where the persistence of the instinct in the infantile fixation does not show through without analysis and therefore is not exposed. If one fears further that by the analysis of the transference, this relation will be preserved, this fact will serve as assurance, that the analysis annuls only the neurotic, infantile characteristics of the transference improperly gained from interchange, but on the other hand, breaks a path to a healthy esteem of the analyst, a highly valuable affection. Riklin puts it in excellent form: "The transference relation is to be dissolved and changed into another relation in which the physician is really what he is, something which an actual relation to the rest of the world and not a relation distorted by the lenses of the transference-glasses brings about." †

Hence the transference can never come to "being in love." Where it comes to view as such, it is to be at once disclosed, though not brusquely, but as psychologically necessary, as illusory in nature and to be sublimated.‡ It is quite in order that the subject may wish to be loved by the analyst but he should gain this love by valuable moral effort whereby he may grow in his love. This positive transference may therefore never be infantile, never excessive tenderness compelling flattery.

* Zbl. II, p. 172.

† Riklin, ü. Psa. Correspondenzbl. f. Schweizer Ärzte, 1912, No. 27, p. 1019.

‡ When it is hard for a beginner to tell a young girl that she is transferring upon him in amorous manner, he thereby betrays his vanity which causes him to forget that he is only an accidental erotic object and is not really meant at all.

There are some persons who fairly exude evidences of love in order to blind the analyst, to guard their secret and to maintain the repression. Thus, the so-called incest may be executed in phantasy on the analyst for the father and this is to be prevented by dissolving the infantile relation. After the dissolution of the false motive, there still always remains gratitude and confidence enough besides, to support a sympathetic relation to the analyst.

The transference should also never lead to dependence. Otherwise, the subject of analysis retreats to his infantile rôle and guards well from becoming healthy and free. The analyst comes into the father- or mother-rôle and the childhood is further played as an ugly farce in the dress of the neurosis or character malformation.

A strong reserve on the part of the analyst is also indicated because the patient likes to cling to him in order not to go out into reality and be compelled to fulfill his life-tasks. If the educator allows him to remain in this rôle, then all is lost. Languishingly, the pupil makes the most enormous demands for affection and avenges himself by holding fast to the symptom. The pampering analyst is an unskillful man.

If the analyst proceeds brutally or clumsily with the breaking of the positive transference, then it changes into its opposite and the libido regresses just so much the deeper. He who lays aside a transference form and has no new one in its place, will inevitably occupy again regressively the old transference way of an earlier barbaric or past cultural stage, says Jung.* The transference is only to be dispensed with when other profitable compensations annul the fear of regression. Stekel thinks it is sufficient that the patient knows that the physician does not despise and does not love him.† I am of other opinion. Most pupils could not accept a pastor who remained unsympathetic upon the confession of the greatest need and would bring to an unemotional confessor of that kind, insuperable repulsion. Certainly, the analyst may not be led so far by his sympathy

---

* Jung, Wandlungen, Jahrb. IV, p. 273.
† Stekel, D. versch. Formen d. Übertragung. Zbl. II, p. 29.

that he would lose the purely objective judgment. In this, I think Freud correct.* The sympathy must be kept in close check in order not to occasion autistic judgments and expose itself to the resistances of the patient. But I think that the latter must assume a large measure of sympathy in his counselor. Who would carry out a long and difficult analysis without inner sympathy? To conceal his good wishes artificially, imposes a dissimulation which must be betrayed and avenged. But of course the analyst should purify all counter-transference by keen autoanalysis and present absolutely nothing except sublimated human friendliness in order that he fall neither into the rôle of a father, injuring the independence of the youth, nor into that of a lover.

To this end, consequently, the analytic physicians refuse every physical examination which might stimulate the exhibition-instinct and refer the patient to another physician in case this is necessary, ordinarily to a specialist.† The educator will not once stroke the hands of the youth or lay his own hands on his shoulder. Upon every opportunity, he will show that he can and will be only a way to a free productive life. If this thought is constantly emphasized and supported by analysis, then it need not be feared that the transference will become too strong and leave the pupil dependent on the analyst.

In order to obtain a sublimated relation to the subject directly, one avoids all unnecessary confidences and relates as little as possible of one's self, one's own needs, weaknesses and fates. Only apparently does one thus bring the other to speak. In reality, one strengthens the resistance. Freud found: ''This technique regularly fails in severe cases in the aroused insatiability of the patient who then greatly likes to reverse the relation and finds the analysis of the physician more interesting than his own. Further, the dissolution of the transference, one of the chief tasks of the treatment, is rendered difficult by the intimate attitude of the physician so that the possible gain at the beginning is finally more than offset. The physician

* Freud, Zur Dynamik d. Übertragung. Zbl. II, p. 436.
† Hitschmann, p. 120.

should be opaque to the analytic patients like a mirror and show nothing except that which is shown to him.'' * The educator should also keep his pupil away from his family and household wherever possible.

Also, in the analysis, the pedagogue seeks to make himself dispensable. He aids to self-analysis and the pupil's own compromise with reality. Thus far, Freud's method corresponds to that of Protestantism and stands diametrically opposed to the Catholic institution of the confessional.

* Freud, Zur Dynamik d. Übertragung, p. 488.

CHAPTER XVIII

RENDERING LIFE-PROBLEMS CONSCIOUS AND COMPREHENDING THEM BY THE AID OF ANALYSIS

IN the initial stage of psychoanalysis, the attention to the past seemed the only condition of the solution. The inhibited person, so it was thought, suffered from unconscious memories; if these were abreacted, then freedom ruled. There followed an epoch, in which the present seemed to be the deciding factor, since the transference created an outlet for the previously dammed-up libido now released by analysis. But also at this point, one could not stop. Freud, Stekel, Jung and all the other psychoanalysts wished under no circumstances to have their patients attached to them but to make them useful for the daily life. Stekel says: ''We must use our mighty influence which we gain over our patients to force them with gentle authority to work. And it is our greatest triumph when the patient takes up his work again and loves it. We should not hesitate to tell the patient the whole truth to his face: 'You will not work.' '' * In this statement, a very important part of the task is without doubt named; but work is not the only end by far. Many neurotics work themselves almost to death, for example, housewives who do not wish to give their husbands their best, their whole love. Just the over-industrious individuals are very often counter-reactionaries who cannot do the one thing which is necessary. We pedagogues know as well as the physician how to esteem work highly and to see its beauty, its hygienic necessity. We pity the man who is shut off from work. But we also know that for a complete life, more than the capacity and opportunity for work is necessary. The harmonious participation in the to-

* Stekel, Nervöse Angstzustände, p. 285.

tality of the world, the conception of the own life-vocation in struggles and sufferings corresponding to the individual law, the best possible realization of the religious-moral ideal, the gaining of correct perspective by denial and self-control, the acquirement of a view of the world and life, satisfying the just claims of the spirit, the proper finding of the object of love, all this is likewise indispensable for a full, well-rounded life. Thus we are compelled to give the future careful consideration as well as the connection to the past and present.

1. The Necessity of the Analytic Attitude Toward Life

It can happen in the analysis that the subliminal remnants of the past are well investigated, a favorable transference prevails, and still the inhibitions of instinct persist. All analysts are accustomed then to judge that the neurotic does not at all wish to be free. If one inquires after the reason for this not-wishing, the views diverge. Freud assumes that the patient does not wish to let his libido flow into reality because he is fixed in infantilism, Jung believes, on the other hand, that the patient may of course be fixed in infantilism but that he is often in that condition because he does not want to come out into reality with his libido or because he does not like to bring about the harmony between inner compulsion and the outer world. According to Freud, the individual bound up in his complexes is drawn back by the infantilism, again become real as a result of an actual conflict; according to Jung, the resistances against the free life-activity in reality or the adaptation to these resistances, drive him back into the infantile stage, therewith to the incest, which however, is not actually meant but has only symbolical significance. Both men, however, are agreed in saying that the neurosis depends on an inner conflict (Freud describes it as between the ego and the libido),* thus not only a difficulty in the outer world but a mental disharmony, which of course is connected with the

* Freud, Ü. neurot. Erkrankungstypen. Zbl. II, p. 301.

attitude toward reality, which causes adherence to the autism of the manifestation.

It has happened to many analysts as to myself that a patient, in spite of careful analysis, remains for a time uncured and somewhat later, without further artificial help, suddenly gets well. This case happened especially often when a removal to other surroundings occurred. One customarily assumes then that the transference not having been dissolved until then, the patient by clinging to the symptom has not been willing to give up the pleasure of working together with the educator or in a negative transference to give up the pleasure of malicious joy in the educator's fruitless work. Such cases certainly do occur.

If we now proceed with Freud from the concepts of the repression and the resistance, we are justified, indeed obliged, to seek another interpretation, especially when we remember what we heard concerning regression and compensation. How would it be if we were to assume that the repression and fixation may have been so removed in those cases where the cure does not directly follow the analytic work, that the forces engaged in the conflict found an adjustment? Thus, we may think that the son dominated by the father-complex, who was tortured by writer's cramp, who got well after leaving the parents' house, may have perceived that he need not fear the father, that he was in a position to conduct his own life, that he could do something worth while according to plans of his own. And therefore he left the infantile fixation. Or he kept himself, as I saw many times earlier, bound religiously by the fifth commandment or such words as: ''The eye that mocketh at his father, and despiseth to obey his mother, the ravens of the valley shall pick it out, and the young eagles shall eat it.'' (Proverbs xxx, 17.) Now he perceives that this saying does not come from God but from the obsessional neurotic spirit of the post-exile hierarchy; he learns to understand more deeply the words of Jesus: ''For this cause shall a man leave his father and mother and cleave to his wife.'' (Mark x, 7) or Mark iii, 32f.: ''For whosoever shall do the will of God, the same is my brother, and my sister, and my mother.'' He recognizes in this test of obedience a higher piety and purer religious experience. Would it not be permissible according to our theoretical principles, to assume that this deeper conception of the problem of life, this clear conscious attitude toward life may have taken from him that fear which drove him to regression into the infantile attitude?

The question of the attitude toward life must be discussed again and again in every thorough analysis. For every dream expresses a relation to reality or certain of its constituent parts and a positive or negative striving. Also, where the attraction of the infantile and unreal is strong, the wish to do this or that with reality cannot be mistaken. Both the wall from which one rebounds into the regression and the force which drives against that wall must be heeded in the analysis. But the strongest barrier and the mightiest instinctive impulse is not contained in every manifestation and its nearest associations. They must often be deduced from these.

Also where the cause of the repression is not directly expressed in the manifestation and associations, it must be recovered in the analysis or at least in the working over of the analytic material. Even from purely theoretical grounds, this work belongs to the full understanding of the declarations of the unconscious. In interpretation, the causal derivation must appear.

A practical interest is added: I found that in the most careful analysis of the past and the transference with my pupil, I came to a standstill. Then I came upon the thought close at hand to a pedagogue, the barrier is in a hated duty which my patient would evade.* I therefore directed his

---

* Even in my first larger psychoanalytic works, I emphasized the offering of ethical-religious regulation of instinct. (Ev. Freiheit, 1909, Sep., p. 31, 1910, p. 24.) I saw ever more plainly that religious and moral needs were released in people. The demands of the genuine Christian religion and morals embraced in the principle of Jesus (love for God, fellowmen and self) are exactly what was revealed to me by psychoanalysis as hygienic according to nature. But one should

attention to this point and with the help of analysis found this stumbling-block, this wall, which caused the relapse. And now it was the pupil's affair to take a clear position to the life-problem. The refusal against the command of a mighty mental impulse then often showed itself as an illusion, a mistake as a result of infantile complex-blending. The cure could then be attained by energetic execution of this striving or by honest renunciation of a dispensable good, by purification of the ideal or forcible cutting through of difficulties.

When Freud asserts that the analysis should only be resorted to when a shorter method does not accomplish the end, he cannot and would not have objected altogether to an analytically prepared elimination of the causes of repression. But one must not overlook the difficulties in doing this. We shall speak of this in the next section.

If the courage for life has broken down, then the knowledge of the causes of the life-inhibitions can only depress. E. T. A. Hoffmann describes very beautifully the powerless dwelling on analytic knowledge: ". . . It seemed to me as if that which we call in general dreams and fancy might probably be the symbolical knowledge of the secret thread which runs through our life, tying it fast in all its conditions, as he may be considered as lost, who thinks with that knowledge to have won the power to pluck out violently that thread and try conclusions with the dark force which rules over us."* The poet here describes an inhibited individual whom the autoanalysis has brought to a penetrating self-knowledge. But on the one hand, the analysis has not probed deep enough, for it leaves a dark controlling force over him, instead of illuminating the forces lying within him, on the other hand, the forces leading to the outer world, especially the transference, are left out of consideration. If the resistances against the sounding of the individual's inmost nature, against the analyst and against the attitude toward reality are overcome

not forget: hygiene gives general rules, it does not tell each what is the best for him in this or that case. So also with religion and morals.

* E. T. A. Hoffman, Die Elixiere des Teufels, Preface.

in sufficient thoroughness, then there comes about the establishment of a useful life-program, even though many dark depths of the unconscious remain unanalyzed.

2. The Treatment of the Inner Harmonization

Even though Freud and Jung differ in theoretical conception, they are agreed that the pupil must be informed concerning the occasion of his regression to the infantile, in order that he may renounce the autistic solution of the conflict. He must be made to see how unworthy is the flight into regression. The ethical difficulties must be overcome by moral forces at the level of reality and the immoral autism replaced by a real achievement. Therein the infantile love-wishes must be sacrificed as in every cure of a neurosis, a moral fact, a renunciation of ease, of cheap pleasure, of unproductive phantasy is needed for the purpose of a higher application of the life-force.

Thus, psychoanalysis reveals to us the necessity and beauty of that idea which finds such exalted expression in the Christian symbol of the cross, in the Christian doctrine of sacrifice. The new life which seems by the law of the inner nature as most valuable goal, is often attainable only by tremendous moral effort, wherein the personality of the analyst can afford a mighty aid. But the struggle will at least be conducted against the real enemy, it will not, as in asceticism and moral-suggestion pedagogy, be conducted against an imaginary enemy, against a mirage. The moral demand, which the analysis discloses, is often incomparably harder to fulfill than the commands of many teachers of morals.

But just in this position toward the moral law, the educator must apply himself with especial care. Freud reminds us that many a neurosis arises from a struggle waged for a moral ideal beyond the strength present. ''The change which the patients strive for, but accomplish only imperfectly, or not at all, has uniformly the value of a progress in the sense of the real life. It is otherwise when one measures with an ethical standard; one sees people become ill as often when they lay aside an ideal as when they wish to attain one.''* Every analyst will admit that an illness very often first begins when a previously practised vice is given up (see above 66, 76, 98, etc.). The disease represents then a compensation which has miscarried. Certainly, however, the regression into unsuitable realization of infantile wishes denotes a source of new mental complications and pathological phenomena, as Freud shows in his article on ''wilde Psychoanalyse'' (wild psychoanalysis).

What is to be done? In the cases mentioned by Freud, the regression was utilizable as the easiest safety valve. A masturbator who becomes ill, perhaps destroyed his strength, in that he was tormented by awful fear of the physical and moral danger of his autoeroticism or wished to escape by violence an obsessing phantasy; if one had held before him more valuable compensations in their beauty and attainability, such as friendship, nature study, scientific enrichment, religion, or if one had first liberated the obsessional idea and thrown back the bolts of the doors to those sublimations, then perhaps this illness would not have resulted. Also in the other cases cited by Freud, a favorable sublimation might have resulted if analysis and transference had rightly lent a helping hand and transported the decisive attack to the ground of the real psychological motives and possibilities.

I mean thus that analysis has on one side to ascertain the existing fixation and on the other, the wishes and possibilities present. It should in the first place show us why an inhibition to development has been present since childhood or a relapse to the earlier stage resulted, thus reveal the recent and old causes of the manifestation. Therein will become visible what kind of forces of attraction entice from the past and what are the forces of repulsion against work, that is, what present shock drives the life-force into the dependence on the unconscious, what task the person in question seeks to escape by this plunge into the regression. But the regression already serves, as we know, the purpose of forging new plans

* Freud, Ü. neur. Erkrankungstypen. Zbl. II, p. 299.

for the future by the aid of the past. This purpose, directed toward the future, is suggested in the manifestation. Even before consciousness can say what meaning it has in mind, indeed often in contrast to its assertion, the mind sketches its plans beneath the threshold of consciousness, which plans show their symbolical signals in the manifestation.

Not every dream contains a whole life-program in outline, as little as one always consciously thinks of his highest purposes in life. But sooner or later, this matter of highest importance comes to manifestation. Nothing could be farther from correct than to consider the tendency discovered by analysis as an authoritative voice of God, an unchangeable life-command. The wish analyzed to-day cannot perhaps bear the light of conscious thinking and by the morrow the life-force may have found another goal which speaks forth from the dream in its secret speech. Perhaps this wish, too, when traced back to its roots by analysis, must be sacrificed as not genuine, unsuitable to the deeper demands. Only that which stands penetrating analysis and the rational adaptation to the possibilities present in reality, reveals the true and actual life-problem.

Thus, one guards against leaving the analytic subject to provisional compensations. One ever seeks for the unconscious motives of the emerging life-demands until one is certain of having found the expression of the innermost life-will. On this journey of exploration, one always has to deal with resistances which stand opposed to the healthy guidance of instinct. The subject of the analysis, however, must always test the material gained by analysis and compare it with the possibilities of reality so that a conscious self-determination, free from the inhibitions of the past, may form the end result of the whole work.

Among the resistances against the analytic finding of the life-program, I name as two of the most frequent: The fear of moral decadence and mental impoverishment as result of the analysis. Both fears rest on errors: The first consideration, Freud parries with the remark, ''the mental and somatic force of a (immoral) wish impulse, when its repression has once failed, proves incomparably stronger when it is unconscious than when it is conscious, so that it can be only weakened by the rendering it conscious.''* That a morally defective analyst can seduce to immorality is not to be denied; but should one make it a reproach to surgery if an unprincipled surgeon performs a criminal abortion? A conscientious educator, however, will demonstrate the laws of morality understood in the highest sense—not merely a questionable interpretation of these laws—as the command of mental hygiene and further the moral impulse. As a matter of fact, many people, who, in spite of desperate effort, must be subject to immoral instincts, have been gained by psychoanalysis for a pure life, valuable in the sense of culture, of personality and of society.†

The second objection also goes lame. Certainly, many great artistic and scientific triumphs spring from the repression. But where a person, as a result of his need, becomes incapable of existence, what good does his genius do him? I have carried out some analyses of artists, constantly with the result that the power of creation increased. Occasionally, for a period, the feeling of desolation appeared, for a new attitude toward life must be won. Then, however, the artistic production prospered so much the better. Further, the manifestations, comprehensible only individually, therefore worthless for society, were replaced by socially suitable, esthetically valuable for-

* Freud, Ü. Psa., p. 59.

† One cannot deny that all persons show a certain ambivalence between the individual imperatives of their natures and the moral demands. Often those unmoral impulses are conditioned by complexes and removable by analysis. If this is not the case—as in the moral imbecile—then the conscience of the analyst decides whether he will leave the consciously-executed unmoral act as the lesser evil as compared with the neurosis and neurotic debauchery. The psychoanalysis gets on well as mere theory and technique with very diverse ethical conceptions. It must get along with frivolous laxity as with strictest austerity as a deeper and freer morality. The means of art are at the disposal of the great master as well as of the morally depraved artist. Obviously we deplore every misuse of psychoanalysis for immoral ends; the analysis in itself is innocent.

mations.* I have never yet seen that an able person experienced a mental deterioration from analysis but very often the opposite. That which the analytic pedagogy eliminates is only the sham and illusion. Truth however is a mother.

If the patient has recognized his holiest imperatives and possibilities determined by his nature, thus, his life-duty, then he must decide what he will undertake. He renounces or executes his wish inwardly. He makes concessions to reality in outright renunciation or conquers self in honorable endeavor. What he does, happens from full conviction with undivided soul. His fixation can be dissolved by his subordinating the egoistic will to the good of the community, but further by giving to self-assertion the victory over the tendency to self-denial. Under some circumstances, only the decisive act tears away the barricade which cuts off the forward march of the instinct.

I learned of the cure of a physician, who, in the analysis, stuck on an obstacle for a fourth of a year until he decided to take a painful step but one necessary to his professional activity. Another subject of analysis was freed in great part from his severe inhibitions, which expressed themselves particularly in obsessional phenomena, as soon as he put away the fear of his strict Catholic parents, which he had harbored for years, and went over to Protestantism.

Freud justly calls attention to the fact that the analyst should not undertake to guide the pupil hither and thither according to wish. ''Not all neurotics,'' he says, ''bring much talent for sublimation; of many among them, one can assume that in general they would not have become ill if they had possessed the art of sublimating their instinct. If one forces them to sublimation excessively and cuts off from them the nearest and pleasantest gratifications of instinct, one usually makes life still more difficult for them than they would have found it otherwise. As physician, one must be content to have won back, not perfection, but some capacity for per-

* Compare my article: D. Entst. d. künstl. Inspiration. Imago II (1913), further the important statements of Rank (Inzest-Motiv).

formance and enjoyment. It is to be considered besides that many persons are rendered ill right in the attempt to sublimate their instincts beyond the limit set by their organization and that in those capable of sublimation, this process is ordinarily executed spontaneously as soon as their inhibitions have been overcome by the analysis.'' * We pedagogues, with our youthful material, are in a far more favorable position. We believe that our boys and girls are still plastic enough to be influenced by ideal models. We carefully guard against compelling, directing and moralizing. We seek, however, to render possible the self-education to unimpeachable moral conduct in life. That we show by word, and I hope by example, the moral demands to be mild and inoffensive in their winning, beneficient beauty, probably does the child good. But the educator should use no violence, lest he create new repressions.

In most analyses, the exploration of the past, the attraction, takes the broadest scope, less often the regulation of the present (the transference) or the laying out of plans for the future. All three tasks are intimately connected. The comprehension of the life-problem corresponding to the immanent law of the personality and performance in reality of the duty embraced in it, that is the highest and last compensation which the analysis, with the help of the transference, must bring to pass. Konrad Ferdinand Meyer gives in these words a classical description of this rebirth from his own experience:

"I was bound by a grievous dream,
I did not live. I lay stark in the dream,
With many thousand unused hours
The present now raged round me.
To awaken green seed from the dark ground,
It needed only the sun's rays and the dew,
I feel how a thousand germs are sprouting.
Day, shine in! and life flow out!" †

The view expressed here signifies a new and difficult application of the analysis in the narrower sense. Originally, an-

* Freud, Ratschläge f. d. Arzt bei d. psa. Behandlung. Zbl. II, 488.
† K. F. Meyer, Ged., p. 139.

alysis applied only to investigating the past, then the transference-analysis was added. Now, the unconscious relations to the future should be analyzed. Thus, the task of present-day analysis has been increased threefold in relation to the original. In reality, in the latter work, lies an abbreviation of the method, because the shock on the life barriers erected by the complex constantly influences the regression anew. In general, neglecting the analysis of the past and the transference and preferring the analysis of the actual conflict is to be guarded against.

The threefold direction of the analysis follows, of necessity, from the psychoanalytic principle of Freud of permitting the patients to speak freely and to investigate their utterances. For every analytic subject reports also of his life problems. Only when one has suggested to him that the cause of his disturbance lies only in the past, will he speak only of that. But just here, lies a particular trick of the resistance and an extremely clever device of the neurotic in opposing the restoration to health. Many patients are actually eager to dig up their past because thereby they best escape the life-duty. Here belong, for example, most lazy, traumatic neurotics who extract great profit from their illnesses. Many of them are glad to allow their past and the transference to be analyzed without the symptoms being disturbed. If one brings up the subject of the life-problem then first begins the decision. Now is the time to give the lazy person the proof by analytic surprising and outwitting that the suffering is wished-for. One should not allow one's self to be deceived in this.

The objection that the neurotic, whose past and transference has been illuminated, orients himself toward the future, certainly holds true in many cases which we have designated as retention types. But in many cases, this is not so. These individuals discover hundreds of tricks, hundreds of new symbolical justifications for retaining the old symptom because the normal outlet of the life-force, which the inner law of life and the external situation demand, is barred. If one does not come upon this dam of the libido, then the regression and

transference must necessarily prove too strong. Every pedagogue is glad when he can avoid both emergency exits, the
one wholly, the other partially. Mere analysis of the past, in
general acts badly on the duration of the analysis and runs
directly contrary to the fundamental principles of Freudian
analysis which, as we know, considers the manifestation as
wishfulfillment, thus imparting to it a forward-looking characteristic.

The quicker it succeeds in guiding the life-force to the
mastery of an actual task, just so much the more are regression
and unmanly transference relieved. Nevertheless, one must
guard against wishing to accomplish this improvement by suggestive compulsion, otherwise the resistance is only increased,
the true healing rendered impossible.

The aim of all analysts is the same: Moral health.
Goethe's saying is applicable to every subject of analysis:
"Where I must cease to be moral, I am of no more value."
(WW., herausg. v. Erich Schmidt, VI, 487.) The difference
exists only in the fact that some believe every one capable
of solving the life-problem for himself after the twofold analysis, others, however, consider threefold exploration toward
all sides as desirable in most cases. Since all are agreed that
not all determinants for cure are necessarily to be found, since
further, all trace the neurosis back to a recent impression, a
present conflict, a present repression, so should one, it seems
to me, at least admit that the analytic explanation of the life-
problem prescribed by the personal nature and relations may
often perform valuable service. I admit that I have turned
my attention thoughtfully to this problem since I have seen
how great advantage this method often offers.

"The free will, I teach, and only to do, should you learn,
for willing is doing." This saying of Nietzsche is also useful
to the analyst for doing is the defensive weapon against exhausting phantasticism. But the will itself must first be
freed. And for this purpose, in severe cases, the analysis is
necessary.

SECTION 3

THE COURSE OF THE PSYCHOANALYTIC TREATMENT

CHAPTER XIX

THE BEGINNING OF THE ANALYTIC EDUCATIONAL WORK WITH ESPECIAL REGARD TO THE OVER-COMING OF THE RESISTANCE

In this chapter, I do not speak of the symptom-analysis which has the manifestation apperceived in brief, and collects associations in order to pass on at once to the interpretation and cure. We come very often by this summary method directly to the goal and gain results which astonish the onlooker almost as miracles. Even cases which appeared extraordinarily grave, were many times brought to order in a very few consultations or indeed sometimes in a single one, so that a life, long unhappy, assumed a turn ethically most satisfactory. Unwished-for suggestion by transference, advice for the elimination of inner conflict and adaptation to the life-problem aided in this.

But this unreliable abbreviation is not to be considered at this time. I want to warn against the opinion that such rapid treatments are the ideal. One often attains lasting cures of the symptom with them but many times also only temporary results. And the most important thing is: the high educational task is only partially performed. One can often in a short time open the eyes for the self-appreciation of the moral task. But all too impatient advance may bring about too violent a shock. It is criminal arrogance to proceed from a "veni, vidi, vici." The physician, from conscientiousness,

490

stands in danger of wanting to advance too rapidly: he wishes to spare his patient the considerable expense of a longer treatment. The pedagogue can easily be tempted to allow the false brilliance of moral counsel to play too early. Not that one should anxiously go out of one's way to avoid a rapid cure. The patient, as well as the analyst, is glad of surprises. But one makes it a duty to replace "cito et jucunde" (quick and pleasant) by good and thorough.

1. THE PREVIOUS PREPARATION FOR PSYCHOANALYSIS

Even at the beginning of the treatment, one follows the rule that the patient should be allowed to talk as freely as possible. It has already been pointed out that the manner and method by which the patient starts in, is important for the diagnosis of his condition. The first statement often reveals, in characteristic form, where the trouble is located.*

A profound hysterical patient said to me right after greeting me: "Give me your word of honor that you will tell my father nothing that I confide to you." Actually, the negative father-complex played the decisive rôle.

Usually, the visitor will say why he has come and tell some of his symptoms. It is worthy of note that many are unable to describe these symptoms in correct, precise manner. Further, many reveal important symptoms only weeks later, to the surprise of the analyst. Most dangerous for the educator are these hidden and intentionally concealed signs of disease, especially the suicidal tendency.

When the case is not a matter of minor affairs, as a nervous tic or moral or religious affairs which do not concern the physician, the pedagogue will first have his visitor examined by a physician and allow him to share the responsibility for the analysis. At this point, one is often in a risky position when one can consult no neurologist skilled in analysis. Our medical practitioners, schooled in a highly one-sided physiology, are inclined greatly to overestimate the organic disturbance.

* Freud (in confirmation of Adler), Bemerkungen ü. e. Fall von Zwangsneurose, Jahrb. I, p. 360.

I, as a layman, would ·not venture to give this judgment if
the great body of psychotherapeutic physicians did not raise
a unanimous complaint over this unfortunate state of affairs.
It is truly pitiful how they attack the host of hysterical troubles
with pills and potions, take the stomach-pump and knife as
aids and treat people as if they were merely bundles of mus-
cle fibres, nerves, tendons and bones. He who, like every orderly and experienced psychoanalyst, esteems medical science
and looks in admiration on its many achievements, is deeply
grieved to see how, under this materialistic practice, not only
is the body maltreated and often injured but also the seat of
the trouble, the mental complication, receives impulses to continue its destruction of moral and intellectual power. With
downright sorrow it must be declared that a multitude of
patients suffer for years, to speak with the Gospel, much from
many physicians, indeed are tortured in unjustifiable manner.
If ''Christian Science'' with its immeasurable exaggerations
did so much damage to the reputation of physicians in many
places, so, not a few of those physicians are guilty who left
the patients in the lurch with their physiological prescrip-
tions, so that the so-called Christian Science offered the suffering ones infinitely more, since it freed them from their
needs and healed them. It should be expressly emphasized
that also among the non-analytic physicians, there are many
excellent psychologists and educators, that many of them
know that the secret of their success lies not in potions and
powders but in the force of their personalities. But that
on the other hand, an infinite amount of harm is done because
of a lack of psychological understanding and pedagogical
skill, must unfortunately· be admitted by all medical authorities who have gained psychotherapeutic experience.

What should one say when an hysterical girl who is tormented by an experience, has her stomach washed out three
times a day with two liters of water for six weeks? (142).
Who will be surprised that the trouble became not a hair better? Or when a woman suffers from symbolical representation of birth-wishes in the form of violent cramps (418),

should one be surprised when, after the painful pelvic operation, not only do the pains persist but also a phobia (fear of burglars) has been added? Or can the pedagogue approve when a conservative neurologist forbids a girl, who suffers from severe anxiety-hysteria and can tell no one of her erotic secrets, to speak and to laugh? Supported by analytic authorities, I allowed myself from the beginning to speak very much with the patient and occasionally also to laugh, and attained at once a pronounced improvement. Or must one stand in astonished admiration when another physician advised the girl in all seriousness, for shaking of the head, to have the throat muscles attacked surgically, the head would then be askew but the shaking would be over. The same hero of the knife would, according to this method, have to cut the muscles of the eyelids, the knees and feet for the tic wandered from place to place while the analysis which had begun but been prematurely interrupted by external mishap, not only eliminated the anxiety and insomnia but also the majority of the tics.

As further difficulty, there is added the fact that many diseases cannot be diagnosticated even by the best physicians a priori as to their psycho- or physio-genesis. Many times, only the analysis gives certain conclusions.

Nevertheless, the pedagogue is advised constantly to work with the physician but he will obviously prefer the physician skilled in analysis. For the hostile physician, he will create by his analytic achievements comprehension for the new pedagogic method. For the rest, he will subordinate himself in all cases where it is a question of the sick, even when he is of another opinion. Hence, he will take only cases in which he does not have to fear the intervention of the physician hostile to analysis. Some people may think that I humble the pedagogue to the physician. But even in regard to medical law and its blessings as in the face of the injurious efforts of quacks with and without religious etiquette,. I consider such discretion the correct thing. In this opinion, I am guided by the experience that the analytic pedagogy, by virtue of its magnitude and effectiveness, will certainly win its field of application without any great difficulties.

Whether one is authorized to do the analysis or if it is a question of healthy individuals, one states to the subject the conditions attached to the carrying out of the analysis. I give as the most important conditions:

1. The subject is obligated to tell as completely as possible all associations which come to his mind, whether these may be unimportant, irrelevant, unpleasant for the pupil or educator or ugly.

One always repeats this supreme rule again when offences against it come to light, which is the case with all patients, even the most agreeable. One shows that the analyst, in exact obedience to Jesus' words, "Judge not" (Matthew vii, 1) will, under no circumstances, censure anything, that the person is not responsible for impulses suddenly appearing or repressed, coming to light in the analysis, that all people, even the holiest and purest, have their base desires without deserving contempt on that account, that the analyst takes nothing as evil even though he be insulted by the patient and treated with sadistic wishes.

2. The subject promises to take no important step during the analysis without informing the analyst of his intention. Thereby one protects his pupils from overhasty acts which are dictated as inferior compensations of the complex. This second rule naturally comes into application only in strongly neurotic persons.

3. If the analyst takes notes during the consultation, not after the session as Freud recommends, the subject should be assured that he is guarded against all indiscretions. If too much resistance is developed, I give the subject the manuscript written in an obsolete stenographic system or give up the taking of notes. The diversion of the attention is not great and further I never felt the strengthening of the resistance. Therefore I can afterwards check up my work more closely and have it tested by other analysts. For the beginner and scientific investigator, I recommend taking notes, for the prac-

ticed educator, Freud's method * of making notes in the evening following the analysis and writing down important dream texts after the analysis.

4. It is very useful to give the pupil a probationary period during which it may be determined whether he is a suitable case for analysis.†

5. The patient is to be warned against impatience. One should never promise to cure in a certain time.

6. If a fee is desired for the psychoanalytic treatment, something which according to Freud's testimony,‡ brings with itself essential advantage for those in need of treatment, it should also be specified that appointments which are not kept will be charged for. The pastor customarily declines an honorarium, at least among his own congregation and usually elsewhere likewise. That, in so doing, the work is often rendered more difficult, I must admit.

Not much dependence can be placed on the expectations brought by patients. Pupils with greatest confidence often refuse very soon, those refractory in the beginning, are often quickly brought around.‖ Stekel finds that individuals who are theoretically well prepared, may be especially disagreeable, since they gain weapons from the analysis to use against disclosing their complexes.¶

2. The Collection of the Conscious Material

If one perceives that no results are to be obtained from a light analysis of symptoms and that the conditions are right for an analysis of the resistance (see below), then one orients himself with the patient concerning the history of the illness, something which usually demands several hours. One informs himself about when the trouble began and what the relations were at its first appearance. In particular, one notices the

* Freud, Ratschläge. Zbl. II, p. 485.
† Freud, Weitere Ratschläge zur Technik d. Psa. Internat. Zsch. f. med. Psa. I (1913), p. 2.
‡ Same, p. 4 f.
‖ Same, p. 3 f.
¶ Stekel, Die Ausgänge der psa. Kuren. Zbl. III, p. 175.

relation to the parents and certain parent-substitutes, for example, teachers, and any erotic complications or conflicts with conscience.

Even now, one pays attention to the complex-indicators which we have studied, especially the physical ones (blushings, twitchings, strikingly soft or loud, quick or slow speech, smiling upon the recounting of severe suffering ("La belle indifference"), symptomatic movements, etc). Mental stigmata, such as striking discrepancies (for example omission of the father, of a period of time) or leaps, peculiar joining of thoughts, grotesque surmises and the like, are carefully noted. No neurotic will report his affairs well-ordered, but ever crisscross in the elaboration of the anamnesis.

In the beginning, one seldom interrupts the speaker, occasionally reminding him of an important connection, telling him of some analogous case in order to show him that one understands his position and to instil confidence. Stekel considers the following a most important psychoanalytic rule: "Use the first hours to gain the patient's confidence and esteem." *

Proceeding from the clinical history, one likes to make a survey of the life history in which special attention is to be paid to the dates, since the patient can seldom relate things in correct chronological order. If however, a manifestation is offered for analysis early, one will gladly stop in passing to weigh it, as in general, the advice given here is not to be followed with pedantic strictness. Every psychoanalyst has his own manner. Still I think I have given not unwelcome and in general helpful advice.

3. The Overcoming of the Resistance

The effort which we set in motion proceeds to the overcoming of various forms of resistance. The fear of rendering conscious the unconscious material, the antipathy for the analyst and the horror for the problem of life must be overcome. From this threefold resistance, there follow three tasks: aboli-

* Stekel, Nerv. Angstzustände, p. 289.

tion of the amnesia, elimination of the negative attitude, purification of the positive transference and comprehension of the
plan of life.* Among the three resistances in the analysis,
especial care is to be devoted to the second. How does this
resistance express itself against the analyst?

We have already (472) said something about this. One
insignificant but diagnostically important symptom, is com-
ing-too-late, which, according to general experience, almost
always betrays resistance. Perhaps the pupil keeps his associations to himself and veils himself in deep silence, many
times under pathological compulsion, or he rebels with immeasurable stubbornness against the most obvious arguments
of the analyst, or he gets mad over a senseless hobby which
does not agree with the rest of his intelligence, or he lies will-
fully, or he revokes for insignificant reasons that which he
accepted on a basis of sufficient proof, or he produces a vast
quantity of manifestations in order to prevent a thorough
working out of any particular one, or he loses himself in ordinary conversation, or he gives up the treatment. He likes
to try to torment the analyst, in whom, he sees the father as
Riklin mentions.†

If the attempt to conquer the resistance is unsuccessful, the
whole analytic effort fails. I am not at all surprised, therefore, that some opponents of psychoanalysis to whom a few
well-intentioned but falsely begun attempts failed, did not
attain their goal and poured the phials of their wrath upon
Freud and his investigation. It came within a hair of happening to one of our most brilliant psychoanalysts: his first
patient, whom he wished to treat according to the new method,
after the beginning psychoanalyst had been introduced by a
professional and been analyzed, refused to speak and for many
hours was absolutely speechless. In his embarrassment, the
physician turned to Freud with an account of the facts in the

---

* Other formulæ are: elimination of infantilism or of anachronism,
overcoming of the involution of the libido (turning-in of the instinct)
or of the isolation caused by repression and attachment, bringing out
into reality, etc.

† Riklin, Aus der Analyse einer Zwangsneurose. Jahrb. II, p. 247.

case; the latter, because of his immense experience, could see through the motive of the resistance and sent his conclusions by letter. And behold, as soon as the physician told his visitor the motive for his resistance, the invisible lock fell from his mouth, whereas all previous efforts had been fruitless. He who has seen something like this occur, has only a mild regret for the scorn of the opponents of Freud's theory of the resistance.

The fact is, that years of experience led to this conclusion, to neglect in severe cases the symptom and direct all attention to the resistance.* If this resistance is broken, the cure easily results. The psychoanalytic treatment has therefore in greatest part become analysis of the resistance.

In order to solve the resistance, one must know how it originated. In great part, it arises from the transference, and indeed from the positive as well as the negative. Often, an identification with father or mother has occurred. The defiance which applies to the father, the fear of him, the disbelief in him, is now set free.† A special cause may perhaps contribute to the transference which cause, it may be possible to discover, or the whole situation may even be disclosed: It is possible for the mouth to serve as sexual symbol so that the closing of the mouth expresses sexual fear. In a case of which I knew, silence betrayed the wish for assurance against perverse activity. It may also happen that an hysterical patient unconsciously sulks: "The mouth serves not only for speaking but also for kissing; if you refuse the latter, so will I refuse the former."‡ The unconsciousness of most motives for resistance is to be borne in mind.

In no case should the educator betray that the resistance vexes him. Most analytic subjects rejoice consciously or unconsciously when they can vex the father, hence when they can vex the analyst, and reckon, as Freud wittily remarks, again and again according to the saying of the little boy: "It

* Freud, Die zukünft. Chancen der psa. Ther. Zbl. I, p. 3.
† Same, p. 4.
‡ Prof. Freud kindly called my attention to this motive.

would serve father just right if I got sick and died." One calmly goes through the various possibilities until the barrier is removed. If the will to health in the patient, the scientific interest in the healthy subject of analysis, is weak, one should defer the treatment until a more favorable time. There are lazy neurotics for whom one would like, in their interest, to allow a worse condition in their suffering, since only then will they really become well and become ready for sacrifice. It is much better for one to refuse those not ready for analysis than that one should bother one's self with them for a long time in vain. The overcoming of the resistance is impossible in catatonics of an advanced stage, while milder introversion often has a favorable outcome, as we have shown in many examples.

Seldom is the resistance so great that no words are obtainable. One merely pays careful attention to the transference symptoms and says to himself that the resistance against the analyst and also against the outer world can signify only the inner resistance against the real comprehension of these or another inner difficulty. If the transference symptom is not analyzed at once, the analysis is hopelessly stranded.

If no association in general will be given, this failure depends, according to Freud, on the fact that the patient is occupying himself with the person of the physician or something belonging to him and he should simply be informed of this state of affairs.*

That which we have said concerning the initial resistance, naturally applies also to the barriers developed during the course of the later analysis.

As a precaution, one should be very conservative at the beginning of the treatment about giving disagreeable interpretations or other communications. One first creates confidence (positive transference), then one allows the patient to gradually find the state of affairs for himself, otherwise, a new flight into the neurosis is easily occasioned.†

* Freud, Zur Dynamik d. Übertragung. Zbl. II, p. 168.
† Freud, Ü. "wilde" Psa. Zbl. I, p. 94.

CHAPTER XX

THE MATERIAL OF THE TREATMENT AND ITS ANALYTIC HANDLING

1. Choice of Subject

(a) By the Patient

Psychoanalysis wishes to educate to freedom. It affords, even during its prosecution, far more freedom than any other psychotherapeutic method, but in so doing, it really makes freedom impose severe autonomous demands. On a basis of extended observation, psychoanalysis has advanced to the insight that the pupil has to choose so far as possible the conversational material which is utilized in analyzing the manifestation. One shows him how unconscious material can be reconstructed out of all possible kinds of information. If he is no dreamer, one tells him how important dreams are, but one is very careful not to make these imperative. "In general, one guards against disclosing a particular interest for the interpretation of the dreams or awakening in the patient the belief that the work must stand still if he brings no dreams. Otherwise, one runs the danger of joining the resistance to the dream production and occasioning a cessation of the dreams." *

If the pupil wishes to tell of a symptomatic act, perhaps a mistake in speaking, one receives it with interest. If he wants to report from his youth, one listens gladly. But if he leaves the rôle of narrator and wishes to hear the view of the analyst, one will be cautious and test exactly how far one may enter into this discussion. One asks one's self whether one is justified in taking from the pupil the responsibility for a decision by advice, whether one already understands his peculiarity

---

* Freud, D. Handhabung d. Traumdeutung i. d. Psa. Zbl. II, p. 110.

sufficiently, whether one may not be enticed away from the analysis by questioning, etc. But so far as possible, one allows the pupil to choose the subjects of conversation.

(b) THE ANALYST'S CHOICE OF MATERIAL

Where the pedagogue finds valuable material which promises an interpretation, he lets the free conversation stop immediately and collects associations to the apperceived object in order to gain an explanation. Of this, we will speak in a moment.

He exercises an influence on the conversational material when it threatens to become superficial chit-chat—but not at once, for even the flat reactions are valuable indicators of the complex. We simply guard against the resistance which would degrade us to trifling.

An arbitrary attack is made upon the constellation on an idea forming a manifestation. Otherwise one would proceed from hundreds to thousands, remain on the surface and lose the interpretation. Thus one asks for associations to such and such a part of the manifestation, to such and such an associated word, now using individual words, now sentences, now a chain of free associations. Now one asks for a crypto-lalia or a cryptogram, now one desires a report on the previous course of the conversations etc., now one has a phantasy spun out, in short, one is never embarrassed for material to be analyzed.

2. THE PROVISIONAL INTERPRETATION

Rather, the beginner may be driven into the corner by very embarrassment of riches, indeed it is very often impossible to thoroughly work through merely the material offered in excessive fulness by the patient himself. Should one give up penetrating into the depths and bestow upon all manifestations an interpretation even though a superficial one? Or should one select a little entity, perhaps a dream, and explore it thoroughly, perhaps in several hours of interpretation?

Freud recommends: "One is always satisfied with the result of interpretation which is to be gained in an hour and does not consider it a loss that one has not completely understood the content of the dream. The next day one does not continue the interpretation-work as matter of course but only when one notices that in the meantime, nothing else has crowded into the foreground with the patient. Thus, one makes it a rule always to take that which first comes into the patient's mind and no exception in favor of an uninterrupted dream-interpretation. If new dreams have been presented, one turns to these more recent productions and makes no reproach against one's self for neglecting the older ones. If the dreams have become too extensive and far extended one renounces a priori a complete solution." *

The important thing in the dream interpretation is always the insight into the instinctive trend. For theoretical ends, the foregoing formulations naturally do not apply. In the interest of science, one will gladly tarry over every detail and ferret out with pleasure the wonderful interweaving of motives. In order to assist the pupil in need of help, we shall so constellate him according to the possibilities that consciousness with its energies of will may touch the point of his unconscious where the instinct is fixed. Whether the parts of the manifestation are so and so many times overdetermined, whether the goal hinted at in the dream occurs once or more than once, whether behind the first existing fixation of instinct which must be overcome, still deeper ones exist, these things are not now the chief concern. We seize first that which is accessible. Perhaps it turns out that it is not sufficient and that we must dig deeper. Patience! Surely this deeper-hidden material will crop out.

We remember that in general no dream can be entirely interpreted (361), indeed that certain dreams cannot be interpreted at all with certainty. In such cases, one waits for further manifestations.

Again I call attention to the advice that one should let the subject of analysis find as much as possible of the interpre-

* Freud, D. Handhabg. d. Traumdeutung. Zbl. II, p. 110.

tation for himself. One cannot expect everything of him. There is only one Freud and it was a long time before he could come. But something of the intellectual pleasure of discovery should be granted every pupil.

One must warn against the expectation of coming to know from one interpretation the whole situation of the pupil viewed from all sides. If one manifestation, for example, shows no trace of homosexuality, this in no way guarantees that such a trace will not appear next time. Only after long observation can one expect to know all sides of the mental make-up. The individual manifestation reveals only the complex most active at the moment.

3. The Discussion of Sexual Material

Formerly, I advised analyzing as if there were no sexuality and simply to wait until the subject of analysis recognized the enemy of sexual repression himself and acknowledged it of his own accord. To-day, I am less timid. Of course one should not frighten the pupil by informing him at once concerning his gross, often perverse, wishes. But one should also not go too far out of the way of a lucid interpretation. Otherwise one awakens the appearance of prudery and arouses resistances on which the analysis may be stranded. At least when one notices that the patient perceives the state of affairs, it is absolutely a duty to meet him in helpful manner and spare him his feeling of shame. The patient perceives much quicker than certain opponents that the discussion of sexual complexes is just as necessary as that of other kinds. It is absolutely absurd to declare the exploration of non-sexual dreams and phantasies as necessary and curative but to reject the analysis of sexual material. The Catholic confessional shows more wisdom in this regard. If one acts timid toward sexual subjects, one does only injury, while by frank interpretation of undoubted sexual material, one removes a burden from the sufferer and renders him grateful. He is glad to speak out freely concerning these things to a man whom he can trust and to be able to obtain instruction.

In this, it is to be emphasized that it is never a question of introducing new phantasies into the pupil but solely one of mastering those ideas already present and active in the unconscious by raising them into consciousness.

The sound tact of the educator who is inwardly free, afflicted neither with prudery nor with frivolity, will certainly find the proper position in this matter.

If anyone is afraid of injuring the pupil by sexual enlightenment and confession, let him look at those who; under the sway of their complexes, are thrown into regular abysses of vice, into perversities of all kinds and are brought by the analysis from their pathological conduct to good ways. Some examples we have given in this book.

I have never seen bad results from a sensible sexual analysis. Of course I consider correct the fundamental principle that the exploration of the sexual past should not penetrate deeper than is absolutely necessary. If one guards against the suggestion that the cause of the neurosis lies solely in the infantile sexual experiences and also directs the analysis toward the obstacles to proper activity of instinct in the present, then the sexual analysis will assume a far smaller extent than at the period of the pure cathartic method or that of the psychoanalysis which expects all healing from abreaction.

To avoid sexuality intentionally, however, is unkind and testifies to a personal fixation.

4. ORDER IN THE PSYCHOANALYSIS

One would expect that a confused medley would result when the pupil tells of his manifestation according to his own pleasure and the analyst interprets more or less according to the time at hand. To external appearances, indeed, such a chaos does exist. But as the tangled associations, like the brush strokes of the caricaturist suddenly resolve themselves into an organic whole, so with the parts of the analysis. Afterwards, one sees a definite arrangement and understands how one discovery makes the next one possible, one interpretation aids further repressed material to an entrance into consciousness.

Following one phase, in which feminine phantasies develop as determinants of a girl's hysteria, there may perhaps come another in which masculine phantasies appear as motives. Then, under some circumstances, autoerotic impulses may appear in the foreground. There results possibly an attempt to bring up once more the first phantasies anew if a satisfying disposition of the life-desire has not been attained, etc.

5. COUNSEL AND COMMAND IN THE PSYCHOANALYSIS

We teachers who are compelled to trouble our pupils with tasks, hear with pleasure that all that kind of demands ceases in the psychoanalysis. It accomplishes nothing to have the dreams written down upon awakening in order to snatch them from oblivion. We know that forgetting also proceeds according to law. If the memory disappears, this shows that the material lurking behind it is not ready for consciousness, the associations are absent and nothing is gained for the pupil.* The practiced analyst probably sees many a dream, the meaning of which he knows, but when he gives the inexperienced patient the explanation supported by experience, the latter will find the explanation violent and arbitrary; he is not convinced and one has done more injury.

Further, meditation over certain periods of life has no value since it does not banish the resistance which comes to expression in the amnesia but rather strengthens it.

The analyst will give counsel only so far as he does not disturb the self-decision. He aids in seeking the temporary dwelling in which the danger of unpleasant difficulties will be as small as possible. He assists in investigating new plans and examining whether they are conditioned on complexes. He calls attention to the unfavorable effects of idleness and when desired, not before, creates opportunities for work, in which he himself does not give or control the work. The analyst should not be a private teacher in school faculties but rather, under certain conditions, work hand in hand with an

* Freud Die Handhabung. Zbl. II, p. 488. Abraham, Int. Ztschr. f. med. Psa. I, p. 194 f.

understanding pedagogue. He should discover the internal and external resistances but not say whether freedom will be gained by renunciation or conquest, reduction of the goal or increased effort. If the patient chooses a useful work which teaches him to taste the pleasure of real endeavor, the analyst will approve of it but be moderate with praise without causing the appearance of negative transference (suspicion of envy, severity, etc.). The responsibility is always to be left to the patient.

He is warned by Freud from the attempt "of turning aside in the treatment into the intellectual field." * There are problem-delvers who throw themselves with ardor upon theories but carefully guard their own fixation of instinct. Every analyst must certainly learn to understand the theory thoroughly and it is good if he has a lively interest in it. But mere reflection over one's own person only injures. Freud allows the patients analytic literature only unwillingly, their relatives none at all, since almost always the resistance is only strengthened.† The chief thing is that the pupil should learn to understand his own condition in the analysis and be inclined to do away with the injurious part of it. Then he himself will give the necessary advice.

* Freud, Ratschläge. Zbl. II, p. 489.
† Jung recommends to a religiously uncultivated person who asks him for reading during the analysis, as the only book, the New Testament.

CHAPTER XXI

THE DURATION AND CONCLUSION OF THE PSYCHOANALYSIS

1. THE DURATION

THE reproach is often made against the psychoanalytic treatment that it takes an enormous amount of time. We educators will be lenient with this fault for we know that an orderly education—and such an one is psychoanalysis—is not to be attained at a gallop.

If it were only a question of the elimination of one or another symptom which had been caused by accidental experiences, then rapid cures would be worth striving for. Or if one has vigorous, able pupils who really know already the right way, for whom the barriers need merely be pushed aside, then rapid cures can occur, very often with definite results. It is an injustice when an opponent of analysis previously mentioned, tells to all the uninformed people, after he has given a caricature of the method, how he cured a psychoneurosis in a half hour (!) and continued: "One thinks now the patient might have fallen into the hands of a psychoanalyst and been analyzed for two or three years." This neurologist must know perfectly well that we too have a multitude of instantaneous cures to show. I have reported in the foregoing chapters a number of that kind of processes which now and then moreover had a highly gratifying moral and religious transformation as a result. But it is distorting the truth to designate such results as the customary ones and it would be foolish to go after a speed record. A prominent neurologist, who enjoyed the highest reputation in practicing the former methods, Prof. J. J. Putnam, testifies in his article, ''Per-

sonal Experiences with Freud's Psychoanalytic Method'':
''It is often asserted that the results of the psychoanalytic
treatment bear no relation to the time applied to the same, and
in this assertion, so much is correct as that the method in its
broadest extent is applicable neither in hospital practice nor
with a large number of patients. So transforming a re-education as is here undertaken, indubitably requires time. . . .
No other treatment achieves so much in so short time.'' *

Thoroughness and constancy, we have to strive for. We
would not only banish the symptom but eliminate the far more
important inner need and set free a maximum of moral energy
and joyous health. That this is not attainable with potions
and electrodes, rest in bed and dietetics, everyone ought to
perceive. Psychoanalysis is the most penetrating method
which can be conceived of. It is not the final goal. It is like
the labor of plowing. The seed must follow. The field itself
must decide for what kind of seed it is adapted. Good things
take time.

Aschaffenburg asserts that other methods do accomplish as
much in the same time as psychoanalysis. How does he explain the fact then that so great a number of patients, who were
treated for years according to other methods and given up as
incurable, found complete health through psychoanalysis, indeed a new life? When Freud, exceptionally of course, used
three and four years in analyses, he was dealing with old
cases which would have been considered a priori incurable by
any other physician. He who reads how pessimistically Oppenheim and many others consider certain nervous diseases
and compares with this what Freud has accomplished, cannot
refrain from astonishment.

The duration of the psychoanalysis depends in the first place
upon the subject. A symptom which appears mild may be
anchored exceedingly deep, be tremendously much overdetermined. Often a whole series of stigmata yields quicker than
a single sign, for example, a nervous tic. More important
than the number of determinants is the degree of resistance,

* Putnam, Zbl. I, p. 535.

the desire for health, the readiness to bring the necessary sacrifice to its attainment.

Because of the resistance, it is also very important how the person of the physician pleases the subject of the analysis. A less skillful and clever analyst often arrives at his goal much quicker than his superior colleague if the patient in question understands the former better, identifies him less with uncomfortable persons, allows his transference to be more happily disposed of. Therefore, it is often quite useful to change analysts although the management of the transference is meanwhile quite difficult.

Further, the number of analytic sessions naturally comes into consideration. Most medical psychoanalysts devote to their patients one hour daily except Sunday. They can therefore treat far fewer patients than other physicians and are compelled to charge higher for their consultations than the latter. For this reason, they must wish for the elaboration of their work, which is indeed only an educational one, by nonmedical pedagogues and pastors. The need is great, the helpers few.

We educators can usually see the patients only once or twice a week. In severe cases, where the pupil is suffering and wants to unburden himself of much material, we must exceptionally sacrifice still more time. In consolation, it may be said that in two successive hours, more can usually be attained than in two separated hours.

Ordinarily, the duration of the treatment cannot be stated. The majority of my cases were relieved in from two to three months, thus without complete analyses, in which connection it should be noted that I have to deal in general with milder maladies. Some patients I kept a year or longer in special pastoral care. This time seems very long. But it is to be remembered that countless nervous patients have to suffer dreadfully for decades, indeed even to the end of life, although they visit one neurologist after another, one sanitarium after another. Further, there ordinarily occurs very soon a decided amelioration during the analytic treatment. Also, the costly nursing in a special institution is here dispensed with. Finally, the cure is a fundamental one and creates a new, beneficent attitude toward life. The deepest, and for the prophylactic instruction, most important insight, is gained only in the late stages of the analysis. Recovery is the enemy of deep investigation. Hence we shall attempt to bring health to the patient as quickly as possible though without forcing. It is beyond doubt that the psychoanalytic technique will undergo many improvements which will shorten its course.*

If the subject becomes impatient, one shows him the extent and difficulty of the task. If he draws back—which by sharp control of the negative transference seldom happens—one lets him go and does not seek to hold him. Ordinarily, he returns again after he has perceived that other methods leave him in the lurch.

2. CONCLUSION OF THE PEDANALYSIS

Every person is unfathomable. The psychoanalysis always remains therefore, as we know, relative. Further, it is not necessary to solve artificially all complications on the other side of consciousness. If a number of threads are cut through, the man can break the rest by his own strength. No one thinks of eliminating all complexes.

An analysis may then be considered concluded when the following three conditions are fulfilled:

1. The analysis of the manifestations can show no more injurious fixations of instinct. Thus, all pathological symptoms must have disappeared for they are all the expression of unsuitable fixation. But further the associations given to normal tests should contain no crass incestuous wishes, no tendencies to introversion, no ardent infantile desires. The anachronisms are never to be entirely overcome but they should no longer have central importance.

2. The transference must have subsided to a modest amount. Of course the discontinuance of the analysis sets free much kindly rapport. Still, the loss becomes unbearable and the

* Freud, D. zuk. Chancen. Zbl. I, p. 3.

longing distracting when the inner change too little prepares the ground for the external separation. Some analysts desire that they become entirely neutral to their patient. I do not consider this good. The self-dependence of the analytic subject should of course never be prejudiced by the picture of the earlier helper in need. But the memory of a well-meaning person belongs to the precious values of life which a normal individual cannot and should not throw overboard. That the analyzed ones show themselves ungrateful, I have very seldom found. Children in particular who have been analyzed, always showed me great attachment and likewise most adults.

3. The ethical situation must be clearly recognized and the necessary things carried out. This compensation is the highest goal of the psychoanalysis. If the inner harmony is established, in execution and renunciation to the moral command and the individual law sufficiently obeyed, then the adaptation to reality becomes suitable. It is free from the worrying, strength-destroying, fevered activity of the complex-tormented neurotic as from the indolence and fatigue of his oppositely influenced companion in fate. Thus the person sufficiently analyzed, experiences with Tasso:

> "I am healthy
> When I can devote myself to my work." *

But it must be a free active work.

The previously repressed instincts are thus made serviceable to the conscious will, the repression of instinct is replaced by control of instinct.

We have heard already (473) that an analytic patient does not wish to free himself sufficiently from his mentor or fulfill his life's duties and therefore clings to his symptom. This shows as we know that the person in question wishes to shirk his life-problem. In such a case, one will inexorably break off the treatment and leave the further education to life which then brings the cure to pass. In this case, the patient usually takes his revenge by not thanking the artificial help but his

* Goethe, Tasso V, p. 2.

"healthy nature" or another physician for the cure.*   Nevertheless, what harm does it do?   A tactful analyst who creates for his pupil an enrichment of the ethical content of life besides health in the medical sense, usually receives much love and gratitude.

* Adler, D. nerv. Charakter, p. 77.   Stekel, Die Ausgänge der psa. Kuren.   Zbl. III, p. 296.

SECTION 4

THE PREREQUISITES OF THE PSYCHOANALYSIS

CHAPTER XXII

THE PREREQUISITES IN THE ANALYST

FROM well-informed circles, the fear has already been expressed that psychoanalysis, if it left the consultation-room of the physician, might be misused for all kinds of mischief. In the hands of improper people, as social sport, tried by frivolous persons, applied by lustful companions for gratification of impure curiosity, it may cause all kinds of misfortune. It may bring moral danger to healthy people and great increase of suffering to the sick when incompetent persons, in mischievous presumption, devote themselves to the interesting method.

I consider these warnings, even though they were spoken by opponents of psychoanalysis, as appropriate and useful. No one acquainted with the powerful effects which the method here presented calls forth, can neglect to warn earnestly against its careless application. He who would venture on the practical application of the pedagogic art created by Freud may do so only in an earnest and exalted responsibility. He will enter upon the work with joy if he feels himself equipped for it and called upon to do it, he will wander with pleasure through the virgin world which is opened to him if he is equipped with the necessary tools. But nowhere is an evil mind so deplorable as in the practice of a difficult, laborious, pastoral training and educational art.

Obviously psychoanalysis cannot be forbidden by legal enactment since it is only a refinement of methods previously used and is delimited as little as the suggestion technique by indispensable rules. It is different with hypnosis.

So much the more will the representatives of a scientific and penetrating pedagogy do everything to protect their method from misuse. We ask therefore what are the requisites, without which, the practice of psychoanalysis is not right?

1. THEORETICAL DEMANDS

He who wishes to practice pedagogically the method of work founded by Freud and elaborated in some particulars by his adherents, must know the results of the previous, enormously extensive studies. It would be imprudent to ignore the work which has been done. He who would do so, notwithstanding, would soon stand before enigmas, for the solution of which he would need the keen vision recognized on all sides even by opponents, the never-failing tendency and acuity of a Freud. Even the experienced analyst often sees himself opposed by difficulties which hard beset him and he is always grateful to counsel with colleagues who have already encountered the same obstacles and fathomed their secrets. Many another therapeutist takes it very easy: he ridicules the analysis, puts the patient to bed, gives hydrotherapy or electrical treatment, gives his little lecture again—perhaps for the two-hundredth time—on the illusory character of the illness, cracks the whip again and calls out his command, and goes forth with the consciousness of the honest man true to his duty. For the analyst, it is not so easy. He must often strain his hunting-sense to the utmost. I cannot agree at all with those who find psychoanalysis easy when it is once learned. I have seen very intelligent people stand months at a time in not a little embarrassment before some peculiar secret of motivation. The counsel of an experienced analyst can often break through the thicket at a stroke.

An exact knowledge of the theory and technique of psychoanalysis is, therefore, an unconditional requisite. How this may be gained, a later chapter will explain.

Still more important than a scientific mind is a healthy

understanding of humanity and a good intention. These alone
help to the knowledge of humanity which is so important. An
impractical man will never become a skillful psychoanalyst.
With women, one often finds particularly sensitive natures
who are wonderfully adapted to analysis. In the exploration
of the first years of childhood, they are without doubt, on the
whole, superior to men.

2. PEDAGOGIC CHARACTER

Psychoanalysis is not a procedure which applies purely and
exclusively to the intellect. , It is psychoanalysis which con-
vinces us of the primacy of the affectivity. The personality
of the educator is at least as important as in any other pedagogic practice, according to the testimony of the most accomplished students, is even one of the most important factors, if
not the most important, in enticing to freedom the fast-fixed
instinct for which the analysis creates latitude. Much depends, therefore, on the character of the analyst. In the
mutual work, he gives much even where he wishes to conceal
and guard against it, from his own experience. The pupil
detects with great keenness the analyst's weaknesses and also
his moral shortcomings. In the unavoidable exaggerations of
the positive transference, the analytic subject will direct his
ethical views according to those of his pastoral adviser. What
a misfortune may happen when the educator is a morally un-
sound man!

One says, to be sure, that the patient should become free
entirely by his own strength, by self-education. This goal
seems well worth striving for. In fact and truth, no analyst
can stand so far in the background that he can be dispensed
with. There is only self-salvation in autoism, for example,
Buddhism. To have before one a healthy, upright man who
has taken hold of life with the necessary amount of courage
and love, causes no decrease in self-determination but rather
renders the personal struggle easier. I think that every
analyst, whether he will or not, must determine thus or so by
his personality. The morally-lax pedagogue becomes seducer,

no matter how zealously he cloaks himself in the mantle of virtue. Hence our obvious demand on the character of the analyzing educator.

3. FREEDOM FROM COMPLEXES

Freud lays great stress on the point that the unconscious of the analyst contributes much, indeed the most, in his cognitive process, to his understanding.* How correct he is, we see in the adventures which every analysit occasionally experiences. It may happen to him that he does not see through a connection, does not understand a phenomenon, and when he tells his colleague of his calamity, he provokes a pleased smile and a solution which recalls Columbus and the egg. In this little defeat, he sees no defect of intelligence, as little as he depreciates the other when the latter turns to him on similar occasions. He institutes a little autoanalysis and usually finds where he should really have found the connection from his experience and as cause of his mental blindness, a complex which agreed with that of the patient. The analyst could not see the latent desire of the other because it was also his own.

Jung told me of a foreign physician who treated a sick colleague, but after some weeks came to a standstill and in spite of all insistence, could make no further progress. However zealously regression and transference were treated, however clearly the complexes lay at hand, it did not occur to them to insert the normal development. Jung found that in all dreams, resistance symbols appeared: the patient ran out of the house or shirked school. This allowed the wish to be determined that he might now solve a problem autistically instead of actually and indeed it concerned the completion of a neglected examination. And why had the colleague been unable to recognize this fact? Because he himself was in the same position as his patient.

Freud has therefore coined the dictum that the analyst can lead his subject only so far as he himself has gone: "The physician (educator) can tolerate in himself no resistances

* Freud, Ratschläge. Zbl. II, p. 486.

which withhold from his consciousness that which is known by his unconscious, otherwise he will introduce into the analysis a new kind of selection and distortion which would be far more injurious than that occasioned by exertion of his conscious attention. It is not sufficient that he himself be an approximately normal person, one should much more impose the demand that he have undergone a psychoanalytic purification and acquired knowledge of his own complexes which would be likely to disturb him in the understanding of the material afforded by the patient. The disqualifying effect of such personal defects cannot be doubted; every unsolved repression in the physician corresponds, according to a happy expression of W. Stekel, to a 'blind spot' in his analytic perception.''*

To the condition of having-been-analyzed, there should be added a happy utilization of his life- and love-forces. Otherwise, the educator easily incurs negative transferences which disturb objective judgment, render impossible the regulation of the transference and introduce uncertainty into the treatment, indeed a weak, changeable attitude. An analyst who believes himself persecuted, is unhappy in love or morally uncertain would be therefore in an extremely difficult position and would do much better, if he does not possess extraordinary self-control, to interrupt his analytic work until his personal relations are arranged.

There are analysts who not only have themselves thoroughly analyzed once but also later occasionally have this done a bit further by a colleague. How then can opponents take offense when they are told that they too are influenced by complexes? For are they not men like the rest of us? Is there a single person who has not his strong attachments and keeps them so far that he will not be analyzed and freed? And who would be absolutely free from complexes?

* Freud, Ratschläge. Zbl. II, p. 487.

CHAPTER XXIII

THE PREREQUISITES IN THE SUBJECT OF ANALYSIS

WE have pointed out repeatedly that psychoanalysis is not applicable to all persons and to all psychoneurotic phenomena. Before one begins so laborious a work, one tests carefully whether it offers sufficient chances.

1. INTELLIGENCE

Superficial analyses can also be carried out on poorly endowed individuals in case no strong resistance is present. The visionnaire mentioned on page 36, who saw her neighbor as an angel, was very deficient in intelligence; further, the girl described on page 86, who suffered from paralysis of the arm, weakness in the leg and twitching of the mouth, was of poor talents and could not be promoted in the folk-school. If the analysis, however, must penetrate deeply, under strong resistance, then the skill of the most able pedagogues should refuse where there is wanting the capacity for combination.

Even with such pupils, a certain result is possible. I freed the boy described on page 159, who was of very poor mental endowment, from the obsession for awakening his brother by sticking his finger in the brother's mouth and reduced the number of attacks. The moral insight also increased. But complete health I did not attain. To-day, I perceive that I also made technical errors: when the answers were not given, I threatened to break off the analysis and compelled communications. I think, nevertheless, that even without those errors, I would not have arrived at the goal.

Unintelligent individuals are treated by consolation and admonition with suggestion—by physicians, with hypnosis.

On the other hand, uneducated people of good minds are generally pleasant to analyze.

2. AGE

Clever educators can analyze children of three to five years, as Freud and Jung have shown. From their observations, one learns to comprehend the conduct in the first months of life. One understands that not only erotic experiences but also change in nourishment, sleeping quarters and other processes presuppose adaptations for which, neurotically predisposed children are not always ready.

In general the rule is: One analyzes children only when it is absolutely necessary to eliminate their fixation of instinct and this not deeper than their trouble renders inevitable.

We know that fixed instinct may itself also under certain circumstances break new useful channels. That which powerfully preserves the complex is often a groundless fear, a continued unfavorable influence from the outside, a persistent refractoriness against a duty imposed by the mental make-up and the external relations. A quieting word of consolation, the righting of a tormenting illusion, an awakening word of encouragement which raises the self-confidence, the expression of recognition and love, can often bring about a freeing of the imprisoned instinct. In particular, a pedagogically proper religious and moral instruction may contribute as much to the overcoming of neurotic phenomena as a false, gloomy, threatening instruction may spoil. The chief thing is that the educator see through the phenomena not analyzed and know their causes.

Girls from fourteen to sixteen years of age are hard to treat in the analysis since their eroticism is not yet purified. Behind decorum, there often lurks boundless desire which is not yet mindful of the earnest moral responsibility and which submits to sublimation with difficulty. Still, cures in this age are also quite frequent.

The upper limit of age when people may be analyzed, Freud placed formerly in the neighborhood of the fiftieth year of life,* since old persons are no longer capable of being educated. Further, it is fearful to contemplate that one had been made a fool of and injured by illusions, for the greatest part of his life, fearful to perceive that the strength for suitable reorganization of life is lost. Yet in mild cases in old people, analyses may be done and cures attained as I showed in one example (noise in the ears, twitching of the cheeks, page 41).

3. MORAL QUALITIES

Moral defectives are analyzable under some circumstances when they perceive that they obtain a gain by the statement of the truth. On the other hand, it is painful for the analyst to see a healed rascal go forth from his work, now more dangerous for the community than when his illness made him an invalid. Fortunately, the diagnosis of moral imbecility (moral insanity) may be made with great certainty before the psychoanalysis is started. I advise pedagogues having individuals who have behind them a series of base conduct, to obtain a diagnosis from a psychiatrist. I have never found that a person analyzed by me became morally worse. On the other hand, I have seen in one young man that after the (incompleted) analysis, he was further addicted to his Don Juanism. A decided improvement appeared during the first months of the treatment when a regular chaos of hysterical troubles, convulsions, obsessional acts, phobias and hallucinations was quickly eliminated. The change for the worse began when I started to admonish him and to interest him in useful works, abstinence, Sunday School, social problems, etc. He immediately put me in the father rôle and resumed his immoral conduct. Of course I did not at that time know the psychology of Don Juanism (329).

Psychoanalysis will always trace back to the original condition and bring into application the educational influences working upon this. Congenital inferiority, it cannot remove.

I consider the psychoanalysis impossible in mendacious persons who see no profit in their cure. Further, with all those

* Freud, Ü. Psychotherapie. Kl. Schr. I, p. 213.

who do not tell falsehoods at all but raise the principle of the least expenditure of effort to the maximum of their action. The wife who, as severe sufferer, is coddled, as healthy person is troubled with burdensome demands, the man to whom pecuniary advantage results from his neurotic incapacity for work, the child who can escape his duties by the aid of a pathological symptom, for example, headache, the lazy student who gets out of an examination by hysterical defects, the son with negative attachment to the father, who brings the latter to despair by his obsessional acts—in short all who prefer a pathological phenomenon to a hard moral task and are not capable of applying their minds to ethical deeds, all these are outside of consideration for analysis. One may exert himself ever so much in their behalf, they will not be saved. Even the most good-natured and sympathetic analyst loses all interest when he has to diagnose this attitude of mind.

In order not to be misunderstood, we emphasize again that many obsessional liars, kleptomaniacs, work-fearers and anarchists are sacrifices to a complex-constellation and in themselves are people of high ethical value. For the educator, the distinction of these two classes of moral inferiority is of immense importance.

To the indispensable moral conditions of an analysis, I reckon a strong will-to-health and the readiness to eliminate the ethical defects lying at the bottom of the disturbance of health, even though great and painful sacrifice of self-esteem, renunciation of sweet anachronisms and the assumption of new burdens is demanded. Nietzsche says very truly: "To make one's self really to new values, that is the most fearful change for a lazy and conservative spirit." *

The analysis makes everyone who yields to it, kind toward the failings of his fellowmen. But it cannot, as Freud rightly warns, lead to the point of pushing everything which makes inferior persons incapable of existence, into the category of disease.†

---

* Nietzsche, Zarathustra I, Die drei Verwandlungen.
† Freud, Ü. Psychotherapie. Kl. Schr. I, p. 212.

With healthy individuals, scientific interest must replace the interest in health, something which it can usually do only in part. The analysis of healthy people is therefore, on the whole, more difficult than that of patients.

4. MEDICAL CONDITIONS

Psychoanalysis is excluded in profound confusion and excitement. It is dangerous in catatonics since under some circumstances, the timid instinct creeps still farther inward and retires from reality. Of course, severe cases of catatonia have been healed by analysis.* Mild introversions, the physician will be glad to trust to the educator skilled in analysis, reserving to himself nevertheless, the supervision of the discharge and assistance in the treatment. Fortunately, one can assert definitely that manic-depressive insanity (circular insanity) and dementia præcox (schizophrenia according to Bleuler, paraphrenia according to Freud) have been cured by psychoanalysis. The pedagogue will guard himself well, however, against treating such severe cases without the aid of a physician. I do not consider it necessary to say more concerning this subject here, for the educator, as already noted, has to obtain direct instruction from the physician for the mental treatment of patients.

5. ANALYSIS OF RELATIVES AND AUTOANALYSIS

The personal relations between analyst and subject may now be briefly mentioned. A condition of being-related always has a highly disturbing influence on the deeper analysis. The analyst's own children, so far as they are accustomed to free conversation with their parents, proceed most easily, as Freud's splendid child-analysis shows, the association material for which was collected by the father.† Aside from this instance, only slight, superficial analyses of relatives can be made.

The autoanalysis comes into consideration preëminently for theoretic purposes. As an introduction into the elements of

* A. Muthmann, Z. Psychol. u. Ther. neurot. Symptome, Halle, 1907.
† Freud, Analyse der Phobie eines 5jähr. Knaben. Jahrb. I, pp. 1–109.

the dream-theory, it is to be highly recommended. A deep autoanalysis is difficult of accomplishment. Even very skilled and clever analysts, in need of analysis, turn to a colleague. Mild neurotic symptoms, as migraine, insomnia, itching of hemorrhoids,. nervous diarrhea, etc., may of course often be eliminated by autoanalysis, but severe phenomena certainly cannot be so removed. As after-treatment in minor troubles or to understand one's own actions better, slight autoanalysis, which does not degenerate into racking one's brains, is indicated.

To pursue the autoanalysis merely as a pastime is a mischievous undertaking. Against a sincere attempt on the part of healthy individuals, there is no objection. They may even get much profit from it. On the other hand, introverted persons easily suffer injury, it may even be conceived that outbreaks of severe neuroses have been occasioned by autoanalyses. From theoretical and practical considerations, therefore, I would advise caution.

SECTION 5

THE PRACTICE OF PEDANALYSIS

CHAPTER XXIV

LEARNING PEDANALYSIS

THIS book thus far serves to introduce the reader to psychoanalysis. There is no intention of replacing the study of the other works covering our field. He who wishes to work most effectively, will first of all procure Freud's works which may be read most advantageously in the order of their appearance.* The works of Freud published in the *Jahrbuch, Zentralblatt* and *Imago* are to be carefully perused. In so doing, one should bear in mind this circumstance: Freud is accustomed, in the later editions of his works, to leave the earlier conclusions unchanged, even where he has modified them. Only seldom does he correct earlier errors in foot-notes. The reader is thus compelled to follow closely the development of psychoanalysis. Only after a knowledge of the whole investigation has been gained, can one be sure of knowing the present theory of the great scholar, which fortunately still admits of much development.

* Only Freud's lectures on psychoanalysis are to be read first. Besides Messmer's excellent article, "Die Psychanalyse und ihre Entwicklung" (Berner Seminarblätter 1912, parts 12–17) Hitschmann's "Freuds Neurosenlehre" gives the best orientation. Unfortunately, the latter is without illustrative cases and is intended principally for physicians. There is an English translation of Hitschmann by Payne, published by the Journal of Nervous and Mental Disease in its Monograph Series, N. Y. Another recent book is Leo Kaplan's Grundzüge der Psychoanalyse, Deuticke, Leipzig and Vienna, 1914. For English readers, there are also Brill's book, "Psychanalysis" (N. Y.), and Jones' "Papers on Psychoanalysis" (London and N. Y.).

524

The other investigations are referred to in full in the periodicals often cited.

Nevertheless, I do not consider it correct to work through too much literature before the personal analytic attempt is made. "Even the physician, who has learned analysis entirely from books without having submitted himself to a thorough mental analysis and having collected practical experiences from patients, cannot be convinced of the truth of the patient's productions; he gains at most a more or less high degree of confidence, which may temporarily approximate conviction very closely, behind which, however, suppressed doubt ever lurks." *

Formerly, the critics complained that Freud presented only assertions and no observations. The complaint was groundless, for in the writings attacked, there is an immense amount of observation material presented. To give more, were superfluous, for he who falls into the old error of the scholar of not wanting to see, can never be convinced by the thousands of corroborations which have been made by hundreds of followers of Freud or Freud's theories. Such fugitives from the facts have only themselves to blame if the development has escaped them and left them in the rear.

The founder of psychoanalysis wrote for such as have eyes and will learn by testing for themselves. The objection that one does not know how this work is to be performed, is incomprehensible to me. I began my first analyses on my own dreams after reading the little brochure of Freud's "Über den Traum" (Concerning the Dream) and found, to my astonishment, the startling statements of that publication in good part substantiated. In most of my experiments, I obtained an interpretation, superficial but nevertheless compelling conviction. The testing of the larger "Traumdeutung" (Interpretation of Dreams) furnished me a deeper understanding; I recognized the necessity of an overinterpretation of those primitive attempts at explanation. Why should not

* Ferenczi, Ü. passagère Symptombildungen während der Analyse. Zbl. II, p. 588.

others also accomplish what so many have already done?

I would advise first utilizing the association scheme of Jung and testing it in the manner described in Chapter XII, 4, in order to investigate the reactions obtained, namely the complex-indicators. This method is the easiest of all but does not lead into the depths, since the journey into the land of the manifestation is always interrupted anew by each new stimulus word.

When one has learned the dream theory, one begins with the intention of testing by the analysis one's own dreams. Even the interpretation of the uppermost stratum affords not a little satisfaction. A supervision by an experienced psychoanalyst is desirable, since he can point out many refinements and disclose many deeper connections.

Further, little mistakes in action, of striking kind (mistakes in speech, in writing, transpositions) may come next. Haunting melodies or words may be honored with a psychoanalytic investigation. Arbitrary, meaningless words or flourishes are to be attacked.

Of such analyses of manifestations, everyone is capable who is not too strongly possessed of the complex-devil.

Further, a slight symptom-analysis where the resistance is quite mild, is not a great task when one is satisfied with therapeutic results and knowledge of the determinants lying uppermost in consciousness.

On the other hand, the analysis of resistance which we cannot avoid in severe cases, presupposes experience and great inner freedom. The most careful description cannot detail the manifold tricks and devices of which one can make use. In order to apply them, it is well if one has himself been in the rôle of subject of an analysis.

For these reasons, it is to be desired that everyone who is going into difficult analyses, should be considerably analyzed by an experienced psychoanalyst. Even in purely scientific disciplines, instruction by competent teachers is considered indispensable. How much more is this requirement demanded in an artistic activity—and psychoanalysis is in great part an artistic mode of work. There are certainly excellent auto-didacticians also in our field, but in general, their way is not to be recommended. Most of them stop much too soon and do not know it, but their pupils suffer the injury. They project themselves into the subjects and do not see the latter objectively.

Especially desirable further is the co-operation of analytic physicians in the treatment of neurotic individuals. It is a mischievous undertaking to begin with the analysis of persons severely ill. Instructive is the example of Aschaffenburg who came upon a sexual complex in a woman suffering from obsessional washing and fear of touching things, but in the excitement which set in, instead of drawing out the pathogenic material, he strictly forbade every thought of sexual experiences and would know nothing of the motives for the anxiety for speaking of the intimate secrets.* With even a modest experience, he would have known that the anxiety expressed a repressed wish (compare anxiety for burglars in the garden, 418, for sticking one's self in the eye, 160). The momentary excitement of the patient threw him into consternation. He acted like a surgeon who, having cut into a swelling and found pus, instead of drawing it off and washing out the wound, strictly forbade taking away the foul stuff and sewed up the wound. Such procedures are reprehensible torture. But what would Aschaffenburg say to a man who would begin his surgical activity with an extremely severe and dangerous operation? Or what would he think of a pulmonary specialist who at once sent a patient away from a sanitarium in the mountains because, immediately after his arrival, febrile phenomena appeared, and told the world that the treatment in the mountains was to blame? Our opponent has only shown, according to the judgment of his colleagues versed in analysis, that one may have an excellent knowledge of old-time psychology and be a useful, conscious-psychologist without understanding psychoanalysis and being able to apply it correctly.

* Aschaffenburg, Die neueren Theorien der Hysterie. Deutsche med. Wochenschrift 1907, No. 44.

When, however, so experienced a psychiatrist can get so excited over the momentary effect of psychoanalysis, how much more must the laity beware of awakening spirits which they cannot banish!

Study, analysis of quite simple manifestations in healthy persons, particularly in one's own self, being analyzed, beginning with quite mild cases, this seems to me the ideal way. To travel this way is to-day, since the new educational method is still but little disseminated, not very easy. It is not denied, of course, that all do not need the same amount of introduction. I know teachers who learned to understand pupils analytically by study alone, and by knowledge of the pathogenic causes, without psychoanalysis, protected the patients against threatening new disasters.

As remarked, in contrast to some who consider psychoanalysis easy,* I consider it a difficult educational method. Many learn it quickly, but in some situations, even the most talented and clever analysts are thrown into embarrassment. For my part, I want also to warn against overestimating the difficulties. Even with modest analytic ability, much successful work may be done, while the most difficult, pathological cases, we leave provisionally to the physician.

* Freud, Kl. Schr. I, pp. 202, 222; II, p. 69.

CHAPTER XXV

THE DOMAIN OF THE PEDANALYSIS

UNDER pedanalysis, I understand in this connection an educational method practiced by professional pedagogues. I am well aware that this definition involves a certain arbitrariness. The analysis performed by a physician on a young person is also a pedagogic one. Even in the name, the difficulty of separating the medical analysis from the professional educational analysis, is indicated.

1. THE RIGHTS OF THE PEDAGOGIC PSYCHOANALYSIS

(A) THE ANALYSIS OF HEALTHY INDIVIDUALS

The treatment of the healthy pupil is solely a matter for the pedagogue. Pedagogy has to decide how far the healthy pupil may and should be analyzed. We have already expressed the opinion that an analysis of youthful persons is only to be undertaken when necessary, hence the healthy youth drops out of consideration. On the other hand, a good bit of psychoanalysis can be done without the youth's knowing it. The clever educator can guess from essays and symptomatic acts, hundreds of important background processes which would otherwise remain hidden, as indeed the knowledge of humanity in general gains an unsuspected enrichment from psychoanalysis.

Little superficial analyses for the purpose of theoretical demonstration will naturally do no harm although it may be asked how far one may go in this direction. It would be bad, if, for instance, pupils of a teachers' seminary were to receive a half-understanding of the analysis and should make foolhardy attempts with this little knowledge. It seems obvious to me that the new educational work must sometime be known to every teacher. That everyone should make practical use of it, is not my intention. An immense field of work is opened to the analyzing education in the salvation of those who are not sick in the medical sense, yet have their lives disturbed and destroyed as a result of continuing unconscious anachronisms. To-day, the analytic neurologist receives many of this class of persons. They treat with wonderful results sons who behave very badly at home and in school, daughters who suffer from fluctuating erotic conditions or female Don Juanism, unhappy marriages, etc., all however, only when no severe constitutional defects are present. In so doing, they attain much better results than professional educators and pastors untrained in analysis, since they receive into their treatment almost entirely only individuals on whom the forenamed have tried their skill. Also, fatal distortions of character, religious abnormalities, ethical monstrosities do not belong so much in the keeping of the neurologist and psychiatrist as in that of the analytic pedagogue.

Likewise to the latter belongs the noble work of prophylaxis. But how can one rightly prevent disease who does not know its causes?

(B) THE RIGHT OF THE PEDAGOGIC ANALYSIS ON SICK CHILDREN

The analytic therapy is, as is admitted on all sides, a work of education. That far, the medical man invades the field of the pedagogue. The treatment of the sick, however, is an affair of the physician. If the pedagogue exercises his office on sick children, it may be asked, whether he does not invade the rights of another profession.

So long as medicine followed, wholly or predominantly, physiological ways, a sharp division was possible. Should the professional educator, today, after the physician himself has become pure educator for a great number of patients, simply withdraw, or does he possess the right also to treat the mental conflicts when a medically pathological trait appears, as he has these same processes to treat exclusively, when—I might almost say accidentally—no pathological sign appears?

I believe that everyone is agreed in the view that physician and educator exist for the sake of the child, not the child for their sake. Consideration for the welfare of the child may thus be the supreme test for the decision of our problem. I will not boast, therefore, that historically, psychotherapy was for thousands of years an affair of the priests and other educators before the medical men engaged in it.

From this standpoint, the following considerations speak for a pedagogic analysis:

1. The great majority of physicians is not so familiar with the child mind as the teacher and pastor. The physician as physician studies people predominantly as physiologist, therewith knowing them according to the physical side; the pedagogue submerges himself early and late in the child mind and thereby adapts himself for the psychoanalysis, on a whole, more easily and quickly than the physician. Of course, the analytic neurologist will also much surpass the educator as student of the mind.

2. In many insignificant pathological symptoms, there is a large educational work to be performed. Hence, since a trespass by one profession upon the other is not to be avoided, the pedagogue commits far less usurpation than the physician.

3. A considerable percentage of all pupils in country and city are neurotics. Admonitions, punishments and promises are rendered of no account by the tyranny of the complexes, while the analysis, by setting the individual free from these inhibiting complexes, can work transformations in the life. Has the teacher now a right to dismiss from educational consideration such pupils, who are often the most valuable ones, the leaders of their classes, when, for example, a little stuttering or writing disturbance is exhibited?

4. The analysis of healthy individuals is best learned on patients, because these show many phenomena most plainly and require the deepest exploration.

5. The teacher sees the neurosis when he understands it,

earliest, and can therefore guard most efficiently against misfortune. He will also, as we shall soon show, direct the sufferer to the physician best adapted for handling this class of cases. When the teachers understand enough of pedagogic analysis, the physicians will receive more analytic work through them, for to-day, much too few patients come into medical care within the period when they may be benefited. It is greatly to be desired that teachers should consult more with the physicians. In the neglect of this consultation, much harm is done by pedagogic ignorance.

6. The power of the physicians could never suffice to eliminate the vast array of neurotic disturbances. In particular, without pedanalysis, numerous poor children lose the benefit of appropriate help, since the physician, for reason of support of self and family, cannot give them his valuable time in sufficient amount, no matter how sympathetic he may be.

2. THE BOUNDS OF THE PEDANALYSIS

The danger and foolishness of a ''wild'' pedagogic analysis has been pointed out many times. I emphasize again the most important points:

1. The educator is often unable to tell whether a psychogenic or physiogenic disturbance is present. Even a clever physician is very often compelled to go to the specialists for a diagnosis. A pedagogue, who, for example, would drive away neuralgic pains, might easily consider every neuralgia as hysteria and apply the analysis in unwise manner. Now, to be sure, this work can do no harm directly, but under some circumstances, it might consume time within which, another treatment, for example, surgical, might be applied with success.*

2. Further, the pedagogue cannot diagnose mental anomalies sufficiently well. Often he does not know whether hysteria or obsessional neurosis, catatonia or some other beginning psychosis is present. The suicide of a patient will be charged to him while the physician is excused when it happens to him.

* Stekel, Zur Differentialdiagnose organischer u. psychogener Erkrankungen. Zbl. I, p. 45 ff.

Further, the psychiatrist recognizes changes for the worse in mental disease earlier than the teacher.

3. THE FUNDAMENTAL CHARACTERISTICS OF THE PEDAGOGIC TREATMENT OF THE SICK

1. In all pathological cases which are not insignificant (analogous to the minor surgery of the barber), the pedagogue obtains the diagnosis from an analytic physician wherever possible and has him authorize the educational work. Dangerous cases, he will gladly renounce.

2. In the further course of the analysis, he will keep in touch with the physician where it is necessary, and in case of need, obtain his advice.

3. The analyzing educator, in his work on patients, never considers himself as rival of the experienced physician but always as pupil, helper and co-worker.

If the educator adheres to these fundamental principles, he has good right to be recognized in his analytic work, not as layman but as professional. To this end, not only his office as professional educator aids him, but also his scientific training. It is beyond question that the psychoanalytic investigation and the elaboration of its technique has much of value to expect from keen-sighted educators and no physician will hesitate to accept this service gratefully.

Our experience agrees fully with the expressions which Prof. Freud has contributed to this book. Aside from him, there have spoken concerning this circumstance only physicians who understand nothing or almost nothing of psychoanalysis. That they are indignant when someone else does something which was denied to them, will neither surprise nor disturb us. A real professional, Riklin, expresses himself thus: "Obviously, we must greet the collaboration of philologists, pedagogues and others with joy. We need them and have the greatest stimulus to expect from them. For psychoanalysis can never be limited to pathology. Further, it is very desirable that the educated world should acquire psychoanalytic knowledge. From the strictly medical standpoint, much is to be expected from this collaboration and a restriction of the neuroses in particular. The principle of the necessary liberation from the parents, the knowledge of the own personality, the conditions of marital competence, etc., must have an unconditional mitigating influence. Besides a prophylactic result, a therapeutic one must also be present. It will be less possible for the conflicts to hide behind the poor masks of the neurosis and happen less often that a patient can terrorize his whole environment. A number of conflicts, for example, those of puberty, will be judged quite differently and be led to rational solutions.

Concerning the practice of analysis by non-physicians (of the physicians who should not do analysis, I have already spoken) the following standpoint may well be taken: There are non-physicians of great psychological acumen and complete comprehension of psychoanalytic questions whose collaboration we very much need: in the assistance of the physician, in the education of neurotic children, etc. For the sake of order, we must wish that the patients treated by these non-physicians should have the diagnosis passed on by a physician schooled in analysis and that the latter should keep in touch with the course of the analytic treatment and help bear the responsibility. Against this formulation, it will be difficult to find an important objection.

To declaim against the application of analytic knowledge in pedagogy and to want to forbid the pedagogue from that kind of conference with his pupils, seems to me unreasonable.'' *

* Riklin, Ü. Psa. Corr. bl. f. Schweizer Ärzte 1912, No. 27, 1020 f.

CONCLUSION

THE RESULTS OF PSYCHOANALYSIS

CHAPTER XXVI

THE PRACTICAL BENEFITS

Two enemies lie in wait for every powerful new movement: the over-valuation of its adherents and the under-valuation of its opponents. Psychoanalysis has encountered both in surprising degree. It afforded its adherents a joyous enthusiasm, which meanwhile found a rather exuberant expression and irritated the opponents unnecessarily. To the writings of this class, belong my own first works, in which, from joy over unexpected practical results and scientific discoveries, I struck a temporarily injudicious and over-affective tone. The greatest error in this was that I, looking through rose-colored glasses, estimated the practical difficulties and theoretical mysteries too low and emphasized them too little; Psychoanalysis is to-day, and in important points, will be for a long time yet, in the stage of testing and proving. I believe that we psychoanalysts should have learned much more from the foresight and modest reserve of Freud. Perhaps some of us sought unconsciously from praise for our work, a compensation for the immeasurably violent attacks on our intellectual and even moral qualities to which we were exposed.

To-day they have become calmer on either side. Far less often than formerly, does the polemic assume an improper tone. There are even one-time opponents who are beginning to test whether Freud may not in the end be right. Bruno Saaler has just published an hysteria-analysis which purifies itself most carefully from having proceeded from the Freudian

535

technique. Against the latter, Saaler even protests that it esti-
mates the ''resistances'' arbitrarily. Nevertheless, the author
attempts to apply the theory of psychoanalysis to a case of
hysteria, and behold, he finds that Freud's fundamental principles of explanation are entirely substantiated and light
thrown into great darkness. Thus, he comes, plainly in spite
of himself, to the confession ''that for the understanding of
certain hysterical maladies, the Freudian theory is in fact indispensable.'' * The student will wonder how Freud's ''arbitrary'' methods can give such correct results that even an apparently little inclined critic must feel himself compelled to
acknowledge their validity. He will wonder further that a
man like Saaler could ignore the therapeutic experiences of
physicians who have analyzed for decades and choose procedures which are in contradiction to his theoretic statement—
I mention only the frequent physical (also gynecological) investigations and daily incidents which must influence the
sexual life of the patients unfavorably. The psychoanalyst
can be satisfied with Saaler's results. We all calculated exactly like him and would to-day be satisfied with this correct but superficial explanation if we had learned nothing in the
last few years. What we are exposed to in the work of the
newly arrived analyst, disappears nevertheless beside the great
service of the author, in whom there is finally given us an investigator who has undertaken the venture of looking the facts
in the face.

That which Freud and his adherents have to regret to-day is
not the contempt for the individual—very seldom is the originator of a mental movement so furiously attacked by the
authorities in wrath and excommunication, so highly esteemed
personally, even by opponents, as Freud. We complain rather
of the contempt for the facts, and find in this, the confirmation of the bitter saying of the gifted Anatole France: ''Les
savants ne sont pas curieux'' (Jung). Still, the signs
multiply that at least those of the investigators still capable of

* D. Saaler, Eine Hysterie-Analyse und ihre Lehren. Allg. Zschr. f.
Psychiatrie u. Psychisch-gerichtl. Medizin, LXIX (1912) p. 866.

learning, are freeing themselves from the previous ontophobia. I therefore consider an agreement with a part of the opposition as imminent.

My explanations, free from emotional restriction, may therefore state openly what education has to expect from psychoanalysis and its never absent synthetic complement.

1. THE CURE OF THE SUBJECTS OF EDUCATION WHO DEVIATE FROM THE NORMAL

A considerable number of pupils with marked pathological symptoms have crossed the preceding pages of this book. Since I have been engaged in analytic pedagogy, I have been filled with astonishment at the enormous percentage of neurotics present in all school classes and of these, indeed, neurotics who are in need of analysis. I shall give only a few groups.

A. PHYSICAL DEFECTS

Bed-wetting, stuttering, disturbances of writing, twitchings, pains in the head and the stomach, neuralgia, intestinal troubles, skin eruptions. We remember that all of these disturbances can also be caused by physiological conditions.

Of the legion of atypical disturbances, I shall not speak further. It is impossible to give all forms of hysterical maladies since their number is unlimited.

B. PSYCHIC DISTURBANCES

In this field, it is more venturesome than in that of the organic, to lay down any boundary between healthy and sick. The separation is closely dependent on subjective impression.

Very frequent abnormalities which the teacher meets, are anxiety and obsessional phenomena. Many pupils are pathologically afraid when they are called upon, or have to recite something. Many betray their anxiety condition by no gestures and are accordingly considered stupid or lazy. In a considerable number of my cases of this class, an easily recognizable transposition and identification was present: the fear of the father, especially where he had interfered brusquely in the love-life of his son, was transferred upon the teacher or the anxiety caused by damming up of eroticism utilized the situation of a mild fear to manifest itself by immense accretions of affect. The examination-anxiety was repeatedly deciphered as repressed wish for verification of potency; I myself analyzed only examination-dreams, which forced this explanation upon me. To the anxiety phenomena, often belong, as we know, also stuttering and writer's cramp.

Among frequent obsessions, I mention stereotyped gestures, ceremonials in walking on the paving stones (touching or avoiding the dividing line between two stones), counting up to certain numbers in marching, division of paving stones into so and so many steps, obtaining oracles, pondering over waking-phantasies, elaboration of secret speech or writing, senseless habits of writing (flourishes, shading of certain loops), laughing upon occasion of serious remarks, obsessional washing, agoraphobia and claustrophobia.

I stop with these typical obsessions which were accompanied by more individual variations. It is unbelievable how many obsessional phenomena are present, even among normal individuals. There are few pupils who do not show a number of such phenomena springing from unconscious trains of thought. Usually, the will can suppress them, and although the attention neglects them, nevertheless, the stigmata caused by them keep cropping out.

The educator can draw very important conclusions from the observation of such obsessional symptoms.

The observations of abulia (deficiency of will) are important. They proceed from the circumstance that the youth is overwhelmed by a conscious or unconscious motive. One of my pupils suffered from bitter reproaches against masturbation which was practiced, on the average, every five weeks. He said to me: "Since I cannot stop that habit, I am a person without will." Analysis was superfluous in this case.

Of all educational problems which demand our analysis, perhaps the one most frequently encountered is the withdrawal of love from persons and objects. This condition involves an introversion, which, in severe cases, leads to mental disease (catatonia, a form of dementia præcox). Milder introversions belong to the tasks of the analyzing pedagogue which yield most gratitude. An immense number of pupils suffer from the condition of their bridges to their fellowmen being broken; hence they fall into melancholia and distaste for life, indeed into danger of suicide. By the aid of transference and the overcoming of the frequently complex-conditioned, illusory denial.of the demands of life, we can successfully turn the instinct which is self-enveloping and depending on infantile fixation, to useful objects. This setting-free of love can often give a life an entirely new, highly pleasing turn and save a soul. Many an incipient Hamlet can be saved from catatonia.

In this connection, the numerous persons who are tired of life should be mentioned; these are most suitable cases for analysis.

Further, the undecided individuals who can bring themselves to no decisive action, for example, choosing a profession, offer good chances for analysis. Usually, these persons are chained by complexes; for them, an image in the unconscious locks the entrance to the life-work.

How strongly the intellectual performances often depend on complex-factors, Alfons Maeder and Otto Mensendieck have first shown * in two excellent little articles. Even the best pupil does nothing when entanglement of the unconscious binds him in chains. Not only is an immense quantity of mental energy lost in the autistic elaboration of the material thereby afforded, but there is also the need of working out his complexes, for constant remolding and distortion of reality. By the analysis, tired and uninterested pupils, who are considered lazy, but are in reality inhibited by fixations of instinct, are transformed into useful, studious pupils who take pleasure in their work. One cannot influence such persons by pun-

* Alfons Maeder and Otto Mensendieck, Diskussionvoten in der zürich. psychanalyt. Vereinigung ü. "Psychoanalyse u. Pädagogik" 1912. Berner Seminarblätter VI, pp. 303–309.

ishment and threats for one merely increases the transposition with the father. Further, transfer to an educational home of freer atmosphere does not solve the complications of their minds even when it effects the removal from the parents so much to be desired.

The most important educational problems are the moral ones. We saw that psychoanalysis in the treatment of moral deficiencies solved many problems which resisted the traditional methods. The analysis cannot make a youth who is constitutionally defective, good. An ethical imbecile is also not to be improved by it. But among the sons and daughters who have turned out badly, there is an immense number who are only a sacrifice to an obsession proceeding from the unconscious and who, in spite of all external and internal effort, all precept and moral instruction, all ascetic practices and fervent vows, all punishments and rewards, fall without salvation to the compulsion to evil and make a wreck of their lives.

I have described the pathological liar (pseudologist) and thief (kleptomaniac), the hater of men (especially parents and brothers and sisters, as well as their substitutes) and of animals, the solitary men who trust no one and hence can make no truly social use of their powers, the quarrelsome, obstinate and eccentric people who, in anarchistic bitterness, scent the father-substitute everywhere and angrily resist it, the crank who, in the leading-string of an infantile complex of inferiority, becomes a disagreeable fool, and in misconstruction of the real relations, constantly throws a block between his feet, the self-torturer who sentences himself in masochistic pleasure-hunger to unfruitful asceticism, and who, because of his inability to utilize the good things of life, properly rationalizes a higher style of life, the grim sadist who executes his inhibited sexual instinct with cruel pleasure upon animals and other people, perhaps even martyring harmless persons to death in the name of Jesus, the fanatic in sport, nature-cures, affairs of morality, etc. From the slight peculiarity of reading-mania or obsessional smoking, up to the crimes of arson and murder,*

* H. Schmid, Zur Psychol. der Brandstifter, Psychol. Abh. edited by

psychoanalysis shows us an immensely comprehensive and
well-filled scale of moral offenses resulting from complexes,
which could be overcome by non-analytic methods in part not
at all, in part only externally. He who has seen in a large
number of cases how psychoanalysis has freed with compara-
tive ease those unfortunates, who, in spite of most grievous
efforts, found no help within or without, can only regard the
pedagogic treatment instituted by Freud, with admiration and
gratitude.

Obviously, we can also influence very strongly, analytically,
the valuation of people and view of the world, so far as these
are dictated by the complex. We all know how little it avails
to bring reason to bear on the ideas of set men-haters, women-
haters and pessimists. The reason is plain: All logical arguments deal at most with the rationalization, not, however, with
the real basis, the complex, from which those ideas proceed
and are of necessity kept fresh. The analyst spares himself
the useless strife. He either applies the analysis where the
affairs demand and allow it, or he refrains from doing anything.

Finally, we possess in psychoanalysis a wonderful instrument for eliminating certain religious inhibitions and bizarre
manifestations.

If we are convinced that in the unconscious, a great part of
those superpowers dwell, which rule our ordinary as well as
our important performances, if we have been taught by experience that the analysis exercises a very strong influence on
those subliminal powers, then we will consider it the duty of
every professional educator to become acquainted with psychoanalysis.

2. Degree of Mental Restoration and Bad Results

We may speak of healing in different senses: A wound may
be well healed if the organism is exactly as powerful and
capable of resistance as before the injury. A facial erysipelas

Jung, Vol. I, pp. 80–179. For my refutation of most of Schmid's statements, see Internat. Zeitschr. f. med. Psa. 111.

is completely recovered from, no symptom, no visible defect, is left behind but the healed patient is still prejudiced, for he is subject in high degree to the danger of a recrudescence. Inversely, a broken bone knits so firmly that the once injured place enjoys greater solidity than before the fracture. No physician can promise that the recovered person will never stumble again and break a limb but he can assert that the probability of a break in the former position is lessened. Finally, we know recoveries which leave the body entirely immune to the preceding disease.

Now, how is the psychoanalytic cure to be understood? Freud's expectations were at first very modest. He did not think of curing the hysteria itself; he thought he must be satisfied with the removal of the individual symptoms. Moreover, in dementia præcox, he held, like Jung, that the analysis was inapplicable. The experience of two decades has exceeded these all too modest assumptions. Permanent cures of hysteria have been observed in immense numbers and even psychoses like dementia præcox (in catatonic, hebephrenic and paranoid forms) and manic-depressive insanity have been cured analytically, even though such outcomes are, for the time being, still rare and further the prognosis in this class of maladies seems so far rather poor.

The thoroughness and permanency of the cure depends on various factors: on the depth of the actual analytic exploration (analysis of the past), on the purity of the attitude toward life (analysis of the future), on the grade of neurotic disposition, on external conditions. In general, one may confidently say: If subject and analyst have worked carefully together, clearly illuminated and vivified the unconscious, distinctly recognized the inner law of life, taken firm hold on reality, then the one-time sick person is in a position to master very hard relations without neurotic relapse. I have often seen individuals, who, before the analysis, were thrown off the track by petty things, bear grievous experiences of life with calm equanimity. The number of relapses known to me is surprisingly small. If a recurrence of the old symptom occurs, a little after-help usually suffices to bring order again.

The analytic cures may be considered in general as actually permanent. In this regard, they surpass very markedly, according to the view of all who know, the cures by hypnosis and pure suggestion.

Even the best methods of treatment have disappointments and bad results. Psychoanalysis offers no exception in this regard. In all stages of the treatment, one may occasionally experience disappointments. Many patients will have nothing to do with the analysis after they have heard of the sacrifices of time and moral effort which the method demands. They were not sincere in wishing salvation. They decide on no second visit and the analyst certainly never invites to one. Others at first seem willing and disclose a part of their complex-material. As the deeper impulses in the series appear, however, they hide in the bulwarks of an insurmountable resistance and turn inward only so much the deeper. Still, this case is less frequent. Others go to pieces on the rocks of the transference. Still others wish at no price to respect the inner imperative and attack the problem of life.

We analytic pedagogues do well to search always for the mistakes within ourselves. But we make ourselves guilty of suspicious mistreatment of self when we set the bad result down to our own account every time. Surely, we all have very much to learn and psychoanalysis still greatly needs careful elaboration, but infallibility we shall never attain.

If we count up the results and failures of psychoanalysis, there still remains a very great pedagogic gain.

CHAPTER XXVII

THE RESULTS FOR PEDAGOGY

THAT education receives from the psychoanalytic investigation a greatly strengthened importance, has already been explained (113f). It may now be pointed out that this consists in an extensive and an intensive increase in value. The former, because the first four or five years of life predetermine with uncommon force the future development; and also the need for education in many neurotic healthy and sick adults comes glaringly to expression. The intensive increase in valuation of education results from the sufficiently proven circumstance that the mental achievements of a whole lifetime, even as far as the attitude toward humanity, choice of profession, artistic, ethical, philosophic and religious endeavors depend, in great part, on educational influences. In order to forestall a harmful misunderstanding, it may at once be added that the higher valuation of educational influences perhaps—we shall investigate the problem—narrow the extent of the voluntary influences upon the pupil and force a fight against ''over-education.''

Also the kind and method of pedagogy, under which we do not understand with Dürr * merely a science, but with Messmer,† theory and practice of education, experiences a change from the analysis. Previously, it devoted itself almost exclusively to the conscious mental life of the pupil; when it also attempted to bring out unconscious or dispositional objects of physical or (rarely) psychical kind, it turned in so doing to the conscious thought, feeling and will and made use of the

---

* Dürr, Einführung in der Pädagogik, p. 16.
† Messmer, Lehrbuch der allgem. Päd. p. 4.

synthesis. If we are now certain that the mental processes go back in great part to unconscious processes and are to be strongly influenced by penetration into the unconscious regions of the mind, indeed that very often alone by such analytic work the desired influencing of harmful tendencies is to be attained, then psychoanalysis becomes an important, in many cases, even an indispensable educational instrument, even though it cannot be applied in practice by all educators.

This is not proclaiming psychoanalysis the only sacred, only justifiable or even only necessary method. As little as ethics, esthetics and metaphysics * may expect an answer to all their questions from it, so little may the science of pedagogy. The former methods and also the experimental ones may calmly continue their efforts. I must, of course, frankly confess that for me the analytic work gained incomparably deeper glimpses into the pupils' minds than all other methods together and that I derived far better counsel in very important cases from the analysis in the management of the educational object than from any kind of text-books, because the latter did not value the weightiest determinants of life or at least not enough.

The pedagogy of the future will without doubt join systematically the analytic method more to the synthetic method than has been possible in this book.

In the present status of the investigation, no one will expect me to state the whole benefit which pedagogy has to gain from the fields of psychoanalysis. What I have to offer are only isolated experiments which may invite productive educators to investigation on their own part.

1. REMARKS ON THE POSITION OF PARENTS TO THE CHILD IN
GENERAL

The psychoanalytic pedagogy lays great stress on prophylaxis. It helps us to avoid an immense amount of misery, of which to-day even the educators, otherwise clever, are unsuspectingly guilty. The importance of prevention was also emphasized in the older education.

* Silberer, Eine prinzip. Anregung. Jahrb. IV, p. 801 ff.

We have heard that the attitude toward the parents very often determines for a lifetime the attitude toward people in general and toward life itself. In almost every pupil who hates the teacher, in many anarchists and haters of religion, we discover a disguised enemy of the father. Such revolutionaries do not mind destroying themselves if only their hate comes to its reckoning. In many a Don Juan, we found the childish remnant of a fixation on the mother.

In the first place, it is desired of parents that they take account of the needs of their children for affection and favor, and gratify it in a reasonable manner. In this regard, I need to state nothing absolutely new but believe by the description of our investigations to be able to lend new weight to the old demands. If the child is treated too tenderly and respectfully, it is threatened by serious dangers: covetousness awakens to a degree plainly characterized by sexuality. The fixation on the parents becomes all too strong when sweetest caresses are handed out without effort on the part of the child.* When the child recoils from the rough external world, he flees, frightened, to the household paradise of the child and creates for himself autistic pleasure by revivifying the one-time joys of childhood. We know that one of the chief sources of the neurosis lies here.

Especially when the child, without valuable achievement, is overwhelmed with affection and recognition in sickness, does it come into serious danger of obtaining surreptitiously by neurotic troubles those sweet pleasures. We have heard of bed-wetting to make the father and mother attentive; we could, however, name a great number of other coercive habits. Too lenient parents, who give their children the best without requiring reciprocal performances on their part, easily ruin their lives.

Almost still worse, nevertheless, works the refusal of affection and recognition. The child must learn to subject his need

---

* Freud, Die zwei Prinzipien des psych. Geschehens. Jahrb. III, p. 6.
Adler, Das Zärtlichkeitsbedürfnis des Kindes. Monatsh. f. Pädogogik u. Schulpolitik, 1908, p. 8 f.

of love to reality. Further, love is, as Freud says in an unpublished analysis, an art which must be learned. If the child is slighted, if one shows him no sympathy, if one does not listen to his wishes and confessions, a repression occurs. The child must withdraw the love, which has developed for the mother as a result of the reception of nourishment and care of his body, from her and if a new carrier of emotion is not at hand, as a grandmother or a teacher, introversion will result from the erotic damming back. We know that herein the danger of distaste for life, hatred of humanity, shut-offness and eccentricity is near, and the moral development, the unfolding of the personality and love for neighbors are seriously endangered. If humanity would be spared the many sadistically inclined teachers, officers and public prosecutors, mean superiors, illhumored philosophers, education must bring the spirit of benevolence more strongly into force.

For this reason, parents must exercise particular care that no feeling of inferiority be aroused. Not only is the feeling of physical defect to be avoided but just as much or indeed more carefully that of incurable intellectual and moral indignity. The belief that the physical constitution is entirely sufficient, is certainly also necessary. If an organic inferiority exists, one shows the child the possibility of compensations. One should not show preference for the boys over the girls, thereby creating a "masculine protest" (Adler) in the latter, which may lead to the neurosis. Bad pupils should be shown the more important censor of the later life and also the high value of proper learning. If a complex of inferiority has already been formed, it absorbs an immense amount of intellectual energy, substitutes unproductive anxiety in place of refreshing pleasure, exchanges the joyous play of free interests for a slavish, tormenting attention to routine. Many a father who wishes to inspire his weak or differently gifted son, who already suffers from repression and fixation, by the evidence of his own achievements, forces him into difficult mental straits and robs him of an enormous quantity of useful mental energy. Thus, it comes about that pupils of supposedly poor endowment, who have been forced by complexes into inhibitions for work, after the analysis prove to be people capable of instruction.

Further, the recognition should be dependent on what may justly be expected and not be excessive. Freud rightly lays great weight on the point that the attraction of the ego-instinct be utilized in the conquest of reality. "Education can be described as incitement to the mastering of the pleasure-principle, to the replacement of this principle by the reality-principle; it will thus afford an aid to the process of development (from pleasure to reality principle) which concerns the ego, to this end making use of the premiums of love on the side of the educators and hence miscarrying when the spoiled child thinks that it already possesses this love regardless, and can lose it under no circumstances." *

In order that the child may have a normal relation to father and mother, both parents must .work together harmoniously. Freud remarks: "The wife ungratified by her husband, is, as mother, over-tender and sentimental toward the child on whom she transfers her need of love and awakens in it sexual pre-cocity. The bad relations between the parents irritate the emotional life of the child, causing him to feel intensively in tenderest age, love, hate and jealousy. The strict education which allows no kind of activity to the prematurely awakened sexual life, assists the suppressing force and this conflict at this age contains everything necessary for the causation of life-long nervousness." † Probably of equal frequency, is the other case of a woman detesting the children of a hated husband. If she wishes to combat her dislike from sense of duty, she falls into the counter-reaction of an over-education which really drives into the neurosis. In such situations, the children should be entrusted to strangers for education. Freud, in oral explanation, presents the thought that a neurosis caused by separation from parents unsuitable for educating the child, is less bad than an entirely unsuccessful education.

* Freud, Die zwei Prinz. Jahrb. III, p. 6.
† Freud, Die "kulturelle" Sexualmoral u. d. moderne Nervosität. Kl. Schr. II, p. 194.

Finally, it is obvious that the life-force should not be restricted by the parents to a condition not to be endured, as a result of the denial of deep-rooted wishes or the utilization of external compulsion. It is better when the highest degree of compulsion which the life and the acquirement of the greatest possible ability render necessary, is applied by strangers. The parents should so far as possible be the liberators, protectors, kind helpers and friends of their children, though not as fostering laziness and sensuality.

Highly important then is the point of view of the gradual separation from the parents. Wise parents educate their children with no more compulsion than is absolutely necessary for the adoption of healthy habits of life. They know that not obedient, but good children form the goal of education. They wish, therefore, not to be overestimated and guard against allowing fear of their persons to grow as a prevailing attitude. They afford their children as much room for expression as possible and loose the reins more and more. He who has seen the infernal wrath of countless neurotics who are ready to destroy themselves merely to torment the father, knows that these statements express no commonplace but an ideal, from the attainment of which, we are for the most part far removed. If the emancipation from the parents in favor of higher considerations once enjoined upon us by Jesus, does not occur, stagnation and regression appear. Even the highly talented Jews and Chinese remain dependent on the father for centuries and experience an ossification of their culture.

Only from the gradual relinquishment of the relation of dependence, can proceed that higher, free piety which gives the father the love of the child and forms a source of blessing for both.

To such education, succeed only parents who are themselves free from complexes. The mistakes of the children are to a certain extent, the reflection of the parents' mistakes. Only the person who is educated and inwardly free, can educate properly. For every other, even the ideal pedagogic introduction is of only modest value.

2. THE POSITION OF THE BROTHERS AND SISTERS

Usually the newborn child is viewed with displeasure by little brother and sister but this applies particularly to giving up to the newly arrived rival, parental affection and material advantages. On this account, the parents should vividly portray the advantages which the intruding mortal brings with him.

It is not good when brothers and sisters are too closely attached to one another. Often, this over-affection betrays an unconscious fixation which makes itself evident in all kinds of ways. We heard of obsessional neurosis as result of father- and brother-sister complex (72), of inability to speak with a strange girl and melancholia accompanying it (266), of inability to transfer the whole love to the husband (296, 385 [Ibsen]), etc.

Where the attachment becomes incestuous, we find in the analysis, as a rule, that the love for the sister, originally and actually applied to the mother, and that for the brother, to the father.

Many prominent men have remained fixed in a love for their sisters. The quarrel of brothers and sisters therefore has its good teleological meaning.

Further, the hate of brothers and sisters often proves to be unfortunate love, as counter-reaction or defence measure against incestuous attachment. We disclosed one brother-hater as sexual misdoer who sought improper pleasure upon the hated one (159). In my investigations into the psychology of hate and reconciliation, I showed another who likewise covered his burning love with his hate. I might present still many other examples for the proposition that extreme hate between brothers and sisters often goes back to love which has remained ungranted, but nevertheless deeply placed and I can testify that all other pedagogic measures are far inferior to the analytic in the treatment of hate between brothers and sisters.

On account of the position which the brothers and sisters

hold toward one another according to our moral law, it is not good for them to associate too long exclusively with one another. If no outside playmates are acquired, a fixation easily arises which leads to the neurosis.

3. TEACHER AND EDUCATOR

Very often the teacher forms a father-substitute for the pupil. If, however, he bears more traits which recall the mother, he becomes identified with her. Hence the pupil transfers the emotions suited to one or both parents upon their representative. If he hates his father, the teacher resembling the father must bear the whole grudge, while perhaps another educator receives the love directed toward the mother. In pathological cases, for example, in tremendous fear (137), the interchange is very plain.

The pedagogue has therefore to say to himself that he enters into the inheritance of his pupil's father or figures as contrasting substitute. If he acts accordingly, he can save himself very many unnecessary disciplinary measures and other unpleasantnesses. Further, he does the pupil good. The young neurotic wishes to conquer the father in the teacher. He does not perceive that he ought to want to learn for himself, he thinks of his mentor and, to his injury, gives himself up to the father-complex.

If the teacher allows himself to be provoked to anger, the pupil has gratified the evil longing of his unconscious. Further, the other educational errors which the pupil detects with keen perception, are provoked in good part by the teacher's unconscious.

Among teachers, there are many who identify themselves with their fathers or would outdo them and have chosen their profession from this cause.* That they are thus in a sad position is evident. There are pedagogues of superior talents who

* Maeder reports of a neurotic teacher who constantly phantasied himself as animal-tamer or general fighting against an army (Psa. u. Päd., p. 297). The man had always wanted to be a soldier. The poor pupils!

commit disciplinary blunder after blunder, who treat pupils totally wrong and derive reproachable educational results from these methods because they are laboring under a negative father-complex. One of our best analysts told of a patient who, as teacher of a secondary school, identified himself with his father, an over-strict officer, as theologian, however, with his mild-mannered mother. The same man, as teacher, treated the pupils with the same cruelty which he had experienced from his father, later as theologian, with feminine gentleness. The mistakes of classes reflect even plainer the complexes of their teacher than the educational deficiencies do the repressions and fixations of their parents.

If we would reform the education of youth, I know no better means than that we teachers undergo analysis. As often as I had the pleasure of analyzing professional colleagues, I observed a profound shock upon the recognition of manifold educational mistakes which had been committed under the influence of complexes.

This inner purification is so much the more important since, according to a statement of Mensendieck, the complexes of teacher and pupil mutually seek one another. If we are ignorant of our own inner entanglements, we act perhaps as unconscious imitators and gratify our ambition but we expose ourselves to the pupil and can with difficulty perceive his highest interests.

The more completely we see through the pupil, so much the more interesting does he become to us. And the more profoundly he perceives himself understood by us, just so much the more influence do we gain over him. He will then no longer attempt to escape a just and necessary command by an unconsciously produced headache, to gain our sympathy by unconsciously arranged sufferings and to pose as victim of overwork when he is lazy.

If the educator is freed from the odium of the unloved father and if he becomes a positive father-substitute, he will utilize this relation repeatedly to guide the pupil to the real tasks of life and free self-reliance. Why should one not let himself be a little idolized by young girls who must turn somewhere with their emotions? But the girl pupils must gain the sympathy of the teacher by worthy achievements. Against hysterical over-sentimentality, which I am accustomed to designate ironically as psychic diabetes, one behaves calmly and gently negatively. Pupils of doubtful morals, one treats with great caution that they may not, realizing a wish, accuse the teacher of gross aggressions.*

It is certain that psychoanalysis also essentially furthers the theoretical educational · results since it lays the correct affective foundation for material study.† The dislike for one or more particular subjects is often successfuly removed by analysis. Maeder ‡ reports of a boy who could not learn mathematics and language because his father urged him particularly to these subjects; in the natural sciences and technique which were connected by him with the beloved mother, he did excellently. The psychoanalysis led the excellent endowment of the boy to the previously hated subjects as well, since it disclosed the father-complex.

To the most powerful analytic deeds of the educator, belongs the elimination of a life-illusion appearing as manifestation. Under this caption, I understand the unconditional devotion to an impossible life-program coming about under subliminal compulsion, or one based on illusion. We know that many individuals get into ruinous place-hunting, proceeding only from external splendor and applause, because they would still an infantile feeling of inferiority. Some suppress themselves for their whole life, because they identify themselves with the father-image. Still other normal individuals

---

* With moral defectives, it may happen that they accuse the analyst of immoral intentions or indeed actions. This happens not alone in the psychoanalytic practice. Morally depraved or hysterical girls have often brought innocent teachers to prison. But it would seem that from the more exact understanding of the transference and the proper handling of this, the analytic method would be much less dangerous in this regard than any other.

† E. Schneider, Psa. u. Päd. Berner Seminarblätter, 1912, No. 11, p. 323.

‡ Maeder, Psa. u. Päd., p. 295.

cling, as Bertschinger showed in his interesting work,* as long as possible to a life-lie until they are driven to flight into the neurosis. Such a life-lie is constantly the counter-reaction against a painful certainty and repulsion of a moral demand. The fanatic for truth and morality sublimates the liar and adulterer in himself, the over-happy individual, who is always talking about his "wonderfully harmonious marriage," his "incomparable health," etc., hides himself and betrays to the one who knows, the inner feeling of unhappiness, but wanders on the dizzy path of danger from the precipice and often squanders a large part of his energy. The analyst helps such blinded persons, who pursue the will-of-the-wisp on the glass ball floating over the abyss, to see their real situation and to replace the longing for an imaginary goal with the striving after an attainable real happiness.

In this way, even youthful anarchists, gunmen, evil-intentioned rascals, woman-haters, apostles of a brutal free-love, world-despisers, world-conquerors, oppressors and similar difficult patients may be made amenable to the educator and allow themselves to be saved by him from tormenting, often life-long persisting, grievous errors.

If one has helped only one pupil in a class to salvation, the effect upon the class is often very strong,† since just such prominent neurotics often give the tone to the class.

4. Authority and Freedom, Asceticism and Indulgence in Pedagogy

From certain sides, some old demands of the Catholic pedagogy have been put forth anew, especially those of subjection to authorities, to asceticism and the forbidding of thought in religious matters.

Asceticism in the sense of the carrying out of artificial renunciation of pleasure and the infliction of pain for the pur-

* H. Bertschinger, Über Gelegenheitsursachen gewisser Neurosen und Psychosen. Allg. Zschr. f. Psychiatrie u. psychisch.-gerichtl. Medizin. Vol. 69 (1912), pp. 588–617.

† Maeder, Psa. u. Päd., p. 295.

pose of strengthening the will, receives a brilliant illumination from psychoanalysis, we have often though to deal with individuals who have been brought into dire mental states and emotional disease by those enforced demands.

Aside from the fact that many of these practices, for example, too early rising, breaking of the night's rest, cause direct exhaustion, I name the following dangers from asceticism:

1. In the ascetic, there develops (masochistic) pleasure in self-torture. I recall the young girl, who, from ascetic motives, poured on a wound the quadruple strength of corrosive prescribed, pretendedly to fix the energy, but who thereby felt a distinct sensation of pleasure. Often this masochistic desire becomes so strong that it leads to self-destruction, as countless women ascetics, Saint Elizabeth in particular, show.

2. The transference of the libido to reality ceases. The ascetic becomes suspicious of real things and introverted. An autistic looking-to-the-future mood takes away the value of the moral relations and tasks, an ardent eroticism changes very often to the ugly form of figures of the future life but at the cost of love for neighbors. Or a stoicism bursts forth which finally, as we have seen in one case, drives to danger of suicide and anxiety, robbing the moral life and likewise the libido.

3. The withholding of proper demands of instinct, for example, in eating, invests the good withheld with a strong overemphasis. The hungry person thinks unduly of food.

4. If asceticism does not attain its goal, there easily results a complete breakdown with self-condemnation and loss of will (abulia). These misfortunes are probably among the most frequent sacrifices to asceticism.

5. The repressed instincts often reappear in the center of the sublimation in the ugliest manner, compare judges of heretics, whose unsatisfied sexual instinct knew how to find satisfaction in sadistic form. Asceticism strengthens the morally disreputable counter-reactions since it prevents the investment of the libido in reality.

6. He who is harsh with himself by asceticism, becomes the same toward others, since masochism and sadism are constantly associated. Pharisees, Dominicans and many other adherents of asceticism are deficient in pity. This corresponds with the fact that the ascetic bears an autoerotic character.

7. Asceticism displaces the moral combat of socially important matters to unimportant private affairs. Thus, an individual may shine autoerotically but be a wight in social-ethical sense.

8. Asceticism wishes to take up with coercion a struggle against the compulsions of complexes and thereby causes grievous tortures without the slightest prospect of results.

Because of all these reasons, I consider asceticism, in the sense named, a dangerous and highly injurious pedagogic measure. That which it cannot achieve with its rack and screws, may often be attained by psychoanalysis without any torture at all. How many pupils who were visited with ascetic demands even to exhaustion and in the masochistic rage of the neurotic, eagerly grasped the opportunity for self-maltreatment until exhausted they broke down, has psychoanalysis saved by its message of salvation and gained for morally valuable lives!

In the place of autoerotic asceticism, psychoanalysis sets up the practice of neighborly love which fights out the moral combat on the floor of reality and helps the dammed-up instinct to sublimation by way of transference. Not the scourge, but love, helps to salvation, not the autoerotic, but the social-ethical panerotic asceticism, if we would still retain the historically important expression for such exercises of the will. Love and service is the best self-education.

The pedagogy of unconditional authority is inglorious in the light of psychoanalysis. He who espouses it, suffers from a father-complex which allows him to be partial to dogmas, priests, sacred writings, scientific quantities, political memories and other substitutes but not to come to true individual life. The pedagogy of subjection is the source of neuroses and counter-reactions. It is the grave of the free, fully developed and fully valued personality.

On the other hand, psychoanalysis teaches us that the happiness of men depends on the suitable investment of the libido capital. It shows us that the introverted, inwardly isolated, love-poor man is sick. It teaches us that we were all created, not like Antigone to hate one another, but to love one another. Hence it joins men in love, thus also in freedom, for freedom lies in the nature of truly moral love. To draw men from introversion, is the aim of the psychoanalytic therapeusis. In its eyes, the introverted individual is like a wander-cell which has escaped from the organism. Thus the analytic pedagogy forms the firmest foundation for the life of the community. It furthers also that only true reverence which is equally removed from self-disparagement and hatred of superiors, the manifestation of the positive and negative father-complex. Thus the psychoanalytic education agrees with F. Th. Vischer who in a happy hour wrote the words:

> "Blindly revered is a great man
> By the good man who can accomplish nothing.
> Not revered is a free man
> By the wight who can see nothing great.
> Freely revered is a great man
> By the man who can do something himself."

It is striking how in psychoanalytic circles, after the beginning when only the demand for allowing as much freedom as possible in education was emphasized, now the demand for strong guidance is also emphasized. To-day, some emphasize with Maeder: "For many children, complete freedom means dilettantism, the beginning of wasting time, of indolence." * "To the natural free development of the child belongs the regard for his need of guidance." † But it is well to remember: "The guiding rôle of the physician (we would say of the analyzing educator) consists not in his allowing himself to be received simply in the series of substitutes for the father

* Maeder, Psa. u. Päd., p. 298.   † Same, p. 301.

(teacher, pastor, elder friend, a popular hero, a great man, the king, a national hero, a great editor or author or artist, later, God or a higher principle) but rather in the furtherance of the development of the original father-image to the individual ideal, i. e., to the ideal which would have been possible for the person in question if he had not been inhibited by the infantile fixation."*

The analyst makes his demands likewise, but he directs the mental energies toward the decisive point and does not throw them away on the shadow pictures of the manifestation and allow them to exhaust themselves there. As has been remarked before, the analysis teaches us to value the helping force of work.

5. PUNISHMENT

I presuppose that the reader considers the aim of punishment to be improvement. The educator who punishes, wishes to amalgamate with the idea of unlawful desire that of a threatening pain and thereby to deter from the same, to make the child prudent by injury (wisdom-giving punishment).† Modern pedagogy emphasizes in general that it depends on the production of shame and repentance.

Psychoanalysis shows us that on one side, punishment or any other method which takes account only of the conscious mental life, cannot possibly attain those moral reactions so long as the unconscious interposes its veto, that on the other side, shame, repentance, most ardent volition do not in the least remove the old mistakes, but on the contrary, strengthen them when the unconscious puts the moral life in chains. Psychoanalysis affords us further the certain proof that the infliction of punishment prevailing to-day and recommended by most text-books on pedagogy, causes much suffering because it does not know and take into account the true instinctive sources of action. The correct attitude of love and of need of mastery

* Same, p. 302.

† Ackermann, Art. "Strafe" in Reins Encykl. Handb. d. Pädagogik, Vol. 6 (Langensalza 1899), p. 919.

is that which rules the moral action and how can punishment guide that primitive force?

Let us take, for example, a boy who suffers from a severe unconscious conflict with his father or one which is fed from the unconscious. He has to give an evil interpretation to the father's best-intentioned advice, the good object of which he immediately recognizes with everyone else. Or let us imagine a youth tormented by a complex of inferiority, what does he care about punishment? Adler gives the following picture of the psychological condition of that kind of people: "To the feeling of inferiority, there correspond traits, like anxiousness, doubt, uncertainty, bashfulness, cowardice and heightened feelings of need of support and submissive obedience. Along with these characteristics are found phantasies, indeed even wishes, which one can classify together as ideas of smallness and masochistic impulses. Above this texture of character-traits, there are regularly—with view of rejecting and compensating—impudence, courage and rashness, tendency to insubordination, obstinacy and defiance, accompanied by phantasies and wishes for the rôle of hero, warrior, robber, in short, ideas of grandeur and sadistic impulses."[*] "The whole instinctive life of the child becomes stimulated and over-intense, vengeful thoughts and death wishes against his own person, as against the surroundings upon the slightest provocation, childish errors and misdeeds are obstinately retained, and sexual precocity, sexual desire, breaks over the child-mind in order to be like the adults, of full value. The power which can do everything, which has everything—that is the father or one who represents him, the mother, an elder brother, the teacher. He becomes the opponent who must be fought, the child becomes blind and deaf to his guidance, misinterprets all good intentions, becomes mistrustful and extremely critical of all influences which come from the father, briefly, he has an attitude of defiance, but has directly thereby made himself dependent on the opinion of others."

[*] Adler, Trotz u. Gehorsam. Monatsh. f. Päd. u. Schulpolitik, 1910, Part 9.

Adler shows further that with such children, under external subjection, the ground of complete obedience is already undermined and the neurosis already in formation. I have shown sufficient examples of this. I-might further tell of a model boy of fifteen who was under the obsession of interpolating in every prayer for the parents a "not" which changed the blessing into a curse; I might also mention the "retarded obedience" which exists in severe emotional troubles (particularly in the obsessional neurosis) when the youth executes by the help of a ruinous illness what the father and father-substitute has demanded of him. The patient with fetichism for clothes described on page 331, who can look at no woman at all without desiring her, is only one of dozens.

What can the most just punishment, filled with the most beautiful lessons, accomplish in the countless individuals who succumb to neurotic obsession? The defiance is only strengthened, the incapacity for adaptation to the demands of life only increased. The explanations of the reasons for the punishment may be ever so plain, the youth remains under the sway of his conviction determined by his complexes: "Say what you will, deep down you intend to do me ill!" Further, many victims of complexes have already said to themselves most which the educator says to them without this making any changes within them. Punishment will therefore only embitter them and strengthen the evil tendency. The sadistic tormentor of animals rejoices, as we saw, when he is chastised and is only strengthened in his cruel inclinations.

Still more clearly does psychoanalysis reveal the folly of punishment for those who are led by it to an ardent desire for a new, pure life but who, as a result of inner attachment, cannot accomplish this. They struggle as we know from our observation of kleptomaniacs and complex-compelled pseudologians, perhaps with the exertion of all their power. But the more they persuade, pray, practice asceticism, so much the stronger are they compelled to do evil which they would not do, to speak with the Apostle Paul.* Punishment causes un-

* Romans vii., 15.

believable devastation there. Hate, self-contempt, melancholia result from such procedures and that which the educator carries out in consciousness of justice and love, the youth feels with perfect right as injustice.

It is surprising ever anew how such complex-goaded misdoers who have been driven by severity into ever-increasing mental distress and finally as true monsters have gained the neurotic's victory over the father, can be brought to the right way by psychoanalysis. The pedagogy desired by us thereby avoids much aimless, yes, pernicious punishment and attains by the sunshine of enlightenment and love what would never have been possible to the assault of chastisement. How many a human life would have taken an entirely different direction if the educators had possessed analytic knowledge!

A word may also be said concerning the execution of punishment. We have shown repeatedly how the punishment of whipping is turned into trauma by awakening masochistic pleasure. We also saw the spectators suffer harm. According to the experience of myself and other analysts, one must reckon with a fairly high probability that there are such persons in every school class to whom the infliction or the sight of corporal punishment does injury. When one sees what a powerful educational instrument a pedagogue, free from bad complexes and possessing exact understanding of the pupils' minds, has, one will not find the demand that corporal punishment be entirely excluded from education, excessive.

From the mental means of punishment, it is to be desired that they do not repressively maltreat the youth's need for self-assertion. How often have I observed "retarded obedience" which represented a cruel revenge on the parents, from the fact that the censure of inferiority had been accepted and built into an obsessional idea by the child! It no longer helped then for the parents to take back their insult and explain: "We did not really mean it, you are a normal person!" The degrading thought had been set free and was not now to be retracted without artificial aid.

6. Sexual Education

We owe to psychoanalysis the discovery of many injurious influences which had previously wrought their effect in the darkness of ignorance. In the first place, we saw deviations of the sexual instinct as enemies of life-happiness and a healthy moral religious development.

The analytically enlightened pedagogy has to take far more earnest account of the sexual excitations of the child than has previously been the case. It forbids excessive fondling, of which ungratified husbands and wives are often guilty. It warns particularly against allowing children after the first year of life in the sleeping-room of the parents and is suspicious of having growing youths in rooms separated from the parents' room by thin walls, for many hysterias and obsessional neuroses, many developed Œdipus complexes undoubtedly go back to overhearing the parents—aside from the actual conflict. Caresses between the parents in front of the children are often to be strictly forbidden.

Supposing that the child could as yet have no incestuous wishes in the literal sense of the word, still, sexual excitements arise which can be continued through regression, to powerful life determinants and to actual pathogenic incestuous phantasies.

Very much to be warned against is the injudicious treatment of bad sexual habits. The most dangerous in this regard is the threat of amputation of the genitalia. In many severe neuroses, we find a castration-complex. I have in mind not only people like the dementia præcox patient mentioned on page 123, whom the castration threat led into anxiety for doves, legs of children and obsessional hiding of the nose, but also persons who, in masochistic desire, practice self-castration for a lifetime by demeaning themselves in general, falling into misfortune, yielding to impotence, becoming incompetent and giving up to a tendency to suicide.

A rational treatment of masturbation must guard against the extremes of frivolity on the one hand and moral fanaticism on the other. The first of these errors has the following results:

1. The energies which in abstinence from suitable primary eroticism should be applied to the service of altruism, friendship, art, love of nature, science, religion and other sublimations, are uselessly wasted.

2. The excessive onanist develops autoerotically, relatively shuts himself off from the surrounding world and becomes introverted. The isolation of self and the indifference of the extreme onanist toward other persons, does not arise usually from the fact that he has an improper secret to hide but from self-gratification and the failure of all erotic longing dependent on this.

3. Freud emphasizes that the sexual behavior is the prototype for all conduct in general. If the onanist becomes accustomed to gaining pleasure by the cheap way of his habit, instead of attaining his goal by the difficult path of suitable courtship, he becomes an unmanly pleasure-seeker who in the rest of his life also avoids the serious tasks and remains a weak-willed, infantile person.*

The other cardinal error consists in moral fanaticism which immeasurably exaggerates the injurious effects of masturbation and combats it with terrible threats. How many boys have been driven by that kind of generally dangerous writings into severe neurosis, indeed into suicide! A pamphlet of Pastor N. Hauri, widely circulated in Switzerland, asserts for example: "When a young man secretly does all kinds of things whereby he stains his body, his health also suffers grievous injury. He becomes tired and sleepy, his mind is weakened, he loses all elasticity and power of will. Ever less can he resist the evil pleasure. Step by step his evil thoughts pursue him to ruin. He loses the joy of work. He becomes in appearance and behavior like an old man and finally any disease may get him which he would otherwise have easily withstood and carries him off in his early years. How many a young man has already

* Freud, 2d Diskuss. der Wiener psa. Vereinigung. Wiesbaden 1912, p. 138. Hitschmann, Freuds Neurosenlehre, p. 18 f.

sunk into an early grave in this way and others have become miserable and sickly or blue and melancholy." *

He who has seen the misery of masturbators who in hot combat were unable to master their sexual instinct, shudders at the thought of the devastation which such awful prophecies must have caused. Hauri's utterances are all the more to be regretted since according to the testimony of every experienced educator and physician, the hints given by him do not by far suffice for most masturbators to find salvation from their difficulty. Warning against evil thoughts, improper books, bad company, idleness, nocturnal revelry, intemperance, untrue assertions over the necessity for sexual activity, admonition to hardening and pious Christian conduct—more than these platitudes, Hauri does not know how to give!—help only a small part of those in need. The rest, who do not know how to help themselves against the enemy, Hauri treats with terrible threats which appear so much the more ugly and distorted since, according to the assurances of the best-informed physicians, over ninety per cent. of all youths have practised masturbation. We saw that very often a neurosis broke out when onanism was discontinued (76, 101, 409, etc.). And should we hurl ourselves with brutal threats upon the boys and girls? A morally earnest educator should not yield himself to such doubtful services as are urged by Hauri out of ignorance.

The conscientious educator clings to the facts. Now it is to be admitted that the injuriousness of masturbation is not estimated alike by all. The modern psychiatrists and neurologists consider the physical effects of masturbation as fairly negligible. Ziehen thinks that at the most, excessive onanism may contribute in certain cases to the origin of psychoses, Aschaffenburg is of the opinion that nervous disturbances either do not, or at least rarely, arise from onanism.† Further, the

---

* N. Hauri, Eine Konfirmanden-Stunde über das 7. Gebot. 4. St. Gallen, 1910, p. 6.

† Aschaffenburg, Die Beziehungen des sex. Lebens zur Entstehung von Nerven- u. Geisteskrankheiten. Münch. med. Wochenschr. 1906, No. 37.

opinions of psychoanalysts are divided. Stekel represents the view that onanism is entirely harmless.* He reports of a man of forty-one years who had practiced onanism for twenty-five years from once a day to six times a day and still remained healthy. Another man well along in the forties, masturbated daily and besides practiced normal coitus daily with extraordinary potency. Nevertheless, there are observations opposed to these which we have mentioned.

How shall we approach the evil? Not with a universal receipt, with uniform suggestions, to invoke heaven and hell. I admit that Hauri's prescription will banish the symptom in very mild cases. But there often arise along with this result, bad after-effects, unhealthy piousness, emotional troubles, etc.

We should investigate each individual case. There is a large number of forms of masturbation. Often, it is joined to obsessional ideas, often, it forms a compensation for homosexuality, often, it is a symptom of shutting-off from humanity or from the female sex, often, the expression of a death-wish, etc.

If it is a case of decided pathological compulsion, which is very often the case, all warning and threatening admonition only strengthens the trouble. All pedanalysts have observed that the obsession becomes just so much the stronger, the stronger the affects are which are directed to combatting it. According to the law of compensation, a greater value must be created for the person struggling against the habit, transference, friendship, hope of winning a pure, joy-bringing wife, close union with religious forces, etc. These compensations serve as diversion when, by appropriate and friendly advice, the counter-will against the evil habit blocks up the previously exercised instinctive function. Already, in the fact that one withdraws the overemphasis from the habit, does one strengthen the power for freedom. Hence it is not advisable to pledge the youth to give up his sin; all the less is it advisable to demand peremptorily immediate total abstinence.

Where a strong network of complexes exists, the prevention

* Stekel, Eine Gegenkritik. Zbl. III, p. 250.

of the peripheral action only causes exaggerated phantasies. And certainly the purely mental masturbation, with its intensive demands on the emotions, is at least as injurious for body and mind as the physical form, especially since it has not, like the latter, a momentary release.

If the intensive onanism is thus, as is very often the case, a manifestation, I consider psychoanalysis as indispensable if the youth is to be freed. There also, I avoid the pedanalysis so long as I can get along with simpler methods. In all severe cases, however, this is not possible. In the analysis, one may attempt to get along with a symptomatic method. One may explore the accompanying phantasies according to their dependence on the past and their relation to the future. I gave an example on page 266.

Another instance may be added: A sixteen-year-old candidate for confirmation confided to me that he had suffered from melancholia for a year. His dreams betrayed that he wished his parents dead. Only after weeks, did he acknowledge daily masturbation which was preceded by the stereotyped idea that a boy, or more rarely, his sister, was spanked on the buttocks. The habit was of about two years' standing. About that length of time, he had suffered from attacks of blushing and pains in his abdomen. The onanism was performed by a climbing exercise in the gymnasium hour. Some weeks later, the youth, during the school recess, rubbed his thighs together under the desk in mastubatory manner when a boy beside him was beaten on the buttocks. The obsessing idea began at once.

Naturally, the school experience revived earlier episodes. The earliest was an experience at play in the fourth or fifth year: In the hall of his home, a wall had been marked with a pencil by an unknown person. The neighbor accused our patient's sister of having done this. The latter, however, took the blame on himself, in no way, however, to save the sister. Since no other reason was apparent, I surmise that he yielded to a masochistic impulse. Soon, the false self-accusation disturbed him. The sister accused the brother but found no credence and received blows on the buttocks, whereupon the brother, as he clearly remembers, felt voluptuous pleasure, while he had witnessed other chastisement without sexual feeling; further, a feeling of guilt set in. Previously, he had felt sexual excitement when he himself was spanked on the buttocks. In later years, the sadistic emotion occurred only when. one of his comrades was whipped because he had done him an injustice.

Thus, the sadistic component was only stimulated to conscious emotional expressions when hate was active. Hate in its turn plainly appeared in our case as repressed incestuous love. In it, lay also the instinctive force for obsession and masturbation. The pedanalytic influence easily succeeded. As pleasant compensation, there came besides the increased joy in life and work, a favorable relation to the sister in place of the previous condition of strife.

Usually, one must employ a more elaborate analysis of resistances and seek to penetrate the mind without any kind of consideration for the special symptom. In such cases, masturbation is a subordinate trace of the mental trouble which causes, outside of this one symptom, a number of far more dangerous disturbances of the moral life. Thus we see the special problem in its great connection to an ethical reorganization in general, and therewith withdraw from it the all too strong investment of the mental life of our pupils. The sexual education can be properly carried on only in the framework of the complete education.

The treatment of perversities must proceed analytically with the same gentleness.

An important part of the pedagogic work discussed here consists in sexual enlightenment. It is recommended by many facts, opposed by nothing worthy of consideration. If the correct instruction is omitted, the following dangers are encountered, to which we have seen many children succumb and from which we have seen many grievous injuries.

1. If the child is not instructed from authoritative side, the

street takes up the task, often in the dirtiest form.* That which should be the object of reverence is painted as ugly and subjected to obscene jests. Thus the sexual life becomes a priori something vulgar and on the parents falls a blemish which allows the mother to appear in dreams and neurotic acts (obsessional love for prostitutes, Don Juanism) as prostitute, the father as libertine. Further effects are often and unconquerable disgust for sexuality, "frigidity," loss of love and many other neurotic pathological phenomena which are suited to ruin a human life.

2. If the correct enlightenment is omitted, false childish phantasies appear in its place, often with sadistic impregnation- and birth-theories connected with perverse procedures, the results of which appear later in disease and perversity.

3. The child whose thirst for knowledge is not gratified by the parents or is put off by symbolical stories, loses confidence in them.†

4. His whole life becomes imbued with obsessional brooding ‡ or inversely, he may lose the craving for knowledge.

For giving the enlightenment, Freud gives the excellent advice: "It happens that the children never originate the idea that one would make for them a mystery out of the facts of the sexual life more than of anything else which is accessible to their understanding. And in order to attain this end, it is necessary that sexual matters should be treated from the beginning in the same manner as other subjects of knowledge. In particular, it is the task of the school not to omit to mention sexual affairs, to give the great facts of reproduction in instruction concerning the animal kingdom in their proper significance and at the same time, to emphasize the fact that man shares all the essentials of his organization with the higher

---

* Compare my presidental address as chairman of the Kantonalen zürich. Pfarrergesellschaft (Verhandlungen d. asket. Ges. 1906, pp. 33–43.

† Jung, Konflikte der kindl. Seele. Jahrb. II, p. 39.

‡ Freud, Zur sex. Aufklärung der Kinder. Kl. Schr. II, p. 156, Leonardo, p. 14.

animals."* Freud adds: "The curiosity of the child will never reach a high grade if it finds satisfaction corresponding to each stage of life. The enlightenment concerning the specific human relations of the sexual life and the reference to the social importance of the same should be added at the close of the instruction in the folk primary school and before the entrance into the intermediate school, thus not later than at the age of ten years. Finally the time of confirmation would be suited, as no other, to explain to the child already enlightened concerning all the physical matters, the moral obligations which are connected with the exercise of the instinct. Such a graduated, progressive enlightenment concerning the sexual life, actually interrupted at no time, for which the school assumes the initiative, seems to me the only one which takes account of the development of the child and hence, fortunately, avoids the dangers at hand." † I might only add to what Freud has said that also from the beginning, the moral side of reproduction, the ethical bond between parents and child, can be emphasized and hence should be.

7. THE MORAL AND RELIGIOUS EDUCATION

Even though psychoanalysis as purely a method of exploration, as we have perceived, may be utilized in the service of any moral or immoral, religious or irreligious purpose, there is no doubt that it mightily assists a healthy moral and religious education.

(A) THE MORAL EDUCATION

The pedanalysis sets up as pedagogic ideal for us the personality fully developed in its proper individuality, hence one that is also socially effective. The personality ideal in the sense of the demand for a human organization realizing the commands of its own nature, inwardly closed, emotionally rich, has kept constantly appearing before our eyes in the course of our investigation. We recognized how much morbid crippling proceeded from the pedagogic violence to the individual neces-

---

* Kl. Schriften II, p. 157.   † Same, p. 158.

sities of life. No psychology and no pedagogy ever proved with such shocking facts the intensity and extent of the grave offence which is committed by the pedagogy of the press and pattern, the pedagogy of educational egoism and short-sightedness.

We have demonstrated further that human happiness and human power are dependent in the first place on the relations to fellowmen, first of all to father and mother and their respective representatives, further upon the capability to sub-limate the primary claims of instinct in the highest fields of the moral life. In so doing, it was shown that the finding of an object of love belonged to the most important tasks of life, be-cause without this, an introversion sets in, which, when it progresses too far, withdraws the libido from all reality and drives it into unproductive phantasies, anxiety, pessimism hostile to life, distaste for life, indeed into severe neurosis and psychosis. The art of proper, morally superior, loving becomes thus the substance of the art of living. But in contrast to sensual indulgence and autistic sentimentality which only testify to internal incapacity for love, we recognized the pro-ductive love which masters reality with the maximal develop-ment of power and adapts itself to it, as the highest moral im-perative in which duty and capacity are united. Self-love without love for neighbors, the absolute egoism, we perceived to be a force hostile to self and destructive to self. Thus were we compelled to postulate the inwardness of the mind, but of the mind lighted with love for one's fellows, in the name of mental health.

We were also forced to the perception that the measure of the realization of the ethical ideal is dependent on the peculiar-ity of each individual and that we should not wish to exact by external pressure the same perfection from all.

The pedagogic ideal recommended by psychoanalysis is not new but new and impressive in its foundation.

Further, the means of education of the psychoanalyst are in good part new. We too utilize the invitation, we desire an achievement corresponding to the individual strength. But we see that the education of to-day is guilty of an immense waste of energy. Most pupils are encumbered with deplorable repressions and fixations, the overcoming of which consumes a large part of the mental energy. To these carriers of ballast, belongs the army of neurotics as also the great part of healthy individuals. No one comes through life entirely free from such injurious burdens. Further, no one thinks of excluding from the world all complex-formation. Everyone must and should bear a certain amount of repression and fixation. Yet not too much! Otherwise the energy disposable for execution of productive performances and for the bearing of unavoidable and healthy troubles of life will be reduced. Sensible, conscious control and guidance of instinct, in place of repression of instinct, is the formal analytic principle of the moral education. Only thereby do we guard against autistic squandering of libido and gain a strong, free, work-enjoying race. Only thereby do we bring about that state of mind, from which alone, the highest mental achievements proceed.

(B) THE RELIGIOUS EDUCATION

The pedanalysis shows us religion from the viewpoint of psychology and biology as well as from that of individual and social hygiene.

In every religion, we find unquestionable sexual forces invested, in the Christian religion, sublimated sexuality. Yet we have already heard (312) how false it would be to consider the evangelic piety simply as sublimated sexuality. Much rather, the results of philosophical thought are derived from the thinking directed by the reality principle, as well as historical knowledge, ethical, esthetic and other functions not to be exhaustively interpreted from the pure libido-movement contained in it. That which sharply differentiates the Christian religion from every other, is a peculiar diversion of the libido into three channels: love for God, love for fellowmen and love for self. Jesus enunciates as chief command—better, as principle of his teaching, the formula: ''Thou shalt love the Lord thy God with thy whole heart and thy neighbor as thyself.'' (Mat. xxii, 37–39; Mark xii, 30 f; Luke x, 27). From the standpoint of the pedanalysis, I consider this principle as positively perfect. Love is thereby recognized and encouraged, and indeed the maximal activity of love, while other religions, in part prohibit love (Buddhism), in part disregard it (Parusism), in part replace it with substitutes. Thus, with Jesus, introversion is happily avoided and the libido saved for reality, morality and culture.

From the pedanalytic viewpoint, the self-love is of high value against suicidal tendencies (compare Saint Elizabeth) and masochistic pleasures. Such ones were ever much beloved: Macarius, in order to escape the temptation of fornication, placed himself entirely naked in a swamp and allowed himself to be tormented by mosquitoes until he looked like a leper and could be recognized only by his voice (Lucius: Die Anfänge des Heiligenkults i. d. christl. Kirche, 363). With the same intention, ''Ammonius tortured his body with a fiery iron until he was entirely covered with burns. Benedict of Nursia danced around in thorn hedges and Evagrius Ponticus allowed his flesh to freeze during a whole night spent in a fountain in the winter time.'' (Same.) The pious Christine of St. Troud (1150–1224) laid herself in the hot oven, fastened herself on the wheel, had herself racked by the wheel and hung on the gallows beside the dangling corpse, buried herself in the grave, suffered from the obsession which is transparent in sexual symbolical sense (page 94) that she must climb roofs, trees and church towers, Margaretha of Ypern (1216–1237) after the cessation of her madness for men, could not bear the presence of a boy but was engaged to Jesus, Christine Ebner (1277–1356) cut a cross in the skin over the heart region and tore it off, wept weeks at a time over Jesus' suffering until her cheeks were sore, until, after two years of horrible self-torture, she fell into sensual visions, in which she felt herself embraced by Jesus and conceived a child by him. Mechtild of Magdeburg (about 1212–1277?), the gifted authoress, felt herself sick from passionate love for the Savior and advised all virgins to follow the most charming of all, the eighteen-year-old Jesus, that he might embrace them; on the other side, however, she became gloomy on account of a harmless laughing or a levity of that kind betrayed to no one, so that the unhappy nun begged piteously and grieved until she again crept into the kitchen "like a whipped dog." (The last four examples are from "Mechtild von Magdeburg, Das fliessende Licht der Gottheit" with the admirable introduction by Mela Escherich, Berlin, 1909.) Heilborn says of the old German mystics: "From antiquity, even with the pious old German theosophists, all pre-sentiments, all self-destructive, lustful, death- and heaven-seeking was overgrown with the over-excitement of sensuality and sensual phantasy excesses. Sensuality and mysticism live in and by one another." *

Who can mistake in these asceticisms which form not by far the most ugly effects of miscarried sexual repressions within the Catholic piety, the victory of masochistic instincts, the intoxicating, voluptuous pleasure from maltreatment of one's own person? Nietzsche rightly names certain forms of asceticism "a holy form of debauchery." †

True Christianity, as living one's life in the highest sense of the word, in contrast to this, is expressed in the words in John xiv, 19: "I live, ye shall live also."

Love for one's neighbors as a main stream for the libido, we saw recommended likewise by the analysis. If the libido is not so guided, there arises at best an elevation of the sexual instinct yet no true sublimation. Many a time, the dammed-up libido has broken out in religion as active cruelty. What person who knows even a little of the psychology of the sexual life, will deny that the Spanish Inquisitor, Petrus Arbues, canonized in 1867, and the whole great army of similar pious monsters, fell into the snares of sadism and in deluded zeal for God, performed only the work of the flesh, of ill-treated sexuality? The history of the Catholic sainthood affords the analytic pathography an inexhaustible material which substantiates the interesting statement of the experienced Fried-

* E. Heilborn, Novalis, der Romantiker, Berlin, 1901.
† Nietzsche, Z. Genealogie d. Moral, 3rd Part, Paragraph 1.

rich von Hardenberg (Novalis): "It is strange that the association of voluptuous pleasure, religion and cruelty has not long ago brought to the attention of men the intimate relationship and common tendency of these." * Psychologically considered, this assertion is absolutely correct. In the religion of the Israelites, we see the sexual debauchery proceed to the temple. The preprophetic religion of Baal allowed father and son to go to the slaves of the temple. The great prophets, as Amos, Hosea, Isaiah, Micah and Jeremiah on the contrary, favored a transformation of the libido into social activity and thus created the first important social religion in which divine pleasure was made dependent on the preservation of social-ethical sentiment. Jesus also voiced this utilization of the libido, but still more decidedly, in that he even preached love for enemies, while Islam with its polygamy, slavery and sensual hope of heaven, clung to a mere elevation of the sexual instinct. Jesus, by his advocacy of a serving love and preaching God's kingdom on the earth, kept religion free from the danger of depreciating the present time by displacing the center of attention into the future.

The love of God is recognized not less by the analyst as a healthful demand. The believer flees to the domain of the ideal, to the heart of the eternal love, when life disappoints him and fellowmen treat him contemptuously and unjustly. In the divine father-love, he, whose longing for help, for ethical salvation is not satisfied by the surrounding reality, finds an asylum. In the love for the Savior, the love-thirsty soul, which finds no comprehension and no return love in his fellowmen, is refreshed. The titanic drama of the work of salvation with its immense contrasts, sin—grace, human depravity—Jesus' conquering love, death—life, affords guilt-laden souls a source of consolation, the sustaining force of which, the irreligious individual can scarcely appreciate. Further, the educated person with deeper thinking and feeling, who bears a mighty desire for the reality of the ideal, will again and again long for

* Heilborn, Novalis, p. 161.

God as the substance and real basis of the ideal and submerge himself in Him when men and nature (in broadest sense) leave him in want.

But if the love for God is not to lead to fanatical excess of passion of plain sexual character, it must be accompanied, as happened in the teachings of Jesus, by love for men and self. Otherwise, it will develop into that system of religious orgies which Margaretha Ebner, Zinzendorf and hundreds of other Christian saints portray. Jesus enunciated as strongly as possible the love for neighbors as the presupposition of all true love for God: an act of brotherly love, the reconciliation, is for him more important than the cultistic performance of the sacrifice (Mat. v, 23, 24).

Of supreme importance, then, is the elaboration of the relation to the father by Jesus. With wonderful acuity, he solved the attachment by sublimating it. We have mentioned some of the places in which Jesus urged the separation from the father as he personally emancipated himself from the mother. The postulate of sublimation is in Matthew xxiii, 9: "Thou shalt call no one on earth, father, for one is thy father who is in heaven." Thereby, Jesus has relieved the harmful fixation and broken the bonds of free personal development.* He has, however, also taken into account the need for paternal protection and reciprocal love.

The need for the mother is given less consideration. Jesus loved his real mother so much that for him a heavenly substitute was superfluous. The Catholics invested Mary and the Church, the Protestants likewise the Church or the Holy Ghost, with mother-attributes.

In Jesus, we find still other thoughts highly important for the pedanalyst. He unburdened the oppressed soul. By abreaction and forgiving of sins, he prepared the healing of neurotic infirmities from within out. Even the belief that those

---

* Hebbel relates very prettily in his "Aufzeichnungen aus meinem Leben" (chap. 5) how religion helped him to cut the mental navelstring which had previously bound him exclusively to the parents. (Stuttgart and Leipzig, p. 582.)

maladies proceed from spirits, draws our sympathy as psychological adaptation, only metaphysically it is false.

Further, Jesus has recognized the tranference with great keenness. Hence he allows himself to love boundlessly. Mat. xi, 28: "Come unto me all ye that labor and are heavy laden, and I will give you rest." Mat. x, 37: "He that loveth father or mother more than me is not worthy of me." Still he does not bind the believers to himself but points them to the Heavenly Father, to the highest religious and moral autonomy of the child of God.

And besides the past and present (abreaction and transference), Jesus takes the future into consideration, instructing in a powerful conception of it.

It is, therefore, not at all absurd for one to find the fundamental characteristics of the pedanalysis marked out by Jesus. Also from other sides, we can consider him as crown witness for the correctness of our theory: He sets free the love banished by the rule of law from the Hebrew religion of his time and guides it to the center of piety. Now, orthodoxy and ceremonialism also cease. The prophets with their social preaching kept the libido in the reality. After the Babylonian exile, national necessity caused enormous repressions. The austere God was feared. The dammed-up libido fled, exactly as in the obsessional neurotic individual, into intellectual achievements and acts difficult of execution,* even into orthodoxy and ceremonialism. Exactly as Freud heals the obsessional neurotic individual by winning back the love and affording it appropriate realization, so does Jesus. He taught to love and thereby destroyed the religious obsessional neurosis.

A great deal more might be said concerning the relations between Jesus' gospel and psychoanalysis. It is enough that we find in him the piety of the healthiest and most profound thinker of men, while Paul and the writings of John represent the piety of the neurotic. Hence even to-day many neurotic individuals are actually most drawn to the latter (neurotics

---

* Freud, Zwangshandlungen u. Religionsübung. Kl. Schr. II, pp. 122–131.

seek one another), while people who are freer from complexes are ordinarily far more attracted by the synoptic piety.

Catholicism renewed the repressions and created a new obsessional neurosis. Dogma and sacrament were its symptoms. Thereby, a grandiose symbolism developed, the regressive character of which is easily perceived. In the Catholic Eucharist, the eating of God meets us as in the eating of the totem animal, the drinking of blood in the Attis mysteries, etc. The life-ideal realized in monks and expressed in the three vows of poverty, obedience and chastity contains the three strongest repressions and renunciations: the renunciation of wealth, self-independence and family. Therewith, the strongest instincts of sex and ego are gagged. For the libido, there is left only the flight into the future life if it is to escape introversion. The father is, in the persons of the Pope and of the spiritual superiors, enthroned in his authority and exercises this authority more strictly than any other kind of father. The three-in-one God loses the personal character and therewith the love-giving power. The obsessional neurosis was unavoidable since love was again in great part excluded.

The Reformation wrought a change for a short time but more in the spirit of Paul than in that of Jesus. Love was soon banished again and a Protestant orthodoxy and exaggeration of ceremony set in. As soon as love again succeeded pietism as the nucleus of the Christian life, the fear of the letter of the Bible, ordinance of the church and ceremony weakened.

Thus the Freudian theory shines brilliantly in the mirror of religious history. Concerning this phenomenon, the future will have much more to say. We are still far from understanding thoroughly the infinitely rich symbolism of Christian ideas and customs. But we know that thanks to Freud's investigation, we are in possession of the key which by hard and earnest work will open the door to these secret chambers.

We already understand why this individual must, as the result of his complexes, join one sect, that individual, another sect, and each find boundless satisfaction in his choice. We know when people are led by psychological necessity to the Catholic Church, when to the Salvation Army, when to the Mormons, when to the Adventists and feel contented there. We understand also the private religions and rites of the individuals analyzed by us. We can say why that neurotic pastor's wife prays to the wind, that youth to the fire, that old man to the phallus, secretly as the highest Godhead. We understand therefore also the relative necessity and healthfulness of sects and abstruse private religions and know that they are not a danger to the churches spiritualized by the Gospel, even though many disposed individuals can certainly be led astray by them to life-impoverishing narrowing of the horizon, neurotic autisticism and moral poverty.

That false religious education in the first years of life, or even later, can inflict grievous injury, should by no means be denied. The pedanalysis warns especially against the following dangers:

Religion cannot be shown merely as dry theory, but should be shown as an experience. It should "embrace the whole inner man so that we make him fresher, fuller of life, more joyful and morally stronger by our religious instruction." It should "encourage the satisfaction which leads to noblest deeds, the heroic pride." The teacher of religion should help the pupils to win a personal view of life in free investigation. He should also strengthen by historical instruction the longing for the future and the determination to fight for it.* He should create the living contact with the creative force which discloses its nature in the ideal and sets the development to the realization of the ideal. God should appear in trusted relation to the youth as loving father, friend, protector, giver of moral, liberating commands and forgiveness. Such religion will turn the libido to the individual and common good, help to prevent the neurosis and psychosis, surround life with a halo and attain a high degree of strength for the real duties of life.

* Compare my article: Religionspädag. Neuland. Eine Unters. ü. d. Erlebnis- und Arbeitsprinzip. Zürich, 1909, p. 6.

To be warned against, is a piety which deadens the intellectual curiosity. This happens when one kills questions by the compulsion of dogmatic tradition or does away with the particular explanation of empirical phenomena with the phrase: "This has God created." Höffding rightly says: "Religion has had great significance for the development of science and will be able to have still more by accentuating the great borderline problems and fixing the conviction that there is a center and that it should be the highest ideal task of thinking to find the same." * As natural science can determine in a painting of Böcklin's the elasticity and composition of the colors, the botanical variety of the wood or canvas on which it is painted, the chemical composition of the pigments, but must be supplemented by an esthetic method of consideration which takes into account the meaning of the picture, so also is the nature investigation to be perfected by a consideration of the value of the laws of the ethical development and evolutionary tendency. Only the religious point of view embraces the comprehensive world picture.

Therein the religious instruction must guard against abstract rationalization. Psychoanalysis shows us the indispensability of the symbol. In the old symbols of the Christian religion, there lurks far more noble content than the theory of faith, so miserably established psychologically, will allow us to believe. Hence, many deep and free religious minds find far more spirit and life in the picture-language of the Bible than in the aqua destillata of critically purified dogmatic formulæ.

But the symbol must be recognized as symbol. Psychoanalysis has clearly shown us anew the right of absolutely free investigation. What is to be hoped for, is a theory of faith which understands how to grasp clearly and sharply the connection between the religious idea and the unconscious. To this end, tedious, deep investigations of living piety and a comprehensive view of life will be necessary.

We have already transgressed the bounds of the psychoanalysis given us by Freud which everywhere discloses impos-

* Höffding, Religionsphilosophie, p. 24.

ing problems in psychology, ethics, esthetics, metaphysics, even though the solution of these problems presupposes still other methods besides itself. My task consisted only in showing the pedagogue what wonderful new paths were open to him if he knew how to use the pedanalysis. Investigating, healing and protecting, the proper professional educator will garner a rich harvest as soon as he has enriched his armamentarium with the new educational method and understands how to apply it with skill. To-day, the need of many pupils is immeasurable and the danger threatening them allows a stormy future to be predicted for them. On the other hand, an enormous amount of pedagogic talent and intelligence lies fallow. May there not be lacking among the pedagogues those whose conscience will drive them in pursuit of an adjustment and who will put themselves as analysts in the service of investigation as well as of helping love! The field is white for the harvest.

INDEX